Springer Series on Ethics, Law, and Aging

Marshall B. Kapp, JD, MPH, Series Editor

2001 **Lessons in Law and Aging**
A Tool for Educators and Students
Marshall B. Kapp, JD, MPH

2001 **Ethics in Community-Based Elder Care**
Martha B. Holstein, PhD, and Phyllis Mitzen, ACSW, LCSW, Editors

1999 **Geriatrics and the Law**
Understanding Patient Rights and Professional Responsibilities,
Third Edition
Marshall B. Kapp, JD, MPH

1998 **Guardianship of the Elderly**
George H. Zimny, PhD, and George T. Grossberg, MD

1998 **Hospice Care for Patients with Advance Progressive Dementia**
Ladislav Volicer, MD, PhD, and Ann Hurley, RN, DSNc

1996 **Older Adults' Decision Making and the Law**
*Michael Smyer, PhD, K. Warner Schaie, PhD, and
Marshall Kapp, JD, MPH*

1995 **Controversies in Ethics in Long-Term Care**
*Ellen Olson, MD, Eileen R. Chichin, DSW, RN, and Leslie S. Libow, MD,
Editors*

1994 **Patient Self-Determination in Long-Term Care**
Implementing the PSDA in Medical Decisions
Marshall B. Kapp, JD, MPH, Editor

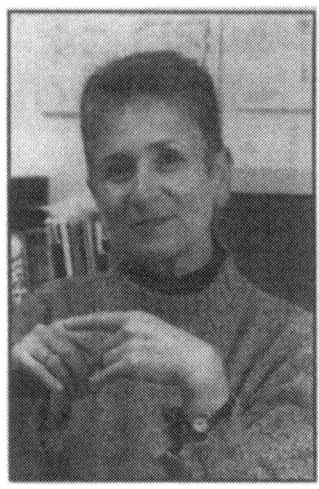
Martha B. Holstein, PhD, is an Associate for Research at the Park Ridge Center for the Study of Health, Faith, and Ethics in Chicago, where her focus is applied ethics in health care and other settings. She holds a PhD from the Institute for the Medical Humanities at the University of Texas Medical Branch and was formerly on the staff of the Hastings Center, Associate Director of the American Society of Aging, and a planner for the San Francisco Commission on Aging. For much of her work life, she has been interested in the bridge between theory and practice; for the past fifteen years this effort has focused on ethics, especially in the area of aging. She has been involved in aging-related issues since 1973 and believes that "doing" ethics is an evolving skill that starts from one's values and stance in the world but does not end there. She also believes that ethical analysis is an engaged enterprise; to try to affect background conditions that help create many problems is the task of the ethicist as citizen. Dr. Holstein writes, teaches, lectures, and conducts training on the subject of ethics and aging.

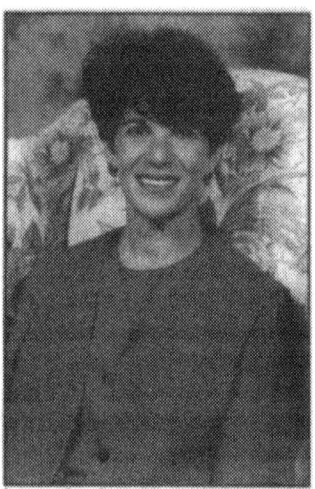
Phyllis Mitzen, ACSW, LCSW, received her MA from the University of Chicago, School of Social Service Administration. She has been at the Council for Jewish Elderly since 1980, where she is currently Director of Development. In her prior role at CJE she managed community-based home-care programs which led her in 1984 to initiate a community ethics committee at CJE. In the 1990's, she chaired the advisory committee to Illinois' community Care Program as it incorporated client-centered concepts into the state run program. The Ethics in Home-Care Project emerged from this work. She has always believed that the problems in home care are too complex and too numerous to be left only to agencies and the state, but that they require reflection by individuals. She has promoted these ideas while serving on home-care boards and commissions. She has written articles, book chapters and has made numerous local, national and international presentations on this topic. In 1995, she was a delegate to the White House Conference on Aging.

Ethics in Community-Based Elder Care

Martha B. Holstein, PhD
Phyllis B. Mitzen, ACSW, LCSW
Editors

Portions of this work were originally published as the Fall 1998 issue of **Generations,** Journal of the American Society on Aging.

 SPRINGER PUBLISHING COMPANY

Copyright © 2001 by Springer Publishing Company, Inc. and American Society on Aging.

All rights reserved

No part of this publication may be reproduced, stored in a retrieval system, or transmitted in any form or by any means, electronic, mechanical, photocopying, recording, or otherwise, without the prior permission of the publisher.

Springer Publishing Company, Inc.
536 Broadway
New York, NY 10012-3955

American Society on Aging
833 Market Street
Suite 511
San Francisco, CA 94103-1824

Acquisitions Editor: Helvi Gold
Production Editor: J. Hurkin-Torres
Cover design by Susan Hauley

01 02 03 04 05 / 5 4 3 2 1

Library of Congress Cataloging-in-Publication Data

Ethics in community-based elder care / editors, Martha B. Holstein, Phyllis Mitzen
    p. cm. — (Springer series on ethics, law, and aging)
    Includes bibliographical references and index.
    ISBN-13: 978-0-8261-2297-1
    1. Community health services—Moral and ethical aspects. 2. Aged—Long-term care—Moral and ethical aspects. 3. Long-term care of the sick—Moral and ethical aspects.
4. Home care services—Moral and ethical aspects. I. Holstein, Martha. II. Mitzen, Phyllis. III. Series.
R725.5 .E885 2001
174'2—dc21   2001020179
                                                                                      CIP

Printed in the United States of America by Maple-Vail

Contents

Contributors ix

Preface xi

Part I. Introduction

1. Elders in the Community: Moral Lives, Moral Quandaries — 3
   Martha B. Holstein and Phyllis Mitzen

Part II. Background/Theory

2. Ethics and Aging: A Historical Perspective — 19
   Brian F. Hofland
3. Bringing Ethics Home: A New Look at Ethics in the Home and the Community — 31
   Martha B. Holstein
4. The Ethical Importance of Home Care — 51
   Mark Waymack
5. An Ethic of Care — 60
   Joan C. Tronto
6. Old Ethical Frameworks: What Works, What Doesn't? — 69
   Mark Waymack

Part III. Organizations/Care Providers/Care Receivers

7. Creating an Ethical Organization — 79
   David B. McCurdy
8. Organizational Ethics in a Nonprofit Agency: Changing Practice, Enduring Values — 94
   Phyllis Mitzen

9. Ethics in Clinical Practice With Older Adults: 98
Recognizing Biases and Respecting Boundaries
Robyn L. Golden and Sallie Sonneborn

10. Ethics and the Frontline Long-Term-Care Worker: A 111
Challenge for the 21st Century
Robyn I. Stone and Yoshiko Yamada

11. When the Helper Needs Help: A Social Worker's 122
Experiences in Receiving Home Care
Nan G. O'Connor

12. Care at Home: Virtue in Multigenerational Households 132
Hilde Lindemann Nelson and James Lindemann Nelson

Part IV. Practice

13. Mapping the Jungle: A Proposed Method for Ethical 145
Decision Making in Geriatric Social Work
David Fireman, Sharon Dornberg-Lee, and Lisa Moss

14. Adult Day Services: Ethics and Daily Life 166
Pat Stacy Cohen

15. Is Home Care Always the Best Care? 187
Daniel Kuhn

16. A Good Death? Finding a Balance Between the Interests 200
of Patients and Caregivers
Stephen Ellingson and Jon D. Fuller

17. Case Managers Meeting to Discuss Ethics 208
Gail McClelland

18. Who's Safe? Who's Sorry?: The Duty to Protect the 217
Safety of HCBS Consumers
Rosalie A. Kane and Carrie A. Levin

19. Addressing Prejudice: A Layered Analysis 234
David E. Guinn

20. Cross-Cultural Geriatric Ethics: Negotiating Our 249
Differences
Harry R. Moody

Part V. Policy

21. The Science and Ethics of Long-Term Care 263
Larry Polivka

22.	Paid Family Caregiving: A Practical and Ethical Conundrum *Martha B. Holstein and Phyllis Mitzen*	276
	The Case Against Paid Family Caregivers: Ethical and Practical Issues *C. Jean Blaser*	278
	Payments to Families Who Provide Care: An Option That Should Be Available *Lori Simon-Rusinowitz, Kevin J. Mahoney, and A. E. Benjamin*	286
23.	Ethics, the State, and Public Policy: From the Inside, From the Outside *June L. Noel*	297

Index   *311*

Contributors

A. E. Benjamin, Ph.D.
School of Public Policy and Social Research
University of California, Los Angeles
Los Angeles, CA

Jean Blaser, Ph.D.
Illinois Department on Aging
Springfield, IL

Pat Stacy Cohen
Accolade Adult Day Care
Oak Park, IL

Sharon Dornberg-Lee, LCSW
Council for Jewish Elderly
Chicago, IL

Stephen Ellingson, Ph.D.
Pacific Lutheran Theological Seminary
Graduate Theological Union
Berkeley, CA

David Fireman, LCSW
Council for Jewish Elderly
Chicago, IL

Jon Fuller, MD
Home Based Primary Care-SFVAMC
Department of Medicine/Geriatrics
San Francisco, CA

Robyn Golden, LCSW
Council for Jewish Elderly
Chicago, IL

David Guinn, J.D., Ph.D.
Park Ridge Center for the Study of Health, Faith, and Ethics
Chicago, IL

Brian Hofland, Ph.D.
Atlantic Philanthropies
New York, NY

Rosalie A. Kane, DSW
Institute for Health Services Research
University of Minnesota
Minneapolis, MN

Dan Kuhn, MSW
Mather Institute on Aging
Evanston, IL

Carrie Levin, Ph.D.
Health Sciences Research and Administration
University of Minnesota
Minneapolis, MN

Kevin Mahoney, Ph.D.
Cash and Counseling Demonstration and Evaluation
Boston College Graduate School of Social Work
University of Maryland
College Park, MD

Gail McClelland, MSW
Milwaukee County Department on Aging
Milwaukee, WI

David McCurdy, D.Minn
Park Ridge Center for the Study of Health, Faith, and Ethics
Chicago, IL

Harry R. Moody, Ph.D.
Institute for Human Values and Aging
Brookdale Center on Aging of Hunter College
New York, NY

Lisa Moss, LCSW
Council for Jewish Elderly
Chicago, IL

Hilde Lindemann Nelson, Ph.D.
Department of Philosophy
Michigan State University
East Lansing, MI

James Lindemann Nelson, Ph.D.
Department of Philosophy
Michigan State University
East Lansing, MI

June Noel, MA
Consultant
Tallahassee, FL

Nan O'Connor, MSW
Self-employed Social Worker
Mt. Pleasant, IL

Larry Polivka, Ph.D.
Florida Policy Exchange Center on Aging
University of South Florida
Tampa, FL

Lori Simon-Rusinowitz, MPH, Ph.D.
Cash and Counseling Demonstration and Evaluation
Center on Aging
University of Maryland
Kensington, MD

Sallie Sonneborn
Center for Applied Gerontology
Council for Jewish Elderly
Chicago, IL

Robyn Stone, Dr.P.H.
Institute for the Future of Aging Services
American Association of Homes and Services for the Aging
Washington, DC

Joan Tronto, Ph.D.
Department of Political Science
Hunter College
New York, NY

Mark Waymack, Ph.D.
Department of Philosophy and Program in Health Care Ethics
Loyola University
Chicago, IL

Yoshiko Yamada
Center for Health Workforce Studies
SUNY Albany
School of Public Health
Rensselaer, NY

Preface

This book is the work of many minds and hearts working both collaboratively and independently, and their commitment to the patients and clients whose lives, we hope, will be better by virtue of the ideas this book presents. Some authors wrote their original articles for an issue of Generations; others have expanded or adapted these original articles, and yet others have written original articles for this book. In our minds it represents the second generation of work in ethics and long-term care, respectfully appreciating the work that has come before but moving off in different directions. This earlier work, stimulated by the bioethical framework that took shape in the acute care setting, centered on such ideals as patient autonomy and informed consent. This book builds upon that critical foundation, and then attempts to expand the repertoire of values and concerns that deserve ethical attention and action. It locates ethics squarely within the realm of practice and so asks us to perceive the ethical terrain expansively and to address problems from a conversational or dialogic perspective. These new directions are thus both substantive and procedural. Its particular focus on home and community-based care itself reflects the major expansion of that sector in the past few years; we express our ethical values in all our relationships of care, concern, and commitment. If this new direction can be stated in a nutshell, it might go like this: an ethics for long-term care spans a large and rich canvas that includes a rethinking of autonomy, wide definitions of respect and dignity, attention to context and particularity, and a focus on everyday matters in addition to moments of choice; bioethics, which includes such important concepts as client autonomy, confidentiality and privacy, and informed consent, only touched upon these issues. The themes of some articles reflect that new expansiveness. Procedurally, the book introduces ways to think about ethical problems that do not rely primarily on principles. Yet, as you shall see, we exercised no editorial veto power over the messages different authors wished to convey.

But all this work is only in its earliest stages. As practitioners, ethicists, and others interested in this area, we must continue to reflect on our practices, question our habitual approvals and disapprovals, and struggle always with the discomfort of ambiguity when really good answers are scarce. We invite readers to join us and the other authors in these intellectually challenging but practically necessary tasks. Resources will not become more plentiful; people will continue to need care in their homes and in the community; and dedicated people will persist in wondering what else they might do to make conditions for clients and patients just a little better.

As co-editors of this book, we thank every author, all of whom answered our requests, took our comments graciously, and responded to them promptly. These authors, all friends and colleagues, have reinforced the important task of joining research and theory to practice; they inform one another. To the working committee of the Retirement Research Foundation for the grant that made much of the co-editors' work possible, we have an abundance of thanks. They not only came to meetings regularly even if it meant being in the car at 5 a.m. but participated in all aspects of the project with enthusiasm and "smarts." The Illinois Department of Aging's Division on Long-Term Care made possible many opportunities for us to meet with case managers, supervisors, and frontline workers. Without their help much would be missing from this book.

We are especially grateful to our organizations—the Park Ridge Center for the Study of Health, Faith, and Ethics for providing an environment in which scholarship can thrive and contribute to practice and the Council for Jewish Elderly for its early recognition that thinking about practice in specifically ethical ways enhances the well-being of clients and supports the care provider. And, more personally, we hope all collaborative efforts can be so blessed as this one. Our friendship not only survived the test of co-editorship but emerged even richer than before.

Martha B. Holstein
Phyllis Mitzen

I
Introduction

CHAPTER 1

Elders in the Community: Moral Lives, Moral Quandaries

Martha B. Holstein and Phyllis Mitzen

> The questions of bioethics and medical ethics are not purely intellectual questions. They are questions of the heart as well as the mind, and questions of social organization, not just the marshalling of arguments. It is harder to reform one's heart or one's society than to improve one's arguments. The sort of disciplined reflection we need on these questions is not merely intellectual. (Baier, 1992, pp. 14–15)

This book, with its focus on the ethics of non-institutional long-term care for the elderly, comes at an auspicious moment for two very different reasons. Applied ethics, the study of how we ought to behave in situations involving human care, is in flux. No longer does it appear sufficient to call upon deductively derived, universal principles and rules to guide action. Contributions from feminism, narrative and moral psychology, and the social sciences have invigorated conversations about "ought" questions and raised doubts about the possibilities for moral certainties (see Waymack, chapter 6, for a discussion of these newer approaches to ethics). It is an exciting, albeit difficult, time as we seek to integrate the new with the old as several chapters in this volume will reveal. Simultaneously, caring for older people outside of institutions is the fastest growing sector of the U.S. health care industry (Feldman, 1997); it seems to be what older people want above all. This wish and its fulfillment, however, can be quite problematic for individuals, for families, and for communities. It is especially difficult for women. Twice as many elderly women as men need care or support if they are to continue residing in the community. Women also provide the greatest amount of formal (paid) and informal (unpaid) care (Arber & Ginn, 1991).

Building upon its important earlier work (see Hofland, chapter 2), the Retirement Research Foundation generously supported the Park Ridge Center for the Study of Health, Faith, and Ethics (PRC) for 2 years in its exploration of an ethics appropriate for home- and community-based care. The PRC had the privilege of convening, for these years, a working group of practitioners and scholars to examine the questions raised in this book. Interviews with care providers, family members, and care receivers further widened our horizon (see chapter 3 for a more detailed description of this project).

In this introduction, we will explore some of what we have learned in this project, recognize the work of the authors who have contributed to this book, and examine the complexities of developing an ethics for community-based long-term care. We do this task modestly, recognizing that our conclusions must necessarily be tentative.

THE HOME AS A SITE OF CARE

Setting a consistent theme, Larry Polivka (chapter 21) challenges policymakers and policy analysts (including himself) to make home care a more viable option for older people needing care. He insists that one more "perfect" study will not "prove" anything more than we already know about home care; while it may add information about cost effectiveness, the moral values at stake are quite clear. In chapter 4, Mark Waymack offers a rich analysis of these moral values. Home is a special place where older people feel less ill than in institutions and where they are able to act, at least to some degree and with help, in ways that cohere with consistent life choices. Yet, even if older people regularly opt for and receive home-based over institutional care, deep moral concerns and value conflicts are not easily eliminated.

One reason for such ethical complications is an underlying problem—the lack of adequate public resources to serve clients in a time of perceived scarcity is often a subtext for much of the ethical anguish that care providers and families face. Home- and community-based care, provided through public programs, are linked to state and federal policy developments that determine the reimbursable service package. Federal cost saving efforts do not bode well for local programs. Constrained resources often limit the level of assistance that older clients receive. At the same time, fiscal accountability transforms often intimate and not always easily defined needs into discrete tasks. A rich account of ethical responsibilities in home care can easily be set aside by the resource constraints and the task-orientation associated with public provision of services. Yet such benefits are necessary for many families. This is one reason (although there are many others) that autonomy has come to have such significant value in home care. It importantly guarantees the participation of the client in decisions about his or her life even though the choices themselves might be quite limited. Autonomy itself can be a lonely substitute for the deeper human relationships that make home care more tolerable as it becomes more necessary. As health care analyst Deborah Stone (1999) tellingly noted: "The more I talked with people, the more I saw how financial tightening and the ratcheting up of managerial scrutiny are changing the moral world of caregiving, along with the quantity and quality of care" (p. 62). So one important—but not easily solved—moral problem is showing that one is accountable for the instrumental tasks in a way that satisfies the funding source without diminishing the human values of caregiving.

Yet, even ample resources cannot eliminate the moral quandaries that arise when painful losses of late life mean looking to others for help with daily needs for food, cleanliness, or elimination. For most of our lives, these "activities of daily living" have been intensely private, at best shared with a few selected intimates. As Nan O'Connor describes in chapter 11, becoming a care receiver is morally perplexing. How does one keep good caregivers? Should one "game" the system to help out a poorly paid worker? How does one face one's own feelings of shame and then anger when the most private acts now demand participation of another? These problems may be mitigated for individuals and families who pay privately for services since more time is available for attentive, empathic care, but the very nature of the situation means that the daily struggle for dignity and self-respect continues.

For most agencies and their employees, making choices about allocating resources is an ongoing struggle. In choosing, there may be no "right" strategies but only marginally acceptable options that serve in the absence of the broader policy changes that we seek as advocates. It may thus be a time when moral imagination can open new possibilities. Can we find voluntary assistance beyond the family? Might a person do with a little less and still be basically okay? Are there any other ways of easing caregivers' anxieties about doing too little when they are doing all that they can do? Can we envision new and different ways of caring for frail and disabled older people? Are there as yet undiscovered ways to balance individual wants/needs with communal needs, a problem that arises both in the macro world of public policy and in the microcosm of adult day health services? Are they necessarily in conflict? Is there something important to be learned from our varied religious traditions about balancing individual and community? June Noel (chapter 23) offers readers a glimpse of how Florida tried to address questions of ethics and resource allocation at a community level. What can we learn from that model?

States with Medicaid home care waivers and other state-funded programs have historically justified providing home- and community-based care on two grounds: It is the preference of elders and it costs less than nursing home care. But often states are also reluctant to develop community care programs because they fear the costs. The potential but unproved "woodwork" effect is one source of anxiety. Families, in general, tend to be remarkably dedicated in the care they provide and count on public assistance only when necessary. States also recognize that for many clients an adequate care plan may cost more than care in a nursing home and for the very impaired client, non-institutional care may always seem inadequate. An "inadequate care plan" creates elemental fears about safety and quality but provokes thinking about the very meanings of safety and also the emerging concept of negotiated risk (see Kane and Levin, chapter 18, and Holstein, chapter 3, for a longer discussion about these themes). Further, what makes a care plan inadequate and who defines inadequacy and on what grounds? The notion of inadequacy returns us to the social question: How many and what kinds of resources is society willing to dedicate not only to provide *some* care for elders with disabling conditions but to provide more than "adequate" care? Will home care and day care services be viable public options for the soon-to-be-aging baby boomers if negative attitudes toward taxation and government services do not change?

THE HOME CARE WORKER

There are other problems. While we often ask about the division of responsibility between family and the state for the client, we less often consider another question: Who cares for the dependency worker? The dependency worker's position is difficult. From the worker's perspective, as Stone and Yamada argue in chapter 10, serious problems emerge with regularity: low pay which compels many workers to have a second or a third job, balancing the needs of different clients, overwhelming feelings of responsibility which often make it difficult to draw boundaries between workers' lives and their work, emotional exhaustion, and poor treatment by the client or the client's family. The almost singleminded emphasis on clients' right tends to diminish an equally important notion, that care workers also deserve dignity and respect.

In many parts of the country there is a shortage of paid home care and adult day service center workers, serious problems with worker turnover, and negative consequences of inadequate training, especially as the home care worker assumes more difficult tasks. Nearly full employment now compounds this problem even further as low-wage service sector jobs give workers new options. When meeting with case managers and supervisors throughout Illinois, the editors encountered a query like this one: Is it better to have no home care aide than one who is only marginally competent or worse? It is difficult to respond when there are no workers available, or no workers available at the minimum wage. Failing a lobbying effort to enlarge state budgets for home care and to renegotiate Medicaid reimbursement rates (and direct such increases to wages for care workers), what else is possible? How does one counter the perspective that "any warm body" can do the sensitive work of caring for older and dependent people? And why are wages and benefits for care workers not central to contemporary debates about health care reform?

In response, some workers are actively unionizing; in other places they are forming worker cooperatives. Both options offer them some autonomy and better pay than they would receive working for an agency. Should remedies for worker stress be implemented, the positive benefits of caregiving (for example, personal fulfillment, some autonomy in regard to hours and pace, rewarding work based on a belief in its value) might prevail and keep workers at their jobs for longer periods of time (Donovan, 1989).

Racist remarks, often directed at the care worker by the client, and sometimes the outright refusal to have someone of "that" race come into my home are not infrequent (see Guinn, chapter 19). While discrimination is both illegal and morally reprehensible, do our ethical obligations to the worker or to the client cease with those affirmations? What steps might we take to address a potentially painful and often explosive issue? Ethical questions that center on workers have only recently gathered attention (see Kane, 1994; McCurdy, 1997). As individuals with moral standing, what are the limits of workers' obligations to, for example, travel to neighborhoods where they fear drug deals and violence on the streets or to homes where they encounter abusive adult children or filth almost beyond their imagination? How can supervisors and case managers support good training, communicate thoughtfully, and provide the "caring" that workers need when, in many parts of the country, case loads are very large and time is a precious commodity?

ACKNOWLEDGING DIFFERENCES

Insensitivity (often because of limited knowledge) about culturally diverse practices among clients in areas that directly affect their dignity and well-being also troubles care providers, the agencies for which they work, and the state that often funds the programs. What is the caregiver to do when her ethical code—and agency requirements—demands informed consent, but her patient's family insists that the patient not be informed of the diagnosis and treatment? This raises the question: Is autonomy a universally held principle enacted in the health care setting through informed consent procedures or is it a more particular moral value that bolsters some Western ideas of what it means to respect a person's dignity? This clash reflects not only external value differences but reaches deep into notions of personhood, family, and community and tests our abilities to empathize and negotiate solutions. Harry R. Moody attends to these concerns in chapter 20.

ORGANIZATIONAL CONCERNS

These issues broach the often-neglected area that David McCurdy's and Phyllis Mitzen's chapters address (chapters 7 and 8). Organizations are not neutral entities. They have moral commitments and moral personalities. Many often have specific codes of ethics but these documents may not, in practice, govern the day-to-day practices that shape an individual's ability to work comfortably, effectively, and indeed ethically. Some organizations, such as the Council for Jewish Elderly (Mitzen, chapter 8), have established organizational ethics committees to address decisions and practices that are problematic. Other organizations focus on caregiving issues; the effort of case managers at the Milwaukee County Department on Aging that Gail McClelland (chapter 17) describes captures this process and the commitment that it requires. Sometimes organizations have established mechanisms not only to discuss specific cases but also to address issues on appeal. The Illinois Department on Aging is one such example. Often-neglected organizational structures, values, and commitments may be some of the central features that shape an individual's ability to behave ethically in his or her work.

FAMILIES AND CAREGIVING

While families—particularly wives, daughters, and daughter-in-laws—have always been at the heart and soul of long-term-care policy in the United States, such caregivers are also caught in webs of conflicting responsibilities and loyalties. Responding to an older person's wish, for example, to die at home, can create devastating consequences for the caregiver as Stephen Ellingson and Jon Fuller suggest in chapter 16. To protect one individual's personal autonomy may deny or limit it for another person. Simultaneously, many family care providers seem to willingly and even aggressively sacrifice their own needs to care for another. While these attitudes and behaviors are most likely linked closely to social constructions of gender, they are also constitutive of how many people understand their identity and moral value and so are not easily set aside. Yet, in our society the caregiver, whether paid or unpaid, rarely receives recognition, especially moral praise. As historian Emily Abel (1995) thoughtfully notes,

> A society that extols the virtues of independence, views old people with dread, and seeks to distance itself from fundamental life events will disparage as unhealthy women who devote themselves to nursing sick and dying elderly people. A major problem for many women is that they are simultaneously encouraged to provide care and condemned for doing so. (p. 62)

Moral flourishing of both caregiver and care receiver is an aim worth seeking. Yet how often that becomes very nearly impossible is a subject that geriatric social workers encounter on a daily basis. In chapter 13, Fireman, Dornberg-Lee, and Moss suggest recourse to a procedural approach to resolving problems that is a good beginning, but the questions one must ask do not always lead to easy resolution.

An important indicator of continuing inequalities in our society becomes readily visible when one looks at who gives care to whom (see Tronto, 1994 and chapter 5). While the woman caregiver may appear to be making an autonomous choice to engage in caregiving activities, it is only by sleight of hand that one can describe her as equally situated and empowered as those individuals who assert that it is her choice (or, as some would have it, her duty). The very needs of the dependent person obligates caregivers in ways that "situate them unequally with respect to others who are not similarly obligated" (Kittay, 1999, p. 76). Only recently have ethicists joined gerontologists in calling attention to problems associated with caregiving; hence the study of gender injustice in caregiving and what it might take to remedy a situation that implicates the American economic structure, the social construction of gender, and other systemic problems requires continued attention in policy and practice (Holstein, 1999; Hooyman & Gonyea, 1995; Okin, 1989). Women caregivers can rarely transfer their responsibilities to others since they lack the resources to pay for help and often get little or no assistance from others in the family. These same women are also bearing the brunt of earlier discharges from hospitals. Since it is unlikely that public spending on caregiving will increase, the one expandable component is the "informal" care of family members, especially women. Yet, what women do is not counted as a cost (England, Keigher, Miller, & Linsk, 1991). Working outside of the market economy, these women (and some men) are often socially and politically invisible. Yet, this informal work, if translated into dollars, is worth more than double the public expenditure of funds (Glazer, 1990; Arno, Levine, & Memmott, 1999).

The point-counterpoint on paid family caregiving (see Blaser, and Simon-Rusinowitz, Mahoney, and Benjamin, chapter 22) analyzes one effort to remedy gender injustice. But, as these articles reveal, it raises other ethical questions that require continued dialogue. Do these solutions solve some problems while creating others? To what extent can policy and programmatic interventions remedy problems that Jean Blaser, for example, identifies? Is there the will or the resources to put interventions in place? What happens when the client is incapable of managing the caregiver?

Worrying about gender injustice and seeking ways to remedy it reflects another trend in ethical thinking—the importance of the family beyond their role as conveyors of their relative's wishes (see Nelson and Nelson, chapter 12). This emphasis on the family serves as a counterweight to the almost single-minded focus on client or patient autonomy that has pervaded the U.S. ethics literature. This work reminds us that few of us live completely self-interested lives; concern for others cannot (should not) be eliminated from our deliberations about and emotional responsiveness to later-life difficulties. Nor should choosing with others in mind simply be one option for the autonomous person. Some scholars have recently insisted that the social nature of the self requires social arrangements that aid its development and continuity and recognize its contribution to our collective moral lives. How would beliefs about moral value and social organization, for example, shift if we took the social self as more adequate than the autonomous self as an account of who we are as people? Adopting such a view of the self does not mean neglecting individual wishes but it does urge us to look beyond autonomy as the central value in our ethical deliberations.

Case managers are often both advocates and gatekeepers who may—perhaps unavoidably—see situations they encounter from a perspective shaped by their own values and experiences (see Golden and Sonneborn, chapter 9). Put into the dual role of caring about the safety and well-being of each client and the overall need to allocate agency resources fairly and in accord with regulations and state requirements, case managers must be alert to what they expect from clients' family members or friends and to their belief systems about the meaning of such terms as safety. While professionals most often reduce safety to physical safety, clients may see have different ideas about risk as they protect their psychological safety (see Kane and Levin, chapter 18; Fireman, Dornberg-Lee, and Moss, chapter 13; Holstein, chapter 3; and Collopy, 1995). Among other questions, one must then ask: Does the client share the care workers' definitions and understandings? To what extent does a case manager try to persuade a client in order to guide or even alter her choices in a direction of professionally defined ideas about safety?

SPECIAL BUT NOT UNCOMMON

Specific illnesses or conditions raise unique problems when caring for elders at home. Dementia, as Dan Kuhn's chapter shows, almost always, once again, raises questions about risk and safety, about patterns of caregiving, about stigma and telling the truth, about dignity and self-maintaining activities (see Kuhn, chapter 15). In many ways, we are only beginning to grapple with the complex ethical issues that Alzheimer's disease raises (see Holstein, 1998, for an entire issue of the *Journal of Clinical Ethics* devoted to ethics and Alzheimer's disease). End-of-life care, for the patient who wishes to die at home, can go smoothly and comfortably but it can also be "messy" (see Ellingson and Fuller, chapter 16). Even in well-intentioned families, it might prove to be too difficult to keep the dying person at home. Here, as with dementia, there will always be less than ideal answers to problematic situations.

THE DAY SERVICES SETTING

The adult day services center has become a critically important adjunct for families who are trying to care for elderly relatives at home. Like home care, day care faces problems of funding, inadequate staffing levels, and a wide mix of patients. In terms of ethics, however, the fact that day services take place in a communal setting gives the aide more immediate access to supervisory personnel than the home care worker has available. This environment permits greater collaboration in anticipating, resolving, and reviewing problems. Yet, difficult situations arise. In chapter 14, Pat Cohen provides an insider's look at what happens within such a center.

MOVING FORWARD

The above discussion outlines some of the familiar ethical and practical problems that arise in home- and community-based care for older people with physical and mental disabilities. These problems challenge us to ask some fundamental questions, namely: What do we really mean when we talk about ethics and *how* should we think through an ethical quandary? Many professionals have been trained to think about ethics as a clash in values or a dilemma of some definable sort; they have also learned to resolve such dilemmas by balancing principles such as autonomy and "do no harm." The key value conflict was generally framed as patient autonomy versus professional beneficence or the directive to do good for the patient. Familiarly known as the "Georgetown mantra," these transcendent and rationally deduced moral values are autonomy, beneficence, non-maleficence, and justice. In this view, balancing these values is the task of ethical analysis. Certain analytical pathways evolved: gather the facts, determine the values of each party, identify the ethical problem, work toward a justifiable solution, and develop a workable plan of action (Haddad & Kapp, 1991). But alone they cannot encompass the particularistic contexts in which actual ethical deliberations occur. Nor do they bring into view the moral qualities of everyday actions that can profoundly shape the quality of an elder's life. Attending closely to public forums, ethics committee meetings, and writing reveals a richer and more complex analysis than the paradigmatic model suggests (see Fireman, Dornberg-Lee, and Moss, chapter 13). Deliberations reflect the diversity of the moral issues we encounter. They also move beyond a basically procedural approach to ask questions about the good—about the basic aims of our practices and the means to achieve these ends.

In our thinking throughout this project, we came to believe that taking ethics seriously is to transcend the resolution of value conflicts in terms of *a priori* rules (see Holstein, chapter 3, for a detailed look at the project and an approach to ethical analysis). As chapter 3 describes, ethics is a part of our everyday encounters with family, friends, colleagues, and clients. It is how our attentiveness and responsiveness becomes part of our caring practices; it focuses on how we respect the client as a person and how we order our relations with other people. We live our morality in our day-to-day lives by exhibiting responsibilities for things open to human care and response (Walker, 1998), hence, much that is ethical occurs in the interstices of our lives when we are hardly paying attention: how we talk to someone, how we greet a client, how we learn about and honor differences. Most of us want to behave in ways that are morally praiseworthy (without having to be Mother Teresa). Ethical language gives us a way to talk about problems that is more expansive and richer than the law or "by the book" policies or procedures and it directs our attention to pressing concerns in our personal lives, in our work lives, and in our society. By reflecting on the following case narrative, we hope the "everydayness" of ethics will become clearer.

HELLO, I'M MRS. PONTE

The Spring Hill Home Care Agency has just sent a home care worker out for the first time to meet a new client. Mrs. Sampson is 88 years old and lives alone in the house she had shared with her husband for over 60 years. The worker, Mrs. Ponte, knows that Mrs. Sampson has three children but that only one lives close enough to visit regularly. Mrs. Sampson's doctor had referred her to the case management agency because it was becoming harder and harder for her to bathe and dress herself and she seemed to be eating little but tea and crackers. They told Mrs. Ponte that the client suffered from osteoporosis and severe, debilitating arthritis. She had a heart condition that was reasonably well controlled by medication but she still got very tired even after mild exertion. Mostly her mind was clear although sometimes she had trouble finding a word or remembering a name. These memory lapses made her anxious although she had no diagnosis of any serious cognitive impairment. Under the Illinois Community Care Program she had qualified for 3 hours of care a day.

Mrs. Ponte arrived at her house at 10 a.m. one spring morning, dressed in a clean new uniform smock and pants. She was surprised to find that the door was unlocked. Mrs. Ponte called out and found Mrs. Sampson sitting in her chair by the living room window. She moved across the living room and stood by Mrs. Sampson's chair. Quite loudly Mrs. Ponte said, "Hi, Rose, I am Mrs. Ponte from the Spring Hill Home Care Agency and in no time at all, we'll get you cleaned up and looking fresh and pretty again. I know how to take care of someone like you. Just you wait and see."

> Mrs. Sampson doesn't say anything but continues to stare straight ahead. Her hands are in her lap, her fingernails are dirty and need cutting but her posture is as erect as it can be given her osteoporosis. You can tell that her dress, though now old and shabby, was once of good quality. A magazine lay in her lap fallen open to an article about Alzheimer's disease.
>
> As she walks around the apartment getting situated, Mrs. Ponte continues to talk to Mrs. Sampson. The first task is to get her cleaned up. So the caregiver checks the condition of the bathroom and finds the tub is a mess; she tells Mrs. Sampson that she's going to clean the tub and then will give her a bath. Like a naughty child, Mrs. Sampson holds her hands over her ears as Mrs. Ponte continues speaking to her. When Mrs. Ponte tries to get her to come to the bathtub, she gets agitated and says she doesn't want to take a bath right then. Okay, Mrs. Ponte thinks, I'll wait awhile even though the water will get cold. Instead she went into the kitchen to begin fixing Mrs. Sampson's lunch. She noticed a funny smell in the refrigerator and began looking around for spoiling food. When she found it, she pointed out to Mrs. Sampson that she is letting food rot in the refrigerator and that eating such food can be dangerous. Mrs. Sampson pointedly ignored Mrs. Ponte.
>
> The situation does not get any better. Mrs. Sampson won't make a move to get to the tub and she barely touches her sandwich. Mrs. Ponte knew that she had followed the instructions that her instructor had given her, that she had done what the care plan had laid out but she seemed to be getting nowhere. Mrs. Sampson still wasn't clean; she hadn't eaten, and the time was running out. Moreover, what about that unlocked door? Mrs. Ponte thought, "What if I left and someone just walked in?" When asked about the unlocked door, Mrs. Sampson said she kept it that way because it was too hard for her to get up to open it if someone rang the bell. She got angry when Mrs. Ponte said that she was going to lock it when she left because she didn't want any strangers breaking into the house.

In thinking about this narrative, you might ask: What was going on? What is ethically important in this story? If Mrs. Ponte had been truly attentive to Mrs. Sampson, what might she have done differently? If you were Mrs. Sampson, how would you tell the story? What do you think Mrs. Sampson was experiencing as cheerful, efficient Mrs. Ponte came into her house? How could Mrs. Ponte have contributed to Mrs. Sampson's efforts to maintain her self-respect and self-esteem? What might she have done to lay the foundations for a trusting relationship? What does it mean to care well? How do we take seriously the moral aspects of giving care: attentiveness, responsiveness? Other questions that we might ask include: What good do we want from our practices? What options can we *imagine* that might ease the situation we are facing? What virtues, like compassion, care, courage, honor do we want to exemplify in our practices and how can we do so in the current environment of home and community care? These questions and concerns do not make it less important to understand Mrs. Sampson's choices when there are choices to be made. Instead they enlarge the moral domain and, by so doing, enhance care.

CONCLUSION

We invite readers to continue thinking with us about the ways in which ethical reflection, especially with an enlarged moral compass, can contribute to the well-being of older clients and patients. In many ways long-term-care settings give us opportunities not available in acute care. We have time to come to know the person and his or her family. We can build trusting relationships and nurture them as the person's condition changes. At the same time, we must learn to live with ambiguity and uncertainty—the situations that arise in long-term care are not easily resolvable even with adequate resources and loving families. This reality does not mitigate the struggle that is inherent in the work we do but it reminds us that there are some problems we cannot solve in altogether comfortable ways.

REFERENCES

Abel, E. (1995). Representations of Caregiving by Margaret Foster, Mary Gordon, and Doris Lessing. *Research on Aging,* 17(1), 63.

Arber, S., & Ginn, J. (1991). *Gender and later life: A sociological analysis of resources and constraints.* London: Sage Publications.

Arno, P., Levine, C., & Memmott, M. (1999). The economic value of caregiving. *Health Affairs,* 18(2), 182–188.

Baier, A. (1992). Alternative offerings to Asclepius? *Medical Humanities Review,* 6(1), 9–19.

Collopy, B. (1995). Safety and independence: Rethinking some basic concepts in long-term care. In L. McCullough & N. Wilson (Eds.), *Long-term care decisions: Ethical and conceptual dimensions* (pp. 137–154). Baltimore: The Johns Hopkins University Press.

Donovan, R. (1989). Worker stress and job satisfaction: A study of home care workers in New York City. *Home Health Care Services Quarterly,* 10(1/2), 97–114.

England, S., Keigher, S., Miller, B., & Linsk, N. (1991). Community care politics and gender justice. In M. Minkler & C. Estes (Eds.), *Critical perspectives on aging: The political and moral economy of growing old* (pp. 227–244). Amityville, NY: Baywood Publishing.

Feldman, P. H. (1997). Labor market issues in home care. In D. Fox & C. Raphael (Eds.), *Home-based care for a new century* (pp. 155–183). New York: Milbank Memorial Fund.

Glazer, N. (1990). The home as a workshop: Women and amateur nurses and medical care providers. *Gender and Society, 4,* 479–499.

Haddad, A., & Kapp, M. (1991). *Ethical and legal issues in home health care.* Norwalk, CT: Appleton & Lange.

Holstein, M. (1999). Home care, women, and aging: A case study of injustice. In M. U. Walker (Ed.), *Mother time: Women, aging, and ethics.* Lanham, MD: Rowman and Littlefield.

Hooyman, N., & Gonyea, J. (1995). *Feminist perspectives on family care: Policies for gender justice.* Thousand Oaks, CA: Sage Publications.

Holstein, M. (Ed.). (1998). Special issue on ethics and Alzheimer's disease. *Journal of Clinical Ethics, 9*(1).

Kane, R. A. (1994). Ethics and the frontline care worker: Mapping the subject. In P. H. Feldman (Ed.), *Generations, 8*(3), 71–74.

Kittay, E. (1999). *Love's labor: Essays on women, equality, and dependency.* New York: Routledge.

McCurdy, D. (1997). Appreciating staff members as moral stakeholders. *Ethical Currents, 48,* 9–10.

Okin, S. M. (1989). *Justice, gender, and the family.* New York: Basic Books.

Stone, D. (1999). Care and trembling. *The American Prospect, 43*(March/April), 61–67.

Taylor, C. (1985). *Human agency: Philosophical papers.* Cambridge: Cambridge University Press.

Tronto, J. (1993). *Moral boundaries: A political argument for an ethic of care.* New York: Routledge.

Walker, M. U. (1998). *Moral understandings: A feminist study in ethics.* New York: Routledge.

II

Background/Theory

CHAPTER 2

Ethics and Aging: A Historical Perspective

Brian F. Hofland

Providing adequate services and care for older adults with disabilities is a great public and private concern in the United States. Efforts to provide services and health care for these elderly individuals bring into sharp focus fundamental value conflicts and ethical dilemmas. As the numbers and percentages of the U.S. frail elderly population continue to grow, these conflicts and dilemmas will take on added urgency. Thus, the current work of Holstein and Mitzen (see chapter 3) in examining the ethics of home care within their "Home- and Community-Based Services for Elders" project is both important and timely. However, their efforts are the direct descendant of a body of earlier work funded by the Retirement Research Foundation that focused on issues of autonomy in long-term care. It is useful to review those earlier efforts to examine where the exploration of ethics in home care began and gain a broader historical perspective of how the conceptualization of and attention to the area has evolved over time.

THE AUTONOMY IN LONG TERM CARE INITIATIVE

For all practical purposes, the field of bioethics began in the 1970s. In 1974 Congress passed the National Research Act establishing the National Commission for the Protection of Human Subjects of Biomedical and Behavioral Research. The *Belmont Report*, published for comment in the Federal Register in 1976 and officially disseminated in 1978, contained a statement of principles to be used for the ethics of human experimentation, but also for bioethical reflection in general. Prior to 1984 there was not much attention or work by ethicists devoted to ethics and aging. What existed had a focus on acute care rather than on long-term care. In 1984, the Retirement Research Foundation (RRF) decided to help fill this gap in attention and knowledge by developing a special initiative in ethics and aging. A key informant telephone interview study of a cross-section of 18 professionals with expertise in ethics and aging (including philosophers, physicians, attorneys, theologians, and social scientists) and consultant meetings with a smaller group of professionals identified two primary possible emphases for the initiative.

One major possibility was "Autonomy of the Elderly Individual," a rubric within which the experts included such issues as informed consent, the decision-making capacity of older adults with cognitive impairment, and the maintenance of personal autonomy, particularly for frail elders. Another major possibility was "Resource Allocation," which dealt with issues of intergenerational justice, means testing, and equity in health care, all within the broad public policy arena. A number of secondary issue categories also emerged. These included "Filial Responsibility," "Education in Ethics and Aging," "Quality of Life for Frail and Ill Older Adults," "Research with Elderly Subjects," "Rights to Sexual Expression in Long Term Care Settings," and "Defection and Evasion in Government Programs for the Elderly."

The Foundation chose a focus on autonomy issues in long-term care. Autonomy, or an individual's self-determination, is a central value of American society. It lies at the basis of ethical principles and is a both a guiding value and an endpoint. The heavily paternalistic flavor to the aging network and long-term-care services provided the opportunity for the special initiative to make a major contribution. "Long-term care" was broadly defined to include the entire spectrum of care for frail or impaired older adults involving both institutional and community-based settings. The Foundation stated its request for proposals in part as follows:

> The Foundation seeks to address the ethical issues implicit in maintaining and enhancing the personal autonomy of elderly individuals in long term care.... The Foundation's goal is to encourage significant advances in knowledge, practice, education and policy.... This effort grows out of the Foundation's continuing interest in maintaining older persons in independent living environments and improving the quality of nursing home care. (Retirement Research Foundation, 1985, p. 2)

The RRF Autonomy in Long Term Care Initiative (the Initiative) was conducted from 1985 to 1990, involving two phases of grant projects and a total budget of $2 million. Twenty-eight individual grant projects were funded. Some of these were short-term projects of 6 months duration. The remaining projects were longer-term projects of one to 2 years. The projects varied a great deal in their focus and included purely conceptual efforts, qualitative and quantitative research, and best-practice and demonstration projects.

The initiative was pioneering also in its mix of overarching and connective activities that helped to build a network and further advance the field of long-term-care ethics. Grantees meeting were held every 6 months. Dr. Christine Cassel, a geriatrician then at the University of Chicago Medical Center and now at Mt. Sinai Medical Center NYU Health Systems in New York City, conducted a "meta-research" study within the Initiative. The meta-research study used the individual Initiative projects as interesting and rich case examples and the investigators as key informants to examine the ethical issues inherent in conducting research in long-term-care settings (Cassel, 1988). A National Focus Group involving representatives of 20 national long-term-care organizations, chaired by Monsignor Charles Fahey of Fordham University, met regularly to both learn about projects and to help shape them.

The particulars of the individual initiative projects will not be described or summarized here. However, special issues of *The Gerontologist* (1988) and *Generations* (1990) provide a useful summary of many of the projects.

SIX LESSONS FROM THE AUTONOMY IN LONG TERM CARE INITIATIVE

There are six major lessons and contributions regarding ethics and aging that were gained from the totality of projects in the Initiative.

1. The importance of interdisciplinary perspectives. To gain a fuller picture in examining ethical issues in aging, the importance of employing interdisciplinary perspectives cannot be over-emphasized. Aging itself is a multifaceted phenomenon. It therefore is logical and natural that to understand the ethical dimensions of a situation within aging, it is helpful to go beyond the perspective of the ethicist/ philosopher and include the perspectives of direct care workers, social workers, case managers, administrators, lawyers, physicians, nurses, social scientists and other relevant professionals. The Initiative served as a forum to bring these professionals together to focus on autonomy issues in long-term care.

2. The lived experience of the elderly needs to be the core of any moral analysis. In conducting an ethical analysis of a situation within aging, it is critical not to forget the realities of the lives of older adults and their direct care workers. It is all too easy to construct elaborate and elegant conceptual models that have little to do with the actual lives of older adults or actual work situations faced by a variety of gerontological professionals. The lived experience of older adults should form the core of any ethical effort in aging, with the moral analysis illuminating those issues. The most successful projects in the Initiative were those that had this core of actual contact with older adults. Even the purely conceptual projects benefited greatly by a grounding in the day-to-day realities of long-term care achieved by direct observation of, interviews with, and formal feedback from older adults and practitioners.

3. Need for collaboration of social science researchers and ethicists. Philosophers examining ethical issues have typically neglected the level of description (the *is*) and have immediately focused on the level of explanation (the *ought*), sometimes followed by prescriptive and proscriptive models for lawyers, clinicians, practitioners and policymakers. There is a need for more basic descriptive data with ethical analysis. Facts cannot settle value questions, but empirical research can help frame the analysis of difficult questions. In turn, descriptive research needs to be focused on key ethical questions. Within a moral analysis in aging, the social sciences can provide the descriptive level of the "is," and ethics can provide the explanatory and prescriptive level of the "ought." Each disciplinary group needs the other. By working together, they can identify the key issues, flesh them out, and illuminate them by moral analysis. A major contribution of the Initiative was the marriage of social science and ethics within individual projects and within the initiative as a whole.

4. Medical ethics does not always capture the ethical nuances and realities of long-term care. Medical ethics focuses primarily on life and death issues and has a relatively short-term perspective. The physician has great knowledge within medical situations. Long-term care focuses primarily on everyday issues and, by definition, has a longer-term perspective. The older adult has considerable and highly relevant knowledge of personal values and preferences within long-term care situations. Care options are often not better or worse, but necessarily involve preferences of the particular older adult.

For example, the needs of a frail older woman may be defined in terms of avoiding falls, if her best interests are defined as avoiding injury and the negative consequences and handicapping limitations that would follow. Here, interventions such as continual supervision by an adult child or nursing home placement would be appropriate. Yet her needs also could be defined in terms of maintaining independence. Here, the removal of interior barriers, such as door thresholds and scatter rugs, and the use of a walker would be appropriate. There is no *a priori* way of weighing the good of security against the good of maintaining independence. In such long-term-care situations, the patient's values and beliefs serve as the basis for defining needs and evaluating the appropriateness of alternative interventions (Hofland, 1988). The Initiative was pioneering in its efforts to go beyond the medical dimensions of ethical issues in long-term care.

5. The importance of everyday ethics. Everyday ethics, as opposed to life-and-death ethics, make up the bulk of long term care and are therefore the part and parcel of long term care ethics. A strong contribution of the Initiative was that many day-to-day ethical issues were examined for the first time, including nursing home admission agreements, the existence and selection of roommates, selection of one's care provider, and scheduling preferences. These everyday ethical issues typically lack the drama of life-and-death matters but also are deserving of attention.

6. Need for focus on applied issues and outcomes of use to practitioners and consumers. Unfortunately, philosophers and ethicists sometimes disdain applied ethics. The Initiative raised applied ethics to a new level. Practitioners often are desperate for practical knowledge and tools to use in difficult everyday ethical situations. The Initiative produced casebooks, training materials, and a wealth of background materials to be used by practitioners and long-term-care ethics committees. Perhaps most importantly, it provided a better conceptual framework and a language with which to parse and discuss long-term-care ethical situations. As one director of a state unit on aging put it, "I always knew that there were these important ethical dilemmas within the services that we provide within the aging network, but I didn't have the language or terms to even frame the issues or ask the questions that needed to be asked. The work of the Autonomy Initiative, particularly that of Collopy (1988), gave me the language and concepts that I needed."

EMERGING ISSUES IN ETHICS AND AGING

Although the Initiative led to many insights and advances, it also had its limitations. What were some of the unaddressed issues in autonomy and long-term care, that generalize to the broader arena of ethics and aging and demand attention now and in the future?

Diversity of Older Persons

Too often ethical analyses in aging invoke a false homogeneous and unitary view of older persons, as demonstrated by the use of the term "the elderly." There is tremendous diversity among older persons in terms of race, ethnicity, religion, gender, and other factors. Different cultures and subcultures view moral and ethical issues differently. Work that is done needs to take this diversity into account. Usually, the ethical research that has been done (including that of the Initiative) used only white, middle-class samples of older adults and resulted in prescriptive or proscriptive recommendations that did not take into account how the analyses might play out differently in other subgroups.

Consumer Self-Direction

Consumer-directed long-term care is a major component in the next generation of work in long-term-care ethics. The disability community's focus on consumer-directed Personal Assistance Services has become more accepted in the aging community (Simon-Rusinowitz & Hofland, 1993). The Robert Wood Johnson Foundation (RWJF) and the U.S. Department of Health and Human Services have jointly funded the Cash and Counseling Demonstration and Evaluation involving the implementation of consumer-directed care programs statewide for persons of all ages with disabilities in four states—New York, Arkansas, New Jersey and Florida. A team of researchers at the University of Maryland is carefully evaluating these major demonstrations. A related effort, the Independent Choices Initiative funded by RWJF, is sponsoring 13 smaller-scale demonstration and research projects designed to expand the knowledge base about consumer direction. In addition, the RWJF's Self-Determination for Persons with Developmental Disabilities has funded sites in 29 states to initiate system changes to improve access to consumer-directed services for persons with developmental disabilities. These efforts adopt a "client knows best" mentality and respect an older client's desire for autonomy, while restructuring services to more directly empower and support that autonomy. As noted elsewhere in this volume (Blaser, and Simon-Rusinowitz, Mahoney, and Benjamin, chapter 22), this restructuring can take the controversial form of payment to family caregivers.

Managed Care

The rapid growth of Medicare managed care invokes both justice and autonomy issues. What treatments are provided to whom? Are the older person's preferences for care and for providers managed away? The recent ethical research of Daniels and Sabin (1997) is noteworthy. It examined the decision-making process used by managed care organizations (MCOs) and other insurers for adding coverage for new technologies, especially those involved in treating the elderly, analyzed the best practices in use, and developed principles for improving the process with special attention to MCOs enrolling Medicare patients.

Daniels and Sabin concluded that four principles were necessary to provide legitimacy and an assurance of fairness to decisions about coverage of new technologies and other limit-setting decisions. These principles are: (1) Publicity. Decisions regarding coverage for new technologies (and other limit-setting decisions) and their rationales must be publicly accessible; (2) Reasonableness. The rationales for coverage decisions should aim to provide a reasonable construal of how the organization should provide "value for money" in meeting the varied health needs of a defined population under reasonable resource constraints. Specifically, a construal will be "reasonable" if it appeals to reasons and principles that are accepted as relevant by people who are disposed to finding terms of cooperation that are mutually justifiable; (3) Appeals. There is a mechanism to challenge and resolve disputes regarding limit-setting decisions, including the opportunity for revising decisions in light of further evidence or arguments; and (4) Enforcement. There is either voluntary or public regulation of the process to ensure that conditions 1–3 are met.

Managed care will continue to present ethical dilemmas for the aging field; further ethical attention to it and creative work is needed.

Need for Emphasis on Community

Autonomy does not trump all other values. In a time of increasing polarization and intergenerational tensions, there is a need to focus on the importance of community and interdependence in the everyday lives of older adults. If the Retirement Research Foundation were to undertake an initiative today in the arena of ethics and aging, it might well focus on this topic. Indeed, in long-term care, one of the paradoxes of autonomy is that older adults are often dependent on others to have their wishes and preferences fulfilled. Moreover, the home care client may have a fiercely protected sense of autonomy, but grow increasingly and dangerously isolated from the broader community as frailty and disability increases (see, for example, chapter 15 by Kuhn).

Meaning of Aging

The traditional conceptualization of retirement is that it is a time to rest after many years of work. As people live into their 80s, 90s and even 100s, and retirement between 60 and 65 years of age continues to be normative, retirement can last 40 years or longer. That is a long time to rest and participate in leisure activities. As one retiree put it, "There are only so many games of golf that you can play!" What then is the meaning of retirement and old age? This in many ways is *the* key question of gerontology today. Are there unique opportunities for continued interpersonal and spiritual growth? The work of Drew Leder (1997, 2000) and Harry R. Moody (1997) has been illuminating in beginning to discuss these critical issues.

USE OF ETHICAL MODELS OTHER THAN PRINCIPLISM

Perhaps the greatest limitation in the work done to date in ethics and aging has been the general failure to use ethical models other than that of principlism. In the important and compelling book, *A Matter of Principles? Ferment in U.S. Bioethics*, DuBose and colleagues (1994) defined principlism as the use of moral principles to address theoretical issues and to resolve conflicts in applied settings. The use of principlism described by Beauchamp and Childress (1983) in *Principles of Biomedical Ethics* has prevailed. The key principles invoked in nearly all moral analyses are beneficence, non-maleficence, respect for autonomy, and distributive justice.

There are many limitations of principlism. It is too narrow in its scope. In focusing so much on principles and the resolution of problems, principlism tends to neglect the personal history and circumstances of the persons who are the focus of the ethical analysis. Culture, traditions, gender and relationships all enormously vary the way that ethical situations should be interpreted and analyzed. Principlism neglects the moral life and moral character of the various agents involved; these are treated as so much "noise" or error variance to be factored out of the ethical equation. There is a great deal of emphasis on individual autonomy and rights, but little emphasis on community and the common good. As Stephen Toulmin (1981) put it, we are left with an "ethics of strangers." In long-term care, this is particularly inappropriate because care providers are usually family members and even where formal services are provided, they take place over long periods of time and a personal relationship often develops between care provider and care receiver.

Principlism is too dominated by philosophy and law, where the relationships are seen as adversarial. This has led to significant problems in the long-term-care arena. For example, guardianship proceedings take place within a probate court where long-simmering family disputes can erupt into a form of family psychodrama that is a costly and inefficient use of expensive judicial personnel and time. These situations often lend themselves to less costly and less adversarial mediation. Similarly, informed consent and advance directives usually are seen as involving the signing of legal documents between adversaries—a product frozen in one moment of time. It would be far better to see informed consent as negotiated consent (Moody, 1988) that involves ample discussion, feedback and a time for questions and answers. Advance directives also would be better seen as a *process* with much communication between relatives or friends and between the signer and his or her key health care professionals. It is the process that is important, not the legal product that is in many ways the artifact of the process.

Principlism also largely excludes religious considerations and theological language from discussions of ethical issues and cases. Professionalism and religion are often seen as mutually exclusive and religious dimensions of an ethical dilemma are sometimes treated by ethicists with something akin to embarrassment. The work of the Park Ridge Center for the Study of Health, Faith, and Ethics has been a major exception and guiding light in overcoming this inappropriate exclusion of religion and theology from ethics. The exclusion of religion is particularly inappropriate in ethics and aging. A Louis Harris poll (Ellor, McGilliard, & Schroeder, 1994) found that 61% of all older persons surveyed had attended worship services at a congregation in the previous month; only 19% had attended a senior center or club within the same period. The religious perspective, far from being a trivial and unimportant dimension, is often one of *the* most important factors in the ethical analysis involving an older person.

DuBose and colleagues (1994) suggested some alternative models to principlism and these are very briefly described below.

Phenomenology

Phenomenology emphasizes the first-hand shared experience of the phenomenon under study by the persons within the situation that is the focus of ethical analysis and the persons doing the ethical analysis. The focus is on how the participants themselves experience and understand their situation and the meaning that they attach to it. By uncovering the meaning that each participant attaches to the situation, the ethicist establishes the groundwork for shared understanding and informed action on ethical issues.

Hermeneutics

In hermeneutics, the relativity of the ethical situation is emphasized. The situation under ethical examination is like a narrative text that is open to many possible interpretations. The hermeneutic ethicist approaches the ethical analysis with a respect for the diversity and divergence of experience and allows that experience to speak its own truths. Hermeneutics invokes a "bottom-up" methodology rather than the "top-down" methods of principlism. Each ethical situation has a wide range of complex and comprehensive readings. The hermeneutic ethicist, in facing ethical dilemmas, helps the participants to interpret and re-interpret their own stories to achieve consensus and mutual understanding.

Narrative Ethics

To a narrative ethicist, the facts of a case are not enough. Storytelling is central in considering and resolving ethical cases, because the storyline of any given ethical situation far exceeds the simple facts. It involves multiple layers of personal, psychological, social and historical meaning. Narrative development involves recognition, formulation, interpretation and validation. It taps into these wider dimensions of meaning of the situation. Because it more adequately resonates with the experience of all of the participants who live through the situation together, narrative ethics is more trustworthy than principlism and provides a richer and more solid base for action.

Casuistry

According to a casuistry model of ethics, the moral and technical aspects of an ethical decision have equal value and there are sharp limits to the extent to which any judgment can be generalized. General ethical theories are useful only to the extent to which they shed secondary light on particular cases. The ethicist as casuist makes use of simple, paradigmatic examples to guide the resolution of more complex cases with their conflicts and ambiguities. Casuistry invokes case ethics to sort out and classify cases into a practical taxonomy. It is a pre-theoretical approach.

Virtue Ethics

Virtue ethics focuses on the character of the participants in an ethical situation and on the kind of person who makes a decision or acts in a certain way. Virtue ethics emphasizes the doctor/patient and caregiver/ care receiver relationship. If the doctor and caregiver are virtuous, they will do what comes naturally and it will be right. Character and virtue are more important than the principles and methods of moral reasoning. Particularly important in virtue ethics are inner realities such as motivations, intentions and attitudes.

CONCLUSION

The chapters in this volume reflect current work in ethics and aging that builds on the lessons learned from past efforts. A variety of interdisciplinary perspectives are presented and the papers are filled with the lived experience of older adults as the core of the ethical analyses and discussion. There is a focus on everyday issues that goes beyond the medical dimensions of home care. The volume represents a collaboration of social scientists and ethicists, yet the focus on applied issues should be helpful to practitioners and older adults alike. Similarly, the chapters help to elucidate many of the emergent issues in ethics and aging. Finally, the ethical work represented here invokes models of ethics other than principlism. Principles are seen as tools for interpreting moral facets of situations and as helpful guides to action. However, the abuses of the past are avoided in that circumstances are not shaped to fit a favored principle within ethical analysis. This volume enriches and expands the earlier work upon which it builds.

REFERENCES

Beauchamp, T., & Childress, J. (1983). *Principles of biomedical ethics.* New York: Oxford University Press.

Cassell, C. (1988). Ethical issues in the conduct of research in long term care. *The Gerontologist,* 28(Suppl.), 90–96.

Collopy, B. J. (1988). Autonomy in long term care: Some critical distinctions. *The Gerontologist,* 28(Suppl.), 10–17.

Daniels, N., & Sabin, J. (1997). Limits to health care: Fair procedures, democratic deliberation, and the legitimacy problem for insurers. *Philosophy and Public Affairs,* 26(4), 303–350.

DuBose, E., Hamel, R., & O'Connell, L. (1994). *A matter of principles?: Ferment in U.S. bioethics.* Valley Forge, PA: Trinity Press International.

Ellor, J. W., McGilliard, J. L., & Schroeder, P. E. (1994). *Let days speak and many years teach: A congregational leaders manual.* Washington, DC: National Council on the Aging, Inc.

Generations. (1990). Autonomy and long term care practice. *14*(Suppl.).
The Gerontologist. (1988). Autonomy and long term care. *28*(Suppl.).
Hofland, B. F. (1988). Autonomy in long term care: Background issues and a programmatic response. *The Gerontologist, 28*(Suppl.), 3–9.
Leder, D. (2000). Aging into the spirit: From traditional wisdom to innovative programs and communities. *Generations, 23*(4), 36–41.
Leder, D. (1997). *Spiritual passages: Embracing life's sacred journey.* New York: Tarcher/Putnam.
Moody, H. R. (1997). *The five stages of the soul.* New York: Anchor Books/Random House.
Moody, H. R. (1988). From informed consent to negotiated consent. *The Gerontologist, 28*(Suppl.), 64–70.
Retirement Research Foundation. (1985). Enhancing personal autonomy of elderly individuals in long-term care: Request for proposals. Park Ridge, IL: Author.
Simon-Rusinowitz, L., & Hofland, B. F. (1993). Adopting a disability approach to home care services for older adults. *The Gerontologist, 33*(2), 159–167.
Toulmin, S. (1981). The tyranny of principles. *Hastings Center Report, 11,* 31–39.

CHAPTER 3

Bringing Ethics Home: A New Look at Ethics in the Home and the Community

Martha B. Holstein

> There is every reason to react with alarm to the prospect of a world filled with self-actualizing persons . . . freely choosing when to begin and end all their relationships. It is hard to see how, in such a world, children could be raised, the sick or disturbed could be cared for, or people could know each other through their lives and grow old together. (Scheman, 1983, p. 240, as quoted in Kittay, 1999)

I arrived in Chicago to work at the Park Ridge Center on February 2, 1996. I barely knew my way around the office when I was privileged to meet social work administrator Phyllis Mitzen from the Council for Jewish Elderly and philosopher Mark Waymack from Loyola University. Knowing something about my background, they quickly included me in discussions about creating an ethics program for providers of home care and adult day services to older people that they and others in Illinois had begun to envision. Originating in the statewide Community Care Program Advisory Committee (CCPAC), the idea was in early discussion phases. This first meeting led to others with the individuals who became the project working committee and its strongest advocates. The Illinois Department on Aging, community service providers, and academic ethicists were among the committee's members. Together we developed a grant proposal, under the auspices of the Park Ridge

Center for the Study of Health, Faith, and Ethics, which the Retirement Research Foundation funded for two years.

This project started with practical ends: case managers and supervisors sought an ethics mechanism to address the myriad of problems that confronted them. Behind that practical need, however, was an unarticulated sense that as yet minimally explored connections between ethics and care could affect their clients' lives and support the state's focus on consumer-centered care (personal communication, P. Mitzen, June 1996). The ethics that many of us had learned, an ethics reflected in many professional codes, could not grapple adequately with this undefined something we were looking for, which is, at bottom, I believe, the fundamental task of morality—to help us (and by extension, our clients) understand and live a good, fully human life (Murray, 1997). Even if the problems that immediately came to mind were often distinctly unglamorous—keeping the client's son from living off her social security check or coping with roach-infested houses—they did not detract from the deeper aims practitioners had for their clients—to help them end their lives with their identity and self-esteem reasonably intact, living with at least a minimum degree of comfort, receiving recognition of their individuality from others, and believing in their own moral worthiness. Practitioners, of course, do not have sole responsibility for these ends. Yet, to ignore them is to impoverish relationships with clients.

If ethics was to be helpful in meeting these aims, which differed substantially from service-oriented care plans, we needed to rethink its parameters both substantively and procedurally. The project working group had good company in the task of critique and reconstruction. The intellectual and practical resources to help in this transformation had surfaced in the literature for some time. Hence, some 15 years after applied ethics entered the field of gerontology (partly as a result of the RRF initiative that Brian Hofland describes in chapter 2), the time seemed propitious to revisit the commonly-accepted scope of "ethics and aging" and the current models of deliberation about ethical problems. Originally developed for the acute-care setting, these models had been transferred and applied to the very different long-term-care setting. Raising questions about these models seemed essential. Were they sufficiently robust to contribute to making a difference in the client's daily life? What were their strengths and limits when applied to the moral complexities that inhered in the actual lives of community-dwelling elders? The experiential world of these elders, often marked by poverty, run-down housing, uncertain neighborhoods, family complexities, advancing age, deteriorating health, pride, and limited opportunities to make significant changes, differed from the ICU or the surgical unit.

Such conditions could be bruising, troubled, and uncertain, although strength too was often apparent. The problems among community-dwelling, though disabled, elders were tied directly to problems of living as the infirmities of age and illness tightened their grip.

The early agenda of ethics and aging adopted issues such as end-of-life care, concepts such as autonomy and informed consent procedures, and principle-based methods for addressing ethical concerns that had dominated the acute-care agenda. But in the community consent was rarely about a single course of treatment and autonomy addressed complex life choices that generally involved others and rarely required the refusal (or acceptance) of a particular treatment option.

For the considerable good that resulted from this particular focus of work in ethics and aging there was also a downside—the unintentional narrowing of issues that came under ethical scrutiny. Deliberations about advance directives overshadowed conversations about other matters of considerable importance, for example, maintenance of a sense of self in spite of loss, or aspirations to continue feeling morally worthy when frailty and need shifted the grounding that had once sustained that sense. The interpersonal aspects of morality tended to overshadow its intrapersonal dimensions (Flanagan, 1996). Other important features of the moral life did not receive adequate attention, for example, the significance of building relationships between care workers and clients or supporting already existing relationships that frailty and need strained. In the ethics literature, elder abuse—real and profoundly troubling—received attention but the often deeply conflictive feelings of concerned family members frequently remained hidden, as did the caregiver's needs for care (see Kittay, 1999, for a discussion of caring for the caregiver). Nor did the ethical agenda examine the gendered nature of caregiving, and the potential for exploitation of both frontline caregivers and care receivers. In the community, younger women, often poor and vulnerable in their own lives, take care of older women who are also vulnerable by reason of age, disability, and income (Holstein, 1999). Caregiving is an object lesson in inequality when dependency needs are not incorporated into thinking about fairness.

Given these complexities, it is no wonder that care providers in the community often feel puzzled about what to do in specific circumstances and feel trapped when no good answers emerge because there may be, in many circumstances, no *really* good answers.

This project's central questions then emerged: If ethical reflection can contribute more fully to consumer-centered care, what are the next steps? How can we assess how to act in difficult or conflictive situations if we do not rely primarily on principles and algorithmic thinking?

THE PROJECT

The project—Home- and Community-Based Services for Elders: An Ethics Resource for Providers—explored these questions through discussions and interviews with caregivers, supervisors, case managers, frontline workers, and, to a lesser extent, with families and clients. From these experiences, it developed a training program that addressed both "everyday" ethics and value conflicts. The project's primary goal was to improve the ability of professional and paraprofessional health care providers to develop ethically responsive ways of being with clients and to address the ethical problems that arise in home and community-care settings. To achieve this goal, the project had the following objectives:

- Identify the ethical issues that occur in home care and adult day services from the multiple perspectives of older clients, their families, health care providers, and home care and day care associations;
- Organize material thematically into case narratives for further study and analysis;
- Create a working group to analyze the cases/stories that the project has collected from each of the relevant individuals and groups and develop practical ways to address them;
- Design a train-the-trainer educational program and test it in the state of Illinois under the auspices of the Illinois Department on Aging;
- Prepare other written material; and
- Disseminate the program broadly.

A project working committee of service providers, Illinois Department on Aging personnel, and ethicists steered the project from its beginnings. My colleague David McCurdy, some project working group members, and I, with the enthusiastic support of the Illinois Department on Aging (IDOA), attended each of the Department sponsored Partners Together meetings for the year 1998 and also its regular meetings for the case coordination units. We also attended meetings of the Day Care Association, the Community Care Program Advisory Committee, and the Elder Abuse Advisory Council. We met with a group of providers at the 1997 Elder Rights conference and stayed in touch with as many people as we could by phone and e-mail. Our informants were primarily case managers, supervisors, and adult day service site directors, who had contracts to provide home care or adult day services under the state's community-care program (CCP), or who worked in the elder abuse unit. (CCP is an entitlement program available to low income older people who meet the program's criteria.) Subsequently, we interviewed frontline home care workers, day center aides, day center clients, and one group of paid family caregivers.

Through self-education, the committee explored different approaches to think about the situations these narratives described. As noted above, the result was a move beyond the model of ethical reflection that centered on weighing deductively derived principles such as autonomy or beneficence (or doing good) as they clashed in specific cases. This model, known as principlism, though serving as an important reminder of critical American values and the voice of the client, had two important limits. It was unable to encompass the broader moral domain in long-term care as we understood it and it circumscribed thinking related to problem resolution. We did not want our ethics to stop too soon. In place of a primary focus on conflictive situations and principlism, we moved toward a more pragmatic, dialogic method of problem solving and a decision to address "everyday" ethics as well as conflictive situations.

Thinking in this enlarged way revealed the importance of seemingly small matters and reminded us (if we needed reminding) how powerful the demands of vulnerability are, but also that we are not infinitely responsible. Division of responsibility and social and religious support ought to be components of the caregivers' caring system; yet, such social responsiveness is often unavailable. Attention to the ethics of daily life also exposed the structural, institutional, and other factors that limited responsible engagement with clients.

A wealth of reflection from different academic directions—the care ethics of many feminist philosophers, the naturalism of some moral psychologists, the critical stance of poststructuralism, and many others—guided our work. In general, such work addresses practical moral reasoning about concrete situations. It calls for skilled moral perception as the starting place for good moral judgments. This work helped situate our thinking within a certain intellectual domain at the same time that it shaped the framework for thinking about ethics more generally and for addressing specific concerns.

Out of this process emerged a 3-hour training program for frontline workers (that can also be offered in three, 1-hour segments), backed by train-the-trainer materials. Committee members and invited consultants closely scrutinized these materials, which were then tested at eight sites in the fall of 1999 and early winter of 2000, with case managers, supervisors, day service center staff, and frontline workers. Revisions were made subsequent to each test program.

IMPORTANT FINDINGS/OUTCOMES

While we recognize that some clients have difficulties with frontline workers, who are among the lowest paid workers in the field of health care, we found the workers' personal accounts of their experiences both informative and moving. The frontline workers we met revealed deep sources of wisdom, an uncommonly strong bond with their clients, and a commitment to their work. One worker seemed to represent the rest when she said, "It takes a special kind of person to do this kind of work and I am that kind of person." A future study involving intensive interviews with frontline workers would provide a better understanding of and remedies for problems that clients and agency staff described—for example tardiness, not showing up, or cajoling clients to sign for more hours than the worker actually worked. The extant literature on frontline workers reveals the many stresses these workers experience that undoubtedly contribute to, without necessarily excusing, these problems (see Stone and Yamada, chapter 10).

The project working committee decided to target the training program primarily to frontline workers, while providing supplemental case and explanatory materials for supervisory personnel, for a specific reason. Frontline workers, who have the most direct contact with clients, also have the most immediate opportunities to make consumer-centered care a greater reality. This ethics program, focusing, in part, on the ethics of everyday life, will enhance that end. Everyday ethics—the way we greet someone, the way we build a trusting relationship, the particularities of caring for and respecting *this* patient as opposed to *all* patients—are those encounters with others that often occur without special notice. Calling attention to these behaviors and explaining their importance can directly affect the quality of life of elderly clients. It is frontline workers whom clients have to trust; for example, they bathe the client in ways that do or do not recognize the potential for shame and demonstrate respect for privacy. Care workers can support and encourage the client's self-maintaining activities and by their actions and words they can demonstrate to the client that she still is a person worthy of respect despite the assistance she needs. They are able to implement plans (developed by agencies, clients, and families) that emphasize not only instrumental tasks like food preparation but caring aims such as compassion, concern, and commitment (Kittay, 1999) that enhance the relationship between worker and client. These everyday aspects of caregiving also serve a preventive function—a good beginning for a caring practice might prevent serious problems from developing in the future. The more familiar focus on ethical dilemmas, though essential, tends to render these everyday encounters invisible. Caregivers and older clients are first and foremost engaged in a relationship that requires attentiveness, responsiveness, and, on occasion, negotiation, to meet the needs of the client without ignoring the needs of the caregiver.

Thus, this project has helped to widen the scope of ethics and aging to encompass certain qualities of being with another person that can easily become neglected in the haste to get tasks done. It demands a great deal from workers because each aspect of their care has an ethical component; yet, the specific actions are simple, so simple that they may go unnoticed unless someone deliberately calls attention to them. To assist workers in thinking about these everyday aspects of caregiving, we highlighted four key questions: (1) How do I go about building and maintaining a relationship of trust with *this* client? (2) How can I respect *this* client and let her know she is a person of worth? (3) How can I care well for *this* particular person? (4) How can I care for myself and feel that I am doing a morally honorable job?

Ethical responsibilities, in their most quotidian aspects, are worked out in the concrete situations of daily life. To answer these questions well, we suggest developing three important skills: attentiveness, clear (and gentle) communication, and appropriate responsiveness recognizing that client and caregiver may bring different values to each experience they face together.

The wealth of information gathered at our community meetings and in interviews provided the "raw" materials for the case narratives that are the centerpiece of the training program. In some cases, the narratives were written out of the direct experiences of workers in the community-care program; others were composites of many stories; still others came from participation on ethics committees of agencies providing home care and day services. We validated the content of these stories in public meetings and at test sites for the training program. These case narratives suggest the importance of understanding both motives for and meanings of actions and offer the chance to explore the different perspectives of each person involved in the situation. They bring ethical analysis very close to the ground by emphasizing the particular features of each situation, features that cannot be ignored in community-based long-term care where decisions are cumulative, situations complex and generally filled with unexplored meanings for clients and families, and rarely involve immediate threats to the client's health.

Case narratives and stories also serve a very important critical function. They allow us to enter in an imaginative but grounded way into the specific phenomenological worlds they describe. Hearing these case narratives and discussing them at the time and later with the project working group gave us some needed distance to analyze them from multiple points of view. Storytelling, according to Hannah Arendt, is a "kind of judgment" because stories reveal the plurality of perspectives and are always open to question (Disch, 1994, p. 4). Stories ground perceptions and enhance the ability to grasp, however obliquely, the motivations, thoughts, and feelings of participants (Murray, 1997; Nelson, 1997; Nussbaum, 1990). Stories revealed varied definitions of problems and the multiple binds that often narrowed possibilities to almost none. These stories raised different voices, facilitated engagement with difference, and provided the substantive information that began the process of making moral judgments. In long-term care, stories can link clients, families, other caregivers, policy, and organizations—all those people and features that influence how we define ethical problems, reflect upon them, and make decisions—into a conceptual whole. In our process, we raised questions about the stories, added new information, noted what made the situations described so difficult, and identified the moral questions that needed to inform discussion.

As the project evolved, a number of questions arose, some of which we could answer; others await further study. What makes caregiving a moral activity and how does it relate to practice? What meaning, especially moral meaning, does caregiving and care receiving have for participants? How can caregivers, care receivers, and family members simultaneously negotiate the need for care and the need for justice? What circumstances create ethically troubling problems? Who defines ethical problems? How can moral imagination expand options to meet the diverse needs of older clients? How do training and personal values and beliefs of each individual shape these problem definitions? Can problems be prevented, delayed, or mitigated through a concentrated attentiveness to the moral qualities of daily life? How does our moral self develop in relationship with others for whom we care? How can we take advantage of naturally occurring situations to enhance the dignity and the self-esteem of clients?

Beyond everyday concerns, the working committee agreed that in conflictive situations, the "resolution" of dilemmas required a denser, richer, and more complex conversation than what had emerged from reliance on principle and rule-based ethics. Watch an experienced ethics committee at work and see how broad the conversation becomes. Even in other chapters in this book, where a commitment to a rule-based approach is strong, observe the way these rules are enlarged and transformed to address particular situations. Yet, the values associated with principle-based ethics are important. They remind us about the dangers of paternalism, the subtle influences of ageism, and the difficult choices we face as individuals and as a society. They are not, however, nearly as rich as our actual behaviors, which respond to the complex situations at hand. "Concepts such as autonomy, safety, and independence are drawn too starkly and too abstractly in the bioethics literature to be adequate to the complex and shifting realities of long-term care decisionmaking" (McCullough & Wilson, 1995, p. 6). Such principles do not project us imaginatively (and practically) into the world of another—the first step in defining moral problems and an important aspect of a caregiver's moral development—and so may limit our moral perceptions.

Themes

Not surprisingly, several issues recurred regularly in our meetings with care workers. The importance of context was one of these themes. Practitioners at all levels experienced the difficulties associated with resource constraints, often expressing chagrin at the perceived inadequacy of the care plan as the result of financial limitations or the difficulty in recruiting workers because wages were low, a problem exacerbated by the strong economy. Competition with businesses, which paid a slightly or much higher wage, made it harder to attract workers.

Another contextual feature—the client's home environment and the danger and dirt workers often perceived or encountered—caused considerable consternation. It also, however, suggested the importance of perspective. Who labeled the conditions of the environment? On what grounds can an agency deny services because of adverse conditions? Alternatively, how bad does it have to be for a worker to say, "No way."

Many workers found family issues particularly troubling. Since care for community-dwelling elders relies heavily on families, if they are present they became part of the client's care plan. Yet, families often disappointed practitioners, if they did not actually frighten them. Did the son keep his mother at home only to collect her Social Security check? What if he doesn't change her clothes or wash her between visits of the care worker? What if families demanded services that were not part of the service package and treated the home care worker like a servant? What should a worker do if she discovers that the client's son is a convicted child molester? What if a case manager learns that a family member has a communicable disease? Should she tell the worker? What should the worker do if families are disruptive, either preventing workers from doing their job or "wrecking" the house? In seeking narratives of "trouble" we rarely heard about the families who try to do too much, who must be encouraged to stop providing care. Yet, we know such families also exist and cause considerable concern to outsiders, including social workers, as described in other chapters in this volume.

On the other hand, workers often develop very close relationships with clients and so learn things that the families might not know. What should they do with such information? There are also more sensitive psychological issues: children are often unable to recognize what the spouse caregiver is experiencing; and therefore, they are unable to support that parent. One man at a day services support group, whose wife no longer recognized him, was unable to "go with" her confused thoughts while his daughter pushed him to do so. "She doesn't understand," he said, "I *am* her husband, not her father or brother."

While the majority of families provide care out of love, concern, and obligation, difficult families are particularly hard on care workers. Part of a caregiver's moral education is to try to understand the enormous burden and conflicting loyalties that even the most loving families who provide care experience. Exhaustion and guilt, rather than harmful intent, may cause many difficulties. The moral issues families raise are particularly sensitive, since family members are intimately intertwined with the client's identity; while appearing disruptive to the worker, families often are essential for the client's well-being.

Other issues focused more specifically on the frontline worker. She often described a feeling of danger, but also expressed concern about isolation and the limited support from her agency (which is also burdened with large case loads) or from other workers since they so rarely had the chance to get together.

Sometimes clients provoked anger by their racist or ethnic slurs or by their demeaning behavior toward the worker. Often they aroused frustrations because they refused to be bathed and would not touch the food the care worker prepared for them. Pay, of course, came up, as did concerns about limited opportunities for future advancement. Underlying these concerns about pay were beliefs that few really appreciated their work. Many workers expressed deep commitments to their clients, laughed together as they recalled the doings of familiar clients, and feared the attachments that made it so hard for them when a client died. Not surprisingly, they sought confirmation that others valued their contributions to the quality of their clients' lives. Their musings recalled moral philosopher Owen Flanagan's (1991) question: "How long can the publicly underestimated and undervalued aspects of moral life survive without recognition and sustenance?" (p. 195). In a society that esteems market success, autonomous actions, and self-actualization there is little place for the simpler moments that make care receiver and caregiver feel joined together in a morally worthy enterprise.

Interorganizational issues troubled many supervisors and case managers. Sometimes goals differed; for example, the elder abuse unit wanted to transfer a client to a nursing home for her safety but the Community Care Program (CCP) wanted to maintain her in her own home. Confidentiality concerns sometimes impeded the ability of agencies to work together as a team to address a client's problems. What do you tell, to whom, and under what circumstances? Thus, practitioners often voiced fears about the possible erosion of trust among agencies serving the same client.

Client issues were broadly defined. Care workers often felt that they had inadequate information about the client or her family. They worried about the client who seemed to resist any services or insisted that a neighbor or a friend was providing all the care they needed. What happens in cases like this when either one ignores—or cannot obtain—the "whole" story, that is, the narrative of the family relationships; the wants and desires of the client; the meaning of services to a client; the needs of the other family members who are there when the home care worker is not? Dementia raised a host of its own concerns, most particularly about safety, which was in general the most frequently voiced concern.

Safety issues posed important but difficult questions: Who decides what is too risky for the client? What does risk mean—environmental dangers, risk from others, risk from the client's own frailty and/or mental or physical condition? Uncertainties often created great stress for care workers. They envisioned their clients alone and endangered, which made the care worker concerned about boundaries—should she call between visits and maybe even stop by?

While professionals generally think about safety in terms of physical well-being, for the older person the struggle to maintain familiar ways of life—in spite of risk—signified a much different meaning of safety. Thus, for many professionals concerns about safety challenges, most fundamentally, the almost single-minded adherence to autonomy usually defined as self-direction, that governs social work practice and contemporary applied ethics. Because of the centrality of safety concerns to long-term care and because it helps reveal the warp and woof of efforts to find meaning in later life, we should look at them in some detail.

Powerfully held beliefs about autonomy could not alleviate care workers' concerns about safety, especially if the client lived alone, if family members appeared to be unreliable, or if the client had dementia. Thoughtful social workers are reluctant to "abandon" clients to their autonomy if they really feel clients are endangered; yet, they are equally uncomfortable seeming to force something on clients, especially if clients do not see their "problem" in the same way that professionals see it. Sometimes dangerous neighborhoods or cluttered, unclean apartments exacerbated safety concerns, but to the client such conditions may simply be home. At other times, distrust of the non-paid primary caregiver provoked such fears. Professionals had difficulty believing that the client's daughter, who worked full time, was providing any care at all. But the client doesn't want to be away from her daughter. Care providers worried about the clients' broken front doors or their sons, who may turn violent at a moment's notice, or so caregivers feared. But the client has lived with both the broken door and the troubled son for many years. Caregivers worry about the client's declining health or her stubborn resistance to accept services into her life—no baths, no food. Her refusal to keep medical appointments causes the care worker to worry that the client's blood pressure is skyrocketing. Doesn't she want to be clean, full, and have her hypertension controlled? Professionals worry that she might get lost if she ventures out of the house or that she might trip and break her hip because of all the accumulated papers and "things" around the house. Even when accepting the client's choice to remain at home, the professional's concern for the client's well-being rarely disappeared.

Clients may be anxious about very different matters. Safety looks different if defined in psychological or physical terms or if one lives in a community or alone (Collopy, 1995). Different perspectives beg professionals to ask what it means to the client when an outside care provider comes into her life to help with some of the most intimate details of daily life, like a bath. How might we recognize what these things we call services mean to her? A client might be willing to risk a fall or even death to stay in the house that she shared with her late husband for fifty years. She wants the freedom to sit in the living room with a cup of tea at midnight or feel the safety of familiar possessions. Case managers, family members, and especially clients often define situations differently; clients may defy living according to a care plan. Sons and daughters, nieces and nephews also worry and experience burn-out as they try to protect the fragile independence of mother or father, aunt or uncle. They, too, are part of the complex narrative involved in negotiating responsibilities and resolving different conceptions of what is really going on.

These competing realities are often the beginning of ethical problems. There is no one agreed-upon narrative that pins down the "real" story; rather it is a story with many beginnings and endings and different perspectives. In long-term care, unfortunately, no "ontologist" can define the "real" nature of the problem (apt phrase from McCullough & Wilson, 1995). We lack the near-certainty of the physician's verdict that if he doesn't operate, our inflamed appendix will rupture, exposing us to severe infection if not death. Variants of the safety story recurred in almost every meeting we held.

As home care becomes less an intimate exchange among relatives and friends (although 80% of care is still provided informally) and more a public benefit, accountability needs have reshaped approaches to care. The human losses that resulted—spontaneous generosity, altruism, a shared history—are often reflected in the words of caregivers and their clients with requests like, "Why can't you just sit and talk to me for awhile, have a cup of tea?" (Stone, 1998). Accountability also defines power relationships; the case manager and the funding agencies, through assessment and monitoring, have much to say about services available to clients.

In the adult day services center, staff struggled with the one and the many—the disruptive client, often beset with his or her own demons, who nonetheless required the attention of staff and disturbed other clients. When, and if, to discharge such clients because they can detract from the security of other clients while absorbing considerable staff time caused tensions among staff. Frequently, sexually motivated behaviors between clients led to confusion about appropriate responses, especially when staff, clients, and families responded differently to the situation. Most often in rural areas, where day service centers assume many responsibilities that home care workers have in urban areas, aides worried about the client who refused to be bathed or the multiple responsibilities of staff and the long bus rides during which clients with dementia often made safety problematic.

Ethical Significance of These Complexities

Ethics is a normative activity that focuses on important "ought" questions: How should I behave in humanly important circumstances over which I have some control? Ethical values differ from other values because they deal with matters of deep significance—how to live and how to be with others. Thus, we must develop a sound approach to making moral judgments about which we have confidence. Since ethics also asks questions about the meaning and purpose of life, identity, and all that flows from having a sense of self—self-respect, self-esteem, agency—we also need to feel justified in the personal choices we make (Flanagan, 1996). We return to the age-old philosophical question: How ought I to live? This definition immediately enlarges our thoughts about ethics.

Ethics is part of the everyday world in which we live, work, and serve clients. It is a part of all of our actions. It is how we show care through our attentiveness and responsiveness, how we respect the client as a person, how we engage in relationships with others. It is about the right and the good and behaving in ways that are morally justifiable. Much that is ethical occurs when we are hardly paying attention: how we talk to someone, how we greet a client, how we learn about and honor differences. It is important to think about these matters so caring goes well even in difficult times.

But it is also about uncertainties, dilemmas, and not knowing what to do. Sometimes care providers will encounter moral conflicts that they cannot easily resolve. Sometimes situations will feel dangerous.

Sometimes it will be hard to understand what the client is experiencing. Caring is a specific kind of ethical activity and, as such, deserves value in society as a whole (Tronto, 1989). Bathing, dressing, and cleaning up the outflow from body orifices are moral activities as well as practice ones, since caring for people in states of deep vulnerability demands keen sensitivities, astute perceptions, responsiveness, and knowledge that is highly particular and attuned to clients' verbal and nonverbal cues. Because caregiving is essentially an activity that relies on trusting relationships, it asks much from both the giver and receiver (if she is able) of care. Recognition of interdependence guides us toward relating to and being with others in ways that help to "sustain good relationships among individuals who are not equal in power and relative dependence" (Carse, 1991, p. 17). Moreover, to acknowledge the ethical significance of caring work, so long devalued or, most often, unnoticed, and the relationships it can nurture, and to highlight its skilled qualities elevates its importance to individuals and to society. It also paves the way for a more finely attended and realistic politics of caregiving (Tronto, 1993).

Thinking Through Complex Situations

Our training program emphasizes the deep moral commitments imposed by caring for people who are vulnerable and rely on us. We also stress that the caregiver, who is often subject to exploitation and to doubts about her own ability to do her job in morally satisfying ways, has significant moral value. But there are times when deep uncertainties prevail. What kind of ethical reasoning can we use to arrive at a satisfying judgment?

The process of decision making that we recommend in the training program takes the moral complexity of long-term care as a given and assumes that uncertainties and ambiguities inhere in most situations we face. In light of those complexities and often with the lack of really good answers, we stress the structured conversational aspects of problem resolution: bringing together key people in a spirit of openness (i.e., willing to listen and even to change their minds) and equality, in which all recommendations, backed by thoughtful reflections/arguments, are placed on the table and discussed until the group can reach a shared decision (which everyone can accept even if it is not their preference). The features of ethical analysis that enter into this conversation include:

- What are the ethical issues at stake? (This step is critical, since it defines the problem one is trying to address and everyone does not necessarily see the problem in the same way.)

- What facts do we need to help us understand what is taking place?
- Are there any important value conflicts? (Remember that often the moral problem is a failure in care, commitment, and concern, a failure to show respect and enhance dignity, or a failure to use power wisely.)
- Can we develop a shared interpretation of the problems and ways to balance the different moral claims and concerns of all?
- What are the options for addressing the situation? (Be sure to include each person's perspective.)
- What are the arguments for and against each of the options? (While "gut" level responses are important, they cannot be the only reasons for taking some action when other people are involved.)
- What choices can everyone involved live with?
- How can you communicate the decision/action in ways that show respect and understanding?

This is certainly the place to remember commitments to client choice, but also the importance of preserving important relationships and values that may have nothing to do with autonomy. The goal is an integrity-preserving compromise (Larmore, 2001).

Since different beliefs and values influence the positions we take on issues, we interpret situations differently, leading to more than one definition of the ethical problem at stake. So with any ethical problem we face, we first must come to a mutual agreement about the problem itself. For example, how great is the risk to the client in the many ways risk is understood, especially since clients, families, social workers, and others often perceive risk differently? Remember the warning—there is no ontologist to define the problem for us as the surgeon can do with the appendix about to rupture. Sometimes the problem is defined by an ethics committee, sometimes within the confines of an agency. What must never be abandoned is the effort to discover the meanings of actions from the client's perspective, especially if clients change their typical patterns of responding. This, the "fact" gathering part of the process, is also marked by questions. What kind of safety, what forms of respect, what kind of care and understanding are clients looking for? Is she thinking about death or feeling neglected and unworthy? Through conversation and with imagination, we might find alternative remedies to support the needs she has at the moment.

The following narrative is emblematic of the kind of issues we encountered in conversations with care workers at all levels.

MRS. STONE AND THE CRUMBLING BACK DOOR

Amanda Stone, at 88, lived in a run-down neighborhood where drug dealing and violence were not uncommon occurrences. But she had lived there for almost 60 years and was convinced that no one would bother her. Drucilla Fittings had been taking care of Amanda for 3 years, but as Amanda's heart condition and osteoporosis weakened her, Drucilla worried even more about her client's safety. She feared that she would trip over the clutter and not be able to get up for hours. And what if she broke a leg or a hip? The day she arrived and found the back door hanging loosely on its hinges just about pushed her over the edge. She and Amanda had a good relationship. They trusted one another and Drucilla knew what to do to make Amanda smile even when she seemed to have little to smile about. (She had few visitors; even her children, who lived nearby, rarely visited.) So the morning that Drucilla saw the condition of the door, she decided to take a closer look around; in fact, she asked Amanda if she could invite the police in to do a complete safety inspection.

Amanda became very agitated. She told Drucilla that she didn't want the police poking around her house. She assured Drucilla that she was safe and told her to quit worrying. After all, she had lived in this house for most of her adult life and, with the exception of one robbery, nothing had ever happened. Amanda tried to reason with her, suggesting that she was not as strong as she had been when she originally moved into the house and that her husband, Jack, was a man no one fooled around with. But she saw she would get nowhere that day. She finished her chores and left but she did not leave her anxieties behind.

This situation was repeated week after week. The door was partially repaired but Amanda's ability to move around the house deteriorated. Drucilla could not get Amanda out of her mind. She called occasionally and when she was in the neighborhood dropped in with some snacks and a few words of conversation. She continued to fret and thought that Amanda would be much better off living in a different place—perhaps assisted living or, at least, going to adult day service programs several days a week. But all she encountered was resistance.

Drucilla told her supervisor, Ruth, about the deteriorating situation. Ruth promised to come out and visit but had not had the chance to do so yet when there was a fire in the neighborhood. Amanda's house was unaffected but it unnerved Drucilla even further.

I'll stop the narrative here but feel certain that most practitioners can fill in the subsequent events that occurred. I will assume that the agency has some kind of an ethics mechanism to which Ruth brings the case. How shall it be addressed? Though it rarely happens, it seems important that Drucilla be present at the discussion. She knows Amanda best and can explain the situation most fully. If Drucilla cannot be present, Ruth should have been thoroughly debriefed by Drucilla. Some questions that call for attention are:

1. What is (are) the ethical problem(s) from everyone's perspective?

   - What does it mean for Amanda to remain in her own home?
   - How real are the dangers that she faces and what are they?
   - What aims for Amanda are appropriate?
   - Besides her home, what would be lost to Amanda if she is forced to move?

2. What values are at stake and how do they support or harm the goals of caring for Amanda?
3. Are there any interventions that might reduce threats and meet these aims?
4. Are there ways to meet the needs that home meets in another, and perhaps physically safer, setting?
5. How can the care worker and the agency best meet the most important aims that Amanda has for her life at this juncture?
6. How should one structure the moral engagement in situations that are marked by circumstances of dependency and inequality?

These questions help fill in the details of the "fact" gathering, problem defining, and option identifying phases of decision-making.

While autonomy is an important factor, these questions extend beyond autonomy versus perceived best interests into a broader domain of considerations if our goal is to have Amanda's deepest wishes and aims met at the same time that Drucilla and the agency feel they are doing their job in protecting Amanda from harm. Persuasion, seeking alternatives, probing for what Amanda most needs and wants are all necessary parts of the thinking work. Instead of trying to resolve a conflict in values where someone wins and someone loses, we are seeking a shared interpretation of problems that balances the different moral claims and concerns of each party. To meet this need, good communication skills are essential. How do we facilitate the hearing and interpreting of what people say or do with insight and understanding? (Moody, 1992). The general outline suggested above will take us through the remainder of an ethical analysis.

This case illustrates a common situation faced by many frontline workers who cared for poor women who lived in poor neighborhoods. It reminds us that deepening disabilities and frailties beset our older clients no matter what we do, that families mostly do the best they can in difficult circumstances but they are not always virtuous, and that caregivers are often very vulnerable themselves. While this story captures a relatively brief period of time, it reflects the process nature of making decisions that may differ sharply from the immediacy of decision making required in acute-care settings. Situations change and therefore renewed focus on what ought to be done occurs frequently in home and community settings. As philosopher Margaret Urban Walker (1998) recently pointed out, these situations of care require a constant readjustment of personal arrangements of accountability so that they continue working for all persons concerned while sustaining relationships. Moral problems signal moments when we must make adjustments and alter understandings of each other and the ways in which we are accountable to one another. This need happens often when we age and it happens with families as well as with paid caregivers.

CONCLUSION

Care for people with dependency needs contains within it important normative and practical demands: concern for the good of others and for the community whose support they require, a capacity for imaginative projections into the position of others and of their situation, attuned responses to others' needs, and flexible attentiveness to changes in the situation. Caring well will also require monitoring our emotional tone—how we do what we do is the foundation of relationship building. Care receivers also value integrity greatly—the consistency of words and actions. Caregivers need also be aware of their own and others' values, fears, capacities and commitments; these factors are important in the interpretation and resolution of ethical conflicts and help us understand the feelings and perspectives of others. Moral judgment becomes a "process of interpreting the moral significance of various courses of conduct . . . both in light of one's own values and capabilities and also in light of one's understanding of others' needs and circumstances" (Meyers, 1994, p. 17). In the end, moral maturity involves a wide range of perceptual, imaginative, rational, emotional, and expressive capacities along with the ability to live with ambiguity and uncertainty. And, lastly, in community care, circumstances that shape the lives of many older clients add to the burdens of behaving in ethically responsible ways. Situations are usually rife with complexity, ripe with often unexpressed feelings, and marked by conflicting values that have little or nothing to do with making choices. Instead, they have to do with getting old in a society that devalues old age, with the different ways families grieve, and how people in families often do what others want because it is a more important value than getting their own way. The tapestry of a whole life is at stake—how to bring to a close the multifaceted experiences that have brought this 85-year-old person to the limits of her living room.

This project, we believe, is the first sustained attempt to reconceptualize the terrain of ethics and aging so that it can more effectively contribute to the goal of consumer-centered care. It has undertaken this reconceptualization in two ways: (1) by grappling with ethical questions that arise in the ordinary exchanges of everyday life where many decisions are made in the absence of any obvious dilemmas; and (2) by introducing dialogic or communicative process as a path to understanding and resolving, where possible, the value conflicts that inevitably arise in long-term care. The next steps are the repeated testing and refinement of this approach in the day-to-day world of home- and community-based care against the intellectual backdrop of philosophical and theological thinking about ethics.

REFERENCES

Agich, G. (1995). Actual autonomy and long-term care decision making. In L. McCullough & N. Wilson (Eds.), *Long-term care: Ethical and conceptual dimensions* (pp. 113–136). Baltimore: Johns Hopkins University Press.

Carse, A. L. (1991). The 'Voice of Care': Implications for bioethical education. *The Journal of Medicine and Philosophy, 16,* 5–28.

Collopy, B. (1995). Safety and independence: Rethinking some basic concepts in long-term care. In L. McCullough & N. Wilson (Eds.), *Long-term care: Ethical and conceptual dimensions* (pp. 137–154). Baltimore: John Hopkins University Press.

Disch, L. (1994). *Hannah Arendt and the limits of philosophy.* Ithaca, NY: Cornell University Press.

Flanagan, O. (1996). Ethics naturalized: Ethics as human ecology. In L. May, M. Friedman, & A. Clark (Eds.), *Mind and morals: Essays on ethics and cognitive science.* Cambridge, MA: The MIT Press.

Flanagan, O. (1991). *Varieties of moral personality: Ethics and psychological realism.* Cambridge, MA: Harvard University Press.

Goodin, R. (1985). *Protecting the vulnerable: A reanalysis of our social responsibility.* Chicago: University of Chicago Press.

Holstein, M. (1999). Home care, women, and aging: A case study of injustice. In M. U. Walker (Ed.), *Mother time: Women, aging, and ethics* (pp. 227–244). Lanham, MD: Rowman and Littlefield.

Kittay, E. F. (1999). *Love's labour: Essays on women, equality, and dependency.* New York: Routledge.

Larmore, C. (2001). *Patterns of moral complexity* (new ed.). Cambridge, UK: Cambridge University Press.

Meyers, D. T. (1994). *Subjection and subjectivity: Psychoanalytic feminism and moral philosophy.* New York: Routledge.

McCollough, L., & Wilson, N. (1995). Rethinking the conceptual and ethical dimensions of long-term care decision making. In L. McCullough & N. Wilson (Eds.), *Long-term care decisions: Ethical and conceptual dimensions* (pp. 1–12). Baltimore: Johns Hopkins University Press.

Moody, H. R. (1992). *Ethics and aging.* Baltimore: Johns Hopkins University Press.

Murray, T. (1997). What do we mean by "narrative ethics"? *Medical Humanities Review, 11*(2), 44–55.

Nelson, H. (Ed.). (1997). *Stories and their limits: Narrative approaches to bioethics.* New York: Routledge.

Nussbaum, M. (1990). *Love's knowledge: Essays on philosophy and literature.* New York: Oxford University Press.

Scheman, N. (1983). Individualism and psychology. In S. Harding & M. Hinlikka (Eds.), *Discovering reality: Feminist perspectives on epistemology, metaphysics, methodology, and philosophy of science.* Dordrecht, Holland: Reidel Pub. Co. Quoted in Eva Feder Kittay (1999), *Love's Labour.*

Scott-Maxwell, F. (1968). *The measure of my days.* New York: Penguin Books.

Stone, D. (1999). Care and trembling. *The American prospect.* No. 43: 61–67.

Tronto, J. (1993). *Moral boundaries: A political argument for an ethics of care.* New York: Routledge.

Tronto, J. (1989). Women and caring: What feminists can learn about morality from caring? In A. M. Jagger & S. Bordo (Eds.), *Gender/body/knowledge.* New Brunswick: Rutgers University Press.

Walker, M. U. (1998). *Moral understandings: A feminist study in ethics.* New York: Routledge.

CHAPTER 4

The Ethical Importance of Home Care

Mark Waymack

> Mid pleasures and palaces though we may roam,
> Be it ever so humble, there's no place like home;
> A charm from the skies seems to hallow us there,
> Which, seek through the world, is ne'er met with elsewhere.
> Home, home, sweet, sweet home!
> There's no place like home! There's no place like home!
> —J. H. Payne ("Home, Sweet Home," 1823)

> It is suicide to be abroad. But what is it to be at home, Mr. Tyler, what is it to be at home? A lingering dissolution.
> —Samuel Becket (*All That Fall*, 1957)

We humans, by nature, have a frail streak in us. As infants and children, we are universally dependent upon the care of others. As adults, we are prone to accidents and disease that can render us dependent upon the care of others. And as we age, we are increasingly likely to require some assistance from others to maintain ourselves. Though it may take a multitude of forms—from a Vanderbilt mansion to a nomad's tent, a ghetto apartment stifling in the summer heat or a split-level somewhere in suburbia—home is where that care is most often delivered.

For most of our social history, other members of the household, the family, have delivered that care in the home. But recent social changes, especially in America, have made this seem more and more difficult or impractical. Social mobility, geographic and economic, has encouraged migration away from any "ancestral home." Consequently, many adult offspring live significant distances away from their aging parents. Furthermore, that distance, geographic and otherwise, has shifted our focus away from the "extended" family and more toward what is termed the "nuclear" family. Furthermore, in the past such care has typically been provided by women—wives, daughters, and daughters-in-law. Yet, the past 2 or 3 decades have seen a sea-change in terms of the work patterns and possibilities for these women. More and more, those daughters and daughters-in-law are employed outside the home; indeed, their income is considered vital to the maintenance of their own homes, not an unnecessary luxury. Therefore, they are less available to provide such home care as they were in the past. Hence, younger generations are now not as able or willing to take frail elders into their homes and provide day-to-day care for them.

One strategy of dealing with the problem posed by frail elderly who are no longer able to maintain themselves safely at home on their own has been to place them in nursing homes—not because of any strictly "medical need," but simply because it was hard to age in a household.

Oftentimes, however, the elderly who were removed from their own homes (seemingly against their will) were unhappy with this move. And families, while unwilling to let their parent suffer unnecessarily at home, were nevertheless appalled at the conditions in the typical nursing home and the subsequent depression and decline of their loved one. "Isn't there a better solution?" they would ask.

Many individuals, though perhaps unable to maintain themselves while living alone in their homes, would prefer to stay there anyway. Moreover, institutional nursing home care, even of mediocre quality, is relatively expensive. Therefore, society increasingly has turned to home care services provided by paid employees as a means to keep frail persons in their own homes. Long an option for wealthier people in our society, many state and local governments have increasingly made such services available to the poor through public funding.

Although home care has sometimes been touted as a way to save money, it is not entirely clear that that is true. Without doubt, institutional nursing home care (often financed by Medicaid for poorer individuals) is expensive. But there are ways in which institutional care is economically efficient. For example, all care recipients are residing under one roof; care providers need not travel from location to location. Furthermore, the concentrated setting of congregate living allows for some economically advantageous specialization of labor. Home care, on the other hand, requires the individual worker to spend considerable time traveling from one client's home to another. Furthermore, that worker is responsible for many different chores at any given location. The visit's time constraints may require that certain tasks be done out-of-synch from an ordinary daily living routine. Finally, because close supervision is impractical, home care is fertile ground for economic fraud and offers the potential for other kinds of abuse as well.

If we acknowledge these difficulties with home care, can we still find good reasons for choosing to commit ourselves to providing adequate, affordable home care for the frail? In this chapter, I shall put forward what I take to be an argument for the moral importance and value of home care: that just as most of us think that some degree of basic health care morally ought to be available to anyone in our society who needs it, so we have a moral obligation to try to meet the home care needs of our frail individuals.

HOME AND THE SELF

Contemporary health care ethics pays little heed to the importance of place to the self. Yet, despite philosophy's relative silence upon the issue, some reflection may allow us to see just how and why place can be of great importance to some individuals' sense of self.

To anyone at all familiar with Western philosophy since the 17th century, it should come as no surprise that moral philosophy, and indeed, philosophy in general, have not made much of an issue of place. At least since Descartes, Western philosophers have tended to equate the self with mind. They have tended to view the mind as the non-spatial, non-material, non-body, thinking thing. The body, on the other hand, is rarely viewed as the self, much less what gives us our identity.

Moral philosophy, taking its lead from this philosophy of mind, has usually grounded its ethical constructs upon this notion of the self—the self as the non-spatial, somewhat abstract, thinking thing. Hence, the body rarely has any essential place in moral theory. Perhaps, as with Kant, it is the body with its urges, desires, and inclinations, that can lead us astray from the moral dictates of rationality; but still it is the mind that is the true self—the body is only the distraction.

Even as the field of medical ethics emerged, borrowing as it has from more abstract moral theory, the body still entered the picture only as one possible field upon which medical ethics dilemmas unfolded. Since bodies belonged to persons (though were not the same as those persons), the moral right to direct the care of that body was vested in its rightful owner. This became the ethics of autonomy in modern health care.

Eric Cassell (1982), however, has persuasively argued that this conception of the self, which we can label as the "Cartesian Myth," is very inadequate. Cassell's particular concern in his seminal article is to illustrate how disease (and even the adverse effects of supposedly therapeutic treatment) can threaten and/or undermine the patient's sense of self. Accordingly, he draws out a rich notion of the many facets of self identity: hopes, fears, plans for the future, familial and social roles, spirituality, and others. Take an accomplished sculptor and give her medical treatment that erodes her ability to sculpt and you may well take away a significant part of her self-identity. Take a dedicated athlete who has built his whole career and self image around his accomplishments in a particular sport, destroy his athletic ability through disease and you may well have seriously diminished his sense of self, causing a crisis of identity. (This is a frequent challenge faced by trauma victims who survive their injuries only to be faced by the realities of paralysis and disfigurement.)

The Cartesian self, and its moral philosophy counterpart, faces other challenges. A persistent thread in the criticisms that feminist moral philosophers have leveled against traditional moral theory is that it overlooks the relational nature of the self. Feminists have chiefly focused upon our relations with other persons, emphasizing familial, personal, and social roles. Although feminist moral philosophy encompasses much more than just the "ethic of care," the ethic of care is a good illustration of this theme. Rather than build ethics around the Cartesian, unimpassioned, intellectual self, deriving moral oughts from our rational nature, the ethic of care sees ethics as an essentially relational enterprise, one that is centrally about maintaining and enriching our relationships, our caring for and about other individuals. The moral self, then, is a self who is essentially among/with/in relationship to others.

Despite their apparent differences, there is this common thread that runs through the critical challenges put forward by Cassell and the feminists: They both place great moral weight upon preserving or rehabilitating the sense of self. Both have also greatly expanded what kinds of things are important in the creation and maintenance of our sense of self.

Now, there is great variability in what different individuals may find important in building their own sense of self, of self-identity—e.g., artistic achievement, intellectual accomplishment, weight-lifting ability, physical appearance, familial roles (mother, father). For at least some (perhaps many) people, an important part of how we identify ourselves will be our home, specifically, our living in our own home.

There are many ways in which home might be of great importance to an individual's sense of self.

First, to have and be able to live in our own home, at least in contemporary American society, is itself evidence of accomplishment and ability. To live in our own home demonstrates that we have sufficient material resources to maintain our own home—a sign of success. To do so also demonstrates a significant degree of functional self-sufficiency—something that many people in this society find admirable.

Second, the self-sufficiency, the functionality, that living at home represents also correlates with a sense of individual autonomy. It is the strength, the power of self-sufficiency that living at home represents or illustrates that reinforces a sense of autonomy. Not only is this my home, but because it is my home I am in charge. It is I who decide how this home will be run.

Third, to live in our own home provides many of us the means to define personal, private space, a space reserved for our self. That we can occupy this space, to the exclusion of others, provides another way of defining our self as distinct from others.

Fourth, especially for individuals who have lived in their home for many years, the home becomes a landscape of memories, memories that can be significant in defining the self: memories of a spousal relationship—a dead husband's favorite chair, the kitchen table where quarrels erupted, the bedroom shared for so many decades; memories of children growing up—the stairs where a son broke his arm, the playroom where so many pictures were colored, the living room where prom photos were staged, the front porch where a daughter and future son-in-law were seen kissing one summer night, and the sofa where a beloved grandchild loves to nap.

A glance around the room, almost any room, can thus help stimulate a flood of memories, memories that are part of one's self-identity. While such stimulants to memory might be pleasant for the revery of the unimpaired individual, think how much more helpful, how restoring they can be for the individual who stands in the early stages of memory loss. For such an individual, a common kind of candidate for institutionalized care, the physicality of being at home can provide a rich stimulus for remembering much that defines the self, much that otherwise might well be lost.

THE LOSS OF HOME AND EROSION OF THE SELF

It should be clear, then, how leaving home can, for many individuals, erode their sense of self.

First, such a removal from home to more institutionalized care has a symbolic meaning. The person being moved and those participating or even simply watching see it as signifying a crucial inadequacy: the individual is no longer able to maintain a home. Admittedly, for some individuals, a home can be an undesirable burden. Inasmuch as they may see it as an undesirable burden, they may freely choose to leave their home, and even see a move as an opportunity to improve their lives. Hence, many "empty nesters" choose to "downsize," leaving behind a larger house that made sense when they were raising a family, but which has now become an obstacle, in terms of either time or money, to the things that they would now like to do. This illustrates the variability in what individuals find to be significant building blocks of their self identity. Suffice it to say, though, that for many Americans this loss of home is not by choice and hence represents a real loss, not a favored choice.

Second, connected to the loss of home, there will be loss of, or at least in a real sense great constraint upon, autonomy. We have long celebrated the Anglo-Saxon tradition encapsulated in such sayings as, "A man is king of his own home" or "A man's home is his castle." These convey the sense of autonomy in its true etymological sense, self-legislating. We lay down the law in our own homes. However, in an institutional setting, such as the nursing home, the resident's ability to "lay down the law" is vastly constrained. Life in such an institution is typically characterized by the rules, the routines, the habits of the institution, not those of the individual. And even where rules of the institution might not intrude, one still resides in "congregate living," and living in such close quarters with others, where there is very little private space (in fact maybe no truly private space), one may be faced with constantly negotiating compromises for the use of public space.

True, the cognitively intact resident will still have say over important decisions regarding medical care. But note what a minuscule fraction of everyday living in a nursing home is comprised of such medical care.

Third, as noted above, the inhabitation of one's home offers a sense of belonging somewhere, a sense that this is one's personal space which excludes others (except through permission given). The possibility for privacy thus could be an important part of self identity. But in the typical nursing home, private space is minimal. Indeed, not only is the privacy of space threatened; often the privacy of personal clothing is lost. The personal space and possessions that home offered are thus largely stripped away in the nursing home; with the result that the sense of self may be greatly diminished. We become less than we were.

Fourth, as noted above, the geography and the furnishings of home often provides the tangible reminders of things past that are yet vastly important for our present sense of self. It is impossible for institutional life to provide such a function. The nursing home will be devoid of such tangible reminders, with the possible exception of one chest of drawers or one night stand, and a few very select photographs. But one or two small pieces of furniture and a couple of pictures can hardly compensate for a lost household of furniture. It is necessarily impossible for the nursing home to provide the stimulus for memory that the geography of one's own home provides. The dining room, where the family ate so many Sunday dinners, is simply not there at the nursing home. The living room where a child took a first step cannot be replaced by the common day room.

What I am arguing is that for very many people, the removal from their homes and placement in a long-term-care facility would be the cause of an erosion, a great diminishment of their selves, a loss of self-identity.

Now, if we accept that Cassell, the feminists, and others are correct in thinking that we have a moral obligation to respond to others when their sense of self is threatened, then it should be quite apparent how home care—providing services that help an individual stay at home who otherwise might have to be removed from home and institutionalized—provides a morally significant and valuable service. Whether or not home care helps society save some money becomes dwarfed, as a question, by the moral service that home care provides in terms of helping the frail, who value their home life, to keep their sense of self, to retain their self integrity, to help them hold the self together for as long as is feasible.

INTRINSIC LIMITATIONS

There are inherent limitations to how even well-financed home care services can achieve many of these desired goals. This is because the necessity for home care, and the intrusion of caregivers into the home, in themselves, undermine some of the self-reinforcing aspects of living at home.

First, note that bringing paid caregivers into the home requires an acknowledgment that a frail individual is no longer capable of maintaining his or her home by his- or herself alone. There is a subtle but important difference between such things as cleaning services that wealthier families, especially two-income households, may use and the kind of services that we are now discussing. When the wealthier households pay someone from outside to perform these services, the understanding is not that the members of this household are not capable of doing these tasks: rather, the understanding is that they deliberately choose not to perform them. But when a frail person accedes to accepting home care services, it is precisely because he or she is now incapable of performing those tasks suitably on his/her own. So acknowledging the need for such home care services also entails acknowledging relative inability. Thus, the admirable self-sufficiency that home occupation represents, to the self and to others, is necessarily undermined though not entirely destroyed.

Second, the intrusion of a paid home care worker into the household represents to some degree an abdication (or usurpation) of autonomy. Not only are home care tasks done according to the worker's schedule rather than the client's; even more significantly, it is the home care workers who now judge what the suitable standards for maintaining the home are to be. It is an outsider who judges whether I am keeping my room tidy enough. It is an outsider who judges whether I am eating properly. It is an outsider who judges whether I am in need of a bath or not. So, though I still reside in my own home, my home is no longer my castle; I am not the exclusive monarch of my private space. The presence and activity of home care workers, therefore, necessarily infringes on my autonomy. Nonetheless, more autonomy surely is maintained in the typical home care arrangement than would be feasible in the typical nursing home setting.

Though there are these sorts of inherent limitations in how home care workers can support the frail individual without undermining that individual's sense of self, of integrity, there are also ways in which the presence of a home care worker, particularly the right sort of worker, can enhance the individual's sense of self. An attentive, patient, humane worker can provide not only cleaning, bathing, and food preparation services; she can also be a human companion. Such companionship can support the individual's sense of self in many different ways. For example, just being there to listen can spark conversation, reminiscing, activities that can help remind frail individuals of who they are. Furthermore, social contact, simply in and of itself, through the recognition of personhood that it entails, can immeasurably help to bolster the sense of self. These are no small accomplishments.

Of course, there may well come a time in any particular case when the limits of the possibilities of home care are reached. Home care is, admittedly, a prop; and eventually that prop may become insufficient to support its structure. Conceptually, this would be when the extent of care needed becomes so great that the limitations discussed above overwhelm the beneficial aspects of home care. Of course, practically, economic constraints of the individual, as well as of society, will also be a limiting factor. When these circumstances are reached, other solutions may have to be sought out.

A MESSAGE FOR HOME CARE WORKERS

Home care workers, we all know, are relatively poorly paid. The working conditions can be demanding, even dangerous. There is a disconcertingly and frustratingly high rate of turnover in the ranks. At least part of an explanation for the pay scale and low social status of the job is the low importance that society has placed upon such work. If such work is conceived simply in terms of housekeeping and a few manual chores, then I suppose such a social judgment might make some sort of sense.

However, if we understand how the activity of sensitive, humane home care workers can be crucial for maintaining the moral sense of self, the sense of integrity, the very self-identity of their clients, then we can easily see the deep moral importance of their work. Without such support, the frail face an impossible choice. Borrowing from and slightly altering the words of Samuel Beckett quoted at the beginning of this chapter, it would be suicide to be institutionalized, but to remain at home without assistance would be a lingering dissolution.

I pray that, if and when I need such help, I can find it.

REFERENCE

Cassell, E. (1982). The nature of suffering and the goals of medicine. *New England Journal of Medicine, 306*(11), 639–645.

CHAPTER 5

An Ethic of Care

Joan C. Tronto

Despite the hospice patient's protestations, May insisted. Slowly, she helped him up to sit with her in the kitchen while she heated up the food that Meals on Wheels had sent for him.

The union meeting at the nursing home had grown more and more angry. In the end, the nurses' aides agreed to strike if more staff were not hired. In their letter to management, they wrote, "We simply do not have enough time to take care of the patients."

The agency head despaired. She had received an angry phone call from a woman whose mother received home-help assistance from her agency. The daughter reported that a five-dollar bill that she had left on her mother's dresser had disappeared after the aide visited yesterday. The administration could fire the aide, but this was the fourth aide she had sent to the household in the past year.

Such vignettes are familiar in caregiving and raise a number of significant questions. But are the questions they raise ethical questions? Often in our culture, *ethical* and *moral* seem to refer to conformity to set principles and precepts: stealing is wrong, do not lie. "Ethics" and "morality" seem to evoke big questions, impossible dilemmas, or conformity to predetermined codes of behavior. By this account, there is no obvious moral issue in insisting that a dying patient continue to be engaged in life, or in staffing levels in a nursing home. This chapter describes a way of thinking about caring that expands our notions of the "ethical" to include many of the everyday judgments involved in activities of caring for ourselves and others. It draws upon a body of recent work in the feminist ethics of care (Benner & Wrubel, 1989; Fisher & Tronto, 1990; Ruddick, 1990; Manning, 1992; Held, 1993; Tronto, 1993; Bubeck, 1995; Held, 1995; Jaggar, 1995; Sevenhuijsen, 1998) to present a more complicated account of ethics, one that tries to restore to the word *ethics* its original meaning—knowledge about how to live a good life. This perspective requires not only a broader interpretation of the nature of ethics, but a more complete account of the nature of care. In making daily and thoughtful judgments about caring, people every day engage in a high moral calling. Our moral sensibilities will be greatly enhanced if we learn to think more thoughtfully about the morality of everyday life embodied in an ethics of care.

A BROAD UNDERSTANDING OF CARE

When Berenice Fisher and I began to explore the nature of care (Fisher & Tronto, 1990), we were surprised that we could find no good and systematic definition of the term. As many commentators have observed, *care* has a dual set of meanings. It refers both to a mental disposition of concern and to actual practices that we engage in as a result of these concerns; for example, a doctor's care involves both an attentiveness and concern and the concrete practices of prescribing medical treatment (Hugman, 1991). Nevertheless, much of the current discussion of care either overemphasizes the emotional and intellectual qualities and ignores its reference to actual work, or overemphasizes care as work at the expense of understanding the deeper intellectual and emotional qualities.

The activities that constitute care are crucial for human life. We defined care in this way: Care is "a species activity that includes everything that we do to maintain, continue, and repair our 'world' so that we can live in it as well as possible. That world includes our bodies, our selves, and our environment, all of which we seek to interweave in a complex, life-sustaining web" (Fisher & Tronto, 1990, p. 40).

Several aspects of this definition of care are noteworthy: First, we describe care as a "species activity," a philosophical term we use because it suggests that how people care for one another is one of the features that make people human. Second, we describe care as an action, as a practice, not as a set of principles or rules. Third, our notion of care contains a standard, but a flexible one: We care so that we can live in the world as well as possible. The understanding of what will be good care depends upon the way of life, the set of values and conditions, of the people engaged in the caring practice.

Furthermore, caring is a process that can occur in a variety of institutions and settings. Care is found in the household, in services and goods sold in the market, in the workings of bureaucratic organizations in contemporary life. Care is not restricted to the traditional realm of mother's work, to welfare agencies, or to hired domestic servants but is found in all of these realms. Indeed, concerns about care permeate our daily lives, the institutions in the modern marketplace, the corridors of government. Because we tend to follow the traditional division of the world into public and private spheres and to think of caring as an aspect of private life, care is usually associated with activities of the household. As a result, caring is greatly undervalued in our culture—in the assumption that caring is somehow "women's work," in perceptions of caring occupations, in the wages and salaries paid to workers engaged in provision of care, in the assumption that care is menial. One of the central tasks for people interested in care is to change the overall public value associated with care. When our public values and priorities reflect the role that care actually plays in our lives, our world will be organized quite differently.

FOUR PHASES OF CARE

Until the world changes, though, an analysis of care can provide us with a useful guide for thinking about how we do our particular caring work and its ethical dimensions—the way in which care is related to what we know about how to live a good life. Such a process can also provide us with a framework for political change. Thinking about the process of care, Fisher and Tronto (1990) identified four phases of care as follow:

Caring About

"Caring about" involves becoming aware of and paying attention to the need for caring. Genuinely to care about someone, some people, or something requires listening to articulated needs, recognizing unspoken needs, distinguishing among and deciding which needs to care about. It requires attentiveness, that is, of being able to perceive needs in self and others and to perceive them with as little distortion as possible, which could be said to be a moral or ethical quality.

Caring For

"Caring for" is the phase in caring when someone assumes responsibility to meet a need that has been identified. Simply seeing a need for care is not enough to make care happen; someone has to assume the responsibility for organizing, marshaling resources or personnel, and paying for the care work that will meet the identified needs. The moral dimension of caring for is to assume, and to take seriously, responsibility.

Caregiving

This phase is the actual material meeting of the caring need. Caregiving requires that individuals and organizations perform the necessary caring tasks. It involves knowledge about how to care. Although we often do not think of it this way, competence is the moral dimension of caregiving. Incompetent care is not only a technical problem, but a moral one.

Care Receiving

This phase involves the response of the thing, person, or group that received the caregiving. Whether the needs have been met or not, whether the caregiving was successful or not, there will be some response to the care that has been given. Care receiving requires the complex moral element of responsiveness. Responsiveness is complex because it shares the moral burden among the person, thing, or group that has received the care, but it also involves the moral attention of the ones who are doing the caring work and those who are responsible for care. In a way, since any single act of care may alter the situation and produce new needs for care, the caring process in this way comes full circle, with responsiveness requiring more attentiveness.

Identifying these four phases of care provides us with a more complex picture of what "good caring" will be. It allows us to recognize that while there may be an ideal form of caring, an integrated holistic process in which those who cared about a problem take responsibility, provide care, and receive thanks when all goes well, to realize this ideal process of caring is highly unlikely. In reality, the process of care rarely occurs in a perfect way.

Several aspects of care make it much more complicated than this account of phases might suggest. In the first place, care is fraught with conflict. Indeed, conflict seems inherent in care. There are more needs for care than can ever be met. Determining which needs are important inevitably involves slighting other needs. At the most personal level, caregivers have needs at the same time that they give care to others, and they need somehow to balance their needs and those of others. At the institutional level, the needs of different clients, groups, and workers may come into conflict with each other. At the political level, a prominent form of political struggle occurs over the recognition of needs, and for individuals and groups to be able to describe their needs (what the political theorist Nancy Fraser [1989] has called a "needs interpretation process").

In the second place, care involves power relations. Care can occur among equals, and some care (called "personal service" by Kari Waerness [1990] and including such cases as doing the cleaning or laundry for others in one's household) is provided by subordinates for people who could otherwise provide this kind of care for themselves. But much care, and much care for the elderly, is what Waerness calls "necessary care": the caregiver has some kind of ability, knowledge, or resource that the care receiver does not have. As a result, there is often an imbalance in power among caregivers and care receivers. Sometimes the relationship between caregivers and receivers becomes a power struggle. Sometimes the care receiver becomes filled with rage. That any party might abuse a caring relationship and take advantage of the others is also possible.

When people recognize that care is a complex process with many components, it becomes possible to avoid either despairing about care or romanticizing it. Care is more likely to be filled with inner contradictions, conflict, and frustration than it is to resemble the idealized interactions of mother and child or teacher and student or nurse and patient.

MAKING CARING JUDGMENTS

The ethic of care, then, both elevates care to a central value in human life and recognizes that care requires a complicated process of judgment. People need to make moral judgments, political judgments, technical judgments, and psychological judgments in their everyday caring activities. Caring, then, is neither simple nor banal; it requires know-how and judgment, and to make such judgments as well as possible becomes the moral task of engaging in care. In general, care judgments require that those involved understand the complexity of the process in which they are enmeshed. Caring involves both rational explications of needs and sympathetic appreciation of emotions. It requires not an abstraction from the concrete case to a universal principle, but an explication of the "full story." Yet, at the same time, those engaged in care practices need to be able to place some distance from their own version of what is happening and other perspectives.

The experience of people working in caring agencies, caregivers, and people who reflect on the caring practices of their everyday lives suggests that using this framework for analysis helps people to pinpoint problems in caring processes and relationships. Using the (probably unachievable) goal of a unified, satisfying process of care as a guide, thinking about care in this more complex way that is linked to morality and ethics allows people to act to improve the situations in which they find themselves. While perfection is impossible, improvement is not; through good caring, people are better able to live in the world.

There are at least three kinds of moral problems related to the practice of care that require reflection. In the first place, problems may arise in thinking about the particular elements of care. In the second place, problems arise from the conflict inherent in care and in the difficulties of integrating the phases of care. In the third place, the context in which caring work occurs also presents moral problems. (Figure 5.1 lists some of the questions that are relevant to explore in thinking about caring.)

A final implication follows from the complexity of the care process and underscores the importance of the "full story" being heard in making judgments about care. Caring should take place in an environment in which all of those engaged in caring—caregivers and care receivers as well as other responsible parties—can contribute to the ongoing discussion of caring needs and how to meet them. No single actors in a care process can assert their own authoritative knowledge in the process. Within the activity of caring itself, actors must continue to be attentive, responsible, competent, and responsive to the others in the caring process.

THE CARE ETHIC, VULNERABILITY, AND CARING FOR THE ELDERLY

Caring is complex, but it is also ubiquitous. Yet we live in a culture that finds it very difficult to acknowledge this fact, for many possible reasons. Perhaps such unwillingness partly stems from a "model of man" that presumes that people are autonomous actors, and so people are unwilling to recognize their own caring needs as legitimate. It may also stem from the unlimited nature of needs, so that when people begin to acknowledge the needs of others they are quickly frustrated by their

Questions that arise from the elements of care:

1. *Attentiveness.* What care is necessary? Are there basic human needs? What types of care now exist; how adequate are they? Who gets to articulate the nature of needs and to say what and how which problems should be cared about?
2. *Responsibility.* Who should be responsible for meeting the needs for care that do exist? How can and should such responsibility be fixed? Why?
3. *Competence.* Who actually are the caregivers? How well do they do their work? What conflicts exist between them and care receivers? What resources do caregivers need in order to care competently? Who pays attention to changes in care receivers' needs?
4. *Responsiveness.* How do care receivers respond to the care that they are given? How well does the care process, as it exists, meet their needs? If their needs conflict with one another, who resolves these conflicts?

Questions that arise from conflict and integration of care:

1. What conflicts exist to disrupt integrated and complete care?
2. How far apart are caregivers and care receivers?
3. How distant from those who give care are those who hold "responsibility"?
4. What connection exists to make those who claim to "care about" a particular problem assume responsibility for it, and pay attention genuinely to its outcome as a caring process?
5. What conflicts emerge between the expertise of those who care about, care for, and give care, and those who primarily receive care?

Questions that arise from the context of care:

1. How are needs understood to define and to shape the nature of the caring process?
2. What forms of power and privilege reside in this care process? How do they shape the nature and adequacy of care? Do they threaten change in current forms of care?
3. What construction of "otherness" (for example, positing "the vulnerable" as "others" who are unlike ourselves) contributes to perceptions of caring?

FIGURE 5.1 Questions that can guide caring judgments.

relative inability to meet all of these needs. Partly, this unwillingness probably stems from a division of the world into public and private realms, in which "caring" is supposed to be done in private, away from public view. And, in part, the unwillingness to recognize the role of care in our lives probably stems from our incapacity to comprehend death. No matter how successfully we care for ourselves or others, human life ends in death.

While the elderly do have particular needs, there is a danger in trying to think about the care needs of the elderly as separate from the broader context—everyone has caring needs. Elderly people care for themselves, and they also care for their families, their friends and neighbors, their communities, and the commonweal. The elderly also receive care from many others. The diversity of practices required to care for elderly people's needs is as great as the diversity of caring for people of other ages. Although some older people are not so, many older people are more vulnerable than they were when they were younger. The processes of aging make some elderly people more vulnerable to some physical and mental incapacities. Elderly people might find themselves in the situation of needing the assistance of others in meeting their needs, and, as a result, may have to change their sense of power in relations of care as they age. Among the elderly, people have different access to resources with which to care for themselves. This fact raises many moral questions about equity in providing for the care of the elderly.

Perhaps what is the most interesting point to notice about the caring needs of the elderly, though, is not so much the nature of the actual needs, but rather the fact that the elderly seem to be "marked" with an assumption that they need more assistance. As a society, our unwillingness to acknowledge our own vulnerability demands the easy solution of identifying particular groups as especially vulnerable, so that we can continue the myth of our own invulnerable autonomy. In a society in which vulnerability is viewed as weakness, those who are perceived to need more care, regardless of the actual situation, are in a more vulnerable position. In fact, many older people do have greater needs for care: health care, physical space, transportation, and housing. Yet as long as these discussions take place in a context in which the elderly are marked as the vulnerable ones, in need of "special" care, we miss our opportunity to see caring in old age as part of a full life process. Embracing care as a part of human life, recognizing its role in creating interconnections and relationships of receiving and giving over a lifetime, may provide us with a way to rethink some of the ways in which we now seem unable to cope with human vulnerability. This is not a problem that concerns only the elderly, it is one that affects everyone.

CONCLUSION

The ethic of care, as feminist theorists have articulated it, provides opportunities for people to analyze their own activities of care as well as to understand the broader place of caring in human life. To return to the examples at the beginning of this essay, conflicts between enraged patients and their caregivers, between management and care workers in institutions, are part of this process. Coming to some resolution of these conflicts is part of the essence of caring activities themselves. It requires thoughtful judgments that involve all who are concerned. Through thoughtful engagement in caring, we can begin to recognize the profound moral dimensions of our everyday lives.

REFERENCES

Benner, P., & Wrubel, J. (1989). *The primacy of caring: Stress and coping in health and illness.* Menlo Park, CA: Addison-Wesley.

Bubeck, D. (1995). *Care, justice and gender.* Oxford, England: Oxford University Press.

Fisher, B., & Tronto, J. (1990). Towards a feminist theory of care. In E. Abel & M. Nelson (Eds.), *Circles of care.* Albany, NY: State University of New York Press.

Fraser, N. (1989). *Unruly practices: Power, discourse, and gender in contemporary social theory.* Minneapolis: University of Minnesota Press.

Held, V. (1993). *Feminist morality: Transforming culture, society and politics.* Chicago: University of Chicago Press.

Held, V. (1995). *Justice and care: Essential readings in feminist ethics.* Boulder, CO: Westview Press.

Hugman, R. (1991). *Power in caring professions.* London: MacMillan.

Jaggar, A. (1995). Caring as a feminist practice of moral reason. In V. Held (Ed.), *Justice and care: Essential readings in feminist ethics.* Boulder, CO: Westview Press.

Manning, R. (1992). *Speaking from the heart: A feminist perspective on ethics.* Lanham, MD: Rowman and Littlefield.

Ruddick, S. (1990). *Maternal thinking: Towards a politics of peace.* Boston: Beacon Press.

Sevenhuijsen, S. (1998). *Citizenship and the ethics of care.* New York: Routledge.

Tronto, J. (1993). *Moral boundaries: A political argument for an ethic of care.* New York: Routledge.

Waerness, K. (1990). Informal and formal care in old age: What is wrong with the new ideology in Scandinavia today? In C. Ungerson (Ed.), *Gender and caring: Work and welfare in Britain and Scandinavia.* London: Harvester, Wheatsheaf.

CHAPTER 6

Old Ethical Frameworks: What Works, What Doesn't?

Mark Waymack

In an insular and unchanging society, there might be no need for much ethical reflection. Perhaps we would each be taught our duties and the punishments for violating them, and we, in turn, would teach them to those who followed us. But the idea of being genuinely unsure of our moral obligations would probably be inconceivable.

American society, of course, is anything but insular and unchanging. The ethnic and cultural demography of our people is in flux. Our technology, including the technology of health care, is in flux. And our social structures and social relationships are in flux.

Home care and home services constitute an area of health care that, though perhaps lacking in high drama, represents vast change in both the technology of health care and the social structures by which such care is delivered. This change has greatly extended the possibility for living at home, but has brought no small measure of moral confusion. How do the ethics of rendering care in someone's own home differ from the ethics of care in a contained institution? What moral rights do providers of home care services have? What is the moral texture of the relationships between recipient of care, family members, and professional service providers? Anyone who has worked in the field knows that these questions are quite difficult to answer.

Indeed, it is largely because of such flux and its resulting moral confusion that the bioethics revolution of the last quarter of this century happened. Confronted by dramatic changes in medical technology, especially noticed in the acute care setting, and changes in our social notion of individual decision-making rights, health care professionals turned to philosophers for help. And moral philosophers, captivated by the unfolding drama of life-and-death choices in the high-technology hospital, willingly responded.

Accordingly, this early foray into health care ethics focused almost exclusively upon the ethical dynamic of the patient confronted with bewildering life-and-death choices in the acute-care setting. What emerged was an ethic that above all emphasized respect for individual autonomy, one of those mythic values of American culture (e.g., Beauchamp & Childress, 1973). Soon, leading acute-care institutions were expected to have ethics policies about such things as resuscitation and "pulling the plug"; and they were expected to have ethics committees to implement such policies and be the protectors of patients' rights.

Eventually, people began to realize that health care was delivered not only in the acute-care setting, but also in the long-term-care institution, so long-term-care ethics was born.

The first generation of long-term-care ethics pretty much borrowed directly from the acute care model. Nursing homes were soon expected to have ethics committees and ethics policies on "do not resuscitate" orders and the like. Some early work tried to argue that ethics in long-term care might have a different complexion. But it was without doubt the anthology *Everyday Ethics: Resolving Dilemmas in Nursing Home Life*, edited by Rosalie Kane and Arthur Caplan (1990), that shook things up. Several key contributed chapters engaged in the watershed process of actually asking nursing home residents what they perceived to be the most significant moral problems. To the surprise of many academics, what nursing home residents themselves considered to be of greatest moral importance was quite different from the moral questions about acute care that had pervaded the first generation of nursing home ethics as conceived in academic institutions.

Still, this second generation of nursing home ethics was born and, though "closer to the ground," it continued to work from a model of health care ethics that lent preeminence to individual autonomy. It took a third generation of nursing home ethics to begin to explore moral values beyond autonomy, values that had more to say in the face of congregate living, limited resources, and dementia (e.g., Agich [1993] and Moody [1992]).

If we are open-minded about our past mistakes, then we may perhaps minimize our chances of repeating them. Our experience with ethics in the nursing home taught us that the problems raised and the issues of greatest concern in the nursing home setting were not necessarily the same as those in acute care. And we also learned that even the prevailing model of health care ethics—the individual autonomy model—was not ideal for addressing many of the ethical dilemmas and tensions experienced in long-term care.

The home care and home services setting is remarkably different from its nursing home cousin, and even more distant from acute care, particularly in the areas of autonomy and family.

Autonomy

In acute care, the patient is a temporary guest in what is to him or her a very alien, high-tech institution. The patient is in crisis and faces bewildering choices. Patients are seriously ill, usually feel alienated by the environment, and are often cared for by physicians and nurses whom they have never before met. It is perhaps natural then that the ethic of the hospital is primarily concerned with bolstering patient autonomy, since patient autonomy is challenged or eroded from numerous directions. In the nursing home, most of the "everyday" ethics have more to do with individual autonomy in the face of congregate living arrangements, arrangements which necessarily compromise individual freedoms. But the home is where the resident is king or queen. It is where people feel most comfortable, most secure in exerting their individual autonomy. Autonomy, therefore, may not require quite as much bolstering as in the acute-care or even long-term-care institutional setting. On the other hand, the recipients of home care services are recipients precisely because they are *not* fully independent; they are most likely frail and in some way dependent. Hence, a home care ethics will have to be sensitive to the ways in which autonomy is (or is not) challenged in its setting. And further, unless ethics is *only* about individual autonomy, we may well expect an ethic of home care to find itself concerned about many important issues other than resident autonomy. We will need, then, more than an ethic of autonomy.

Family

In both the acute-care and the nursing home settings, family may well play a significant role. When the individual is cognitively incapacitated (and in the absence of explicit advance directives), ethics typically recommends looking to the family to take an important role in decision making, and we may also encourage them to provide emotional support. Family is rarely expected or encouraged to provide any of the actual care in these institutions. But in the home care setting, the care that is provided is in some sense care that has traditionally been provided by family. Furthermore, even in the presence of home care service providers, family typically still play a significant role, often providing the bulk of the hours and work of care. Family may even live alongside the care recipient and, in some arrangements, family members are even paid to provide the kind of care that they might have been traditionally expected to provide on their own, simply as family members. Hence, there is quickly a blurring of roles and responsibilities between family and paid care providers.

We have in some sense created a new social role. Yes, in the past the wealthy always had access to such "in home" care. But such care was clearly a privilege enjoyed by few and grounded in an employer-employee relationship. Now, however, we have made at least some moves in the direction of recognizing home care as something to be available to classes outside the wealthy. But we have yet to think through the ethics of this new social arrangement. Should such service be a market commodity for those who have willing insurers or moderately deep pockets of their own? Or should such service be viewed more as a social right? But if a social right, then subsidized to what extent and by whom?

Is there some special moral obligation of the agency (and worker) to the recipient of care? Or is this simply another strictly free-market business relationship?

To what extent can the recipient of care dictate behavior to the provider? Can the provider be required to obey the recipient's commands, even when they place the recipient at great risk? What is the ethics of the relationship between the provider and the family?

In addition, other problems arise that seem unique to the home care field: While the employer at the institution—the hospital or nursing home—can and should be held responsible for maintaining a safe workplace, the employer at a home care agency seemingly has little ability to provide such safety. Home care workers daily go into dangerous neighborhoods, and even into dangerous homes, to provide services. They are placing themselves at risk. What rights do the workers have?

If we are truly to assist home care and services workers, their employers, and their clients by clarifying, articulating, and perhaps in some real sense improving the ethics of this field, two lessons, in particular, should be kept in mind:

First, we—the academics, the writers, and in particular the "ethicists"—should not presume ahead of time to know what the most pressing ethical issues in home care are. Rather, we must work closely with the people who are receiving home services, those who provide those services, and those who manage those providers, to learn from them what they perceive the ethical difficulties to be.

Gleaning this information is not necessarily as easy as it may sound. Obstacles stand in the way. For example, the recipients of care as well as the providers of care typically lack special education in the concepts and language of ethics. Hence, while they may feel quite acutely the pangs of ethical difficulties, they may lack the conceptual or vocabulary resources to articulate exactly what is at issue. Hence, the skills of a talented facilitator to listen, to tease out, and to clarify may be indispensable. But this facilitator must be careful not to "lead" the other person in his or her descriptions of the ethical difficulties, to unconsciously lure the other into framing the ethical problems in the ways that the facilitator has already conceptualized the matter. We must remain open to what those working in the field desperately want to tell us.

Second, once these "phenomenological data" have been collected, those of us who are trying to articulate an ethics of home care and home services must bring our ethical tools to bear. But here we must be careful not to get boxed into the rather single-minded ethic of individual autonomy that is so prevalent. Moral philosophy has broadened considerably since the early 1970s. And there are several new models of moral reasoning—perspectives on morality—that may prove to be of particular value in understanding the complex ethics of home care and home services.

Feminist ethics, for example, has brought fresh criticisms of the atomistic concept of the individual that underlies much of the ethic of individual autonomy. First, feminists' moral philosophy has been much more sensitive to the social realities of the position of women (and minorities) than has traditional moral philosophy. This thinking is more often alert to how socialized gender roles and expectations may actually constrain or hamper the will of an individual. Talk about autonomy, for example, may well suit a population of well-educated, middle- and upper-income white males who feel fully empowered and capable of exercising autonomy; but for many women, economic dependency and social conventions reinforce feelings of constraint and powerlessness rather than feelings of empowerment. The feminist perspective, therefore, may be much better suited to perceiving instances where the aged, dependent, frail recipient of care is (in subtle or not-so-subtle ways) being used or coerced by family in a home care setting. The feminist perspective is also chary of devotion to a one-principle system of ethics. In its stead, feminist moral philosophers have explored an ethic of relationships, including family and caregiver relations. Included in this broad family is the ethics of care. These perspectives on care and relationships, rather than abstract principles, may prove far more illuminating as we peer into the home care setting.

Another possible conceptual resource is communicative ethics, an ethical theory that emphasizes ethical decisions as the outcome of a dialogue in which everyone is heard. Especially important here is that the voices of those who are typically at the margins of society—the poor, the frail, the dependent, the disadvantaged—are heard and respected. This perspective could be of immense value in the home care setting, as its brings to the fore the highly interactive and interdependent nature of home care. Is everyone's voice being heard—not only that of the client, but also those of the family, the case workers, and the agency? This is morally crucial, as each and every one of these individuals is in some sense a participant in the delivery of care. Issues like risks, responsibilities, and limits can all be brought out into the open as concerns for dialogue.

A third neglected perspective is that of narrative ethics. This perspective emphasizes the narrative structure of moral knowledge and moral education. We noted earlier that for several reasons, it is of great importance that we progress in home care ethics by learning from case workers in the field and from their clients to determine how they perceive the moral issues, typically by listening to their case-based stories, their narratives. Furthermore, as was also noted earlier, if an ethic of home care is to be constructive in the end, it has to be formulated and presented in a way that can be readily understood and appropriated by clients and workers in the field. Narrative ethics, by presenting the story, offers an educational strategy that can be highly effective.

Finally, the complexities of these relationships in home care would seem to suggest that any ethic that would do those relationships justice will be somewhat complex. Having one, two, or even a small handful of "basic principles" may either distort the reality of the ethics or else be so vague as to be unhelpful. Yet the more complex the articulation of this ethic, the more difficult it is to teach such an ethic and to hold others accountable to it. And this challenge is especially compounded in the home care and home services field, where low social status of the job and low economic rewards attract a relatively poorly educated workforce and encourage a distressingly high turnover rate. Ethical standards or guidelines only work if people know about them and understand them. But if the ethics education is complicated and time-consuming, then before our efforts can bear their fruit in more ethical practices, the overwhelming majority of our workers in the field are likely to have moved on to other jobs, and we will be confronted with a new crop of ethically undertrained workers. Thus, however complex we academic types find the ethics of home care and home services to be, we must strive to condense moral reflection into something that can be easily taught, easily learned, and actually practiced.

We are near the beginning of this project. Kane and Caplan (1993) offered an anthology that was in many regards a first foray into the field. But more needs to be done. It will not be quick; nor will it be easy. And though it may not be full of drama and glitz, like an "ER" television show, the effort to provide an ethical framework for home care practice may have an enormous effect on the lives of countless workers and recipients of care, family, and supervisors, day in and day out. Let us do the best that we can.

REFERENCES

Agich, G. (1993). *Autonomy and long-term care.* New York: Oxford University Press.
Beauchamp, T., & Childress, J. (1973). *Principles of biomedical ethics.* New York: Oxford University Press.
Kane, R., & Caplan, A. (Eds.). (1990). *Everyday ethics: Resolving dilemmas in nursing home life.* New York: Springer Publishing.
Kane, R., & Caplan, A. (1993). *Ethical conflicts in the management of home care.* New York: Springer Publishing.
Moody, H. R. (1992). *Ethics in an aging society.* Baltimore, MD: Johns Hopkins University Press.

III

Organizations/ Care Providers/ Care Receivers

CHAPTER 7

Creating an Ethical Organization

David B. McCurdy

It is easy to overlook the moral role of the community-based agency or organization—whether for-profit or not-for-profit—that provides home care, adult day care, or related services to elders. The limited attention so far paid to the ethical problems of offering such care has largely focused on the individuals who provide care and on the difficult choices they face. This focus, important as it is, may ignore the substantial power of an organization—even a "mom and pop" community care agency—to influence individual attitudes, decisions, and practices for good or ill. Organizations—human service agencies among them—can be very complex entities, incorporating intricate patterns of human interaction and interdependence (Herman, 1997) and that nebulous phenomenon known as organizational "culture" (O'Reilly, 1989; Schein, 1992), all of which shape individuals' predispositions and behaviors in both obvious and subtle ways. From this perspective, creating an "ethical" organization is neither a small nor an unimportant task.

Even so, some organizational denizens would consider the accomplishment of this aim a "no-brainer." They view "ethics" and the tasks of creating an ethical organization as a straightforward venture requiring the same efficient approach as other administrative projects: First, develop a code of conduct or ethical behavior. Don't waste time "reinventing the wheel"; borrow from another organization's code if it seems to fit. Second, make sure that all staff members are aware of the code and receive a copy of it. Require all recipients to "sign off" on receiving and reading the code. For good measure, have those in management positions verify in writing that they are not engaging in unethical conduct. Finally, monitor compliance with the newly established procedures. Adherence to this process should create an ethical organization, or permit an administration to certify that the organization was ethical to begin with. Case closed.

Others perceive creating an ethical organization as a daunting, if not impossible, project. They spy a wealth of potential ethical issues—not only those inherent in the direct provision of services, but also those arising in relationships with other organizations (including governmental agencies) and in internal relationships (including those between management and line staff). They recognize the multiplicity of constituents and interests involved, and they sense that assessing and addressing organizational culture is an unavoidable dimension of the task. Beholding the scope of the challenge and the obstacles involved, they may feel overwhelmed—and may wonder whether the results will be worth the effort required.

Yet a third group would emphatically endorse the last-named reservation of the second group. For them, efforts to address organizational ethics are a fool's errand. They speak from the skeptical perspective of personal disillusionment with organizations they have known. For them, the problem is not the complexity of organizations, but the reality that organizations lack the motivation, will, and nerve to address ethical issues effectively or consistently. Though this group's perspective may be wrapped in cynicism, it is really the product of a frustrated idealism that expects much of any organization of which they are a part—and is repeatedly disappointed by the ambiguous (at best) morality that the organization actually displays. Unhappy experience has taught them that any effort to improve an organization's ethics is doomed to failure. It is better, they say, to carry out one's own responsibilities as ethically as possible—sometimes by ignoring the organization's policies and practices in order to do the right thing.

While each of these views has its more or less evident limitations, each also glimpses some important truths about ethics in organizations. The "fool's errand" view is alert to the perennial organizational gap between "talking the talk" and "walking the walk." This gap's persistence suggests a need to establish realistic expectations—without abandoning the standards and aspirations against which ethical progress is measured. The "daunted" view rightly sees that analyzing and addressing issues of organizational ethics is indeed a complex task, one that is not for the faint of heart—or the casually committed. It recognizes the importance of changing organizational culture, not merely formal policies and procedures. Finally, whatever its flaws, the "no-brainer" view senses that it *is* possible to make headway in creating an ethical organization. This approach recognizes that administrative commitment and a well-articulated plan, one that provides for evaluation as well as implementation, are critical to establishing a sustainable ethics process.

WHAT IS AN ETHICAL ORGANIZATION?

Creating an ethical organization requires some agreement on what it means to be such an organization. Some would argue that it is actually misleading to speak of an ethical *organization,* for such language suggests that the organization itself could be ethical apart from the individuals who constitute it. If we want an ethical organization, according to this argument, we should first make sure that the organization hires ethical people. Once employed, those individuals must step up to the moral challenge and fulfill the ethical responsibilities they have. In short, "individuals bear responsibility" for the ethical nature of their organizations; it will not do to claim that the *organization* can somehow "lead individuals to do good or evil" (Potter, 1996) or that the organization can be guilty of unethical behavior apart from identifiable individuals who lead it and staff it.

While this notion of the ethical organization has its merits, it is also one-sided. It seems to assume that an organization is—or should be—led and staffed by "moral heroes" who are strong enough to withstand any dubious influences of peer pressure and organizational climate. This view overlooks the fact that organizations consist of highly interdependent relationships in which not only individuals but groups (homemakers and case managers in home care, for example) influence each other in myriad ways (Herman, 1997).

Thus, while individuals have an indisputable moral responsibility in organizations, people also need their organization's moral support. Organizations can support individuals in doing good and right things—and they can hinder such behavior, discourage it, or even foster its opposite. Developing "mechanisms" (Schyve, 1996) to address ethical issues is critical to becoming a more "ethical" organization. These mechanisms can help to assure a consistency of behavior that transcends idiosyncratic differences, day-to-day inconsistencies, and even the weakness of character of individual practitioners.

To some, the test of an ethical organization is whether it establishes standards for the conduct of its affairs and for the conduct of the individuals it employs, then monitors "compliance" with those standards. In this understanding, the term "ethical" means "conforming to a set of rules or a code of conduct." Such conformity or compliance may be a necessary characteristic of an ethical organization, particularly in an era when the federal government has adopted the legal model of "corporate compliance" to combat fraud and abuse in many industries, including health care (Guinn, 2000; Boyle et al., 2001). Moreover, it is conceivable that states could adopt a similar model for the purpose of recouping allegedly misspent or ill-gotten state funds. But even if compliance is necessary, it is not a sufficient model for organizational ethics. By itself, it reflects a too-limited understanding of the terms "ethics" and "ethical."

In a broader view, an ethical organization is one that is also *continually reflective* about its moral responsibilities. Ethics in this broader sense involves a continual asking and learning about the issues that should be addressed, the values that should be considered, and the voices (internal and external) that should be heard and attended to (Tronto, 1993; McCurdy, 1997). It involves a recognition that, ethically speaking, we seldom (if ever) "get it" once and for all, that changing circumstances often require us to rethink our ethical approach, and that new issues have a way of taking us by surprise unless we are paying regular attention to the ethical landscape (Goodpaster, 1998).

Thus, above all, the ethical organization is one that is continually alert to and reflective about ethical questions, with an eye to establishing—where possible—standards or accepted ways of approaching issues, while also recognizing the provisional, perpetually reviewable nature of the standards and practices that it develops. Further, the ethical organization seeks over time to identify and address ethical issues in all the significant areas of its life and practice. Organizations in home care and community-based care will no doubt begin with issues that arise in their relationships with the elders who receive services and with the elders' families.

The organization that is serious about becoming more ethical will not limit its attention to such issues, however. Over time it will examine its relationships with other agencies, including vendors, prospective partners, and—especially in home care and adult day care— governmental agencies. Its ethics agenda may also include internal issues that can arise, such as the appropriate allocation of its resources and various aspects of staff relations and other human resource issues. Once existing issues are recognized and addressed, the organization may begin to focus on "preventive ethics" as it grows increasingly able to anticipate and address problems at early stages—or even before they arise (Forrow, Arnold, & Parker, 1993).

CREATING AN ETHICS-CENTERED GROUP

Although the organization and all its members share responsibility for ethical conduct in all the organization's relationships, the old saw, "If everybody's responsible, nobody's responsible," still applies. Somebody or, even better, some collective body needs to serve as a focal point and an initiating resource for ethical attention, reflection, and action in the organization. The ultimate organizational accountability for attention to ethical issues may rest with an individual, such as an administrator, and indeed it is vital that strong support for ethics come from the organization's top leadership (Hamel, 1997). But if ethics is to pervade the organization, it is also vital that a designated ethics-centered group, such as a committee or "forum" (Millspaugh, 1998), be established early on in the ethics improvement process.

The very process of forming an ethics group and publicizing its existence can serve a variety of purposes. If the group consists of representatives from all layers of the organization and from all disciplines or departments, the combination of vertical and horizontal representation signals that ethics is indeed for everyone, that all disciplines and levels among personnel are valued as potential contributors to the ethics process, and that their concerns will be taken seriously. Beyond the symbolism of such a message, inclusive representation increases the practical likelihood that people throughout the organization will hear about ethics, and about the ethics forum and its activities, from peers who are part of the group. From a long-range perspective, the creation of a body to consider ethics concerns lays the foundation for the growth over time of a genuine "moral community" of ethics-interested persons within the organization (Bioethics Consultation Group, 1992; Hamel, 1997). Such an inclusive process would fulfill an underlying premise of an ethics forum's very existence: involving multiple perspectives and voices, minds and hearts, in ethics concerns is better than having only one perspective (an ethics "czar"), or a small number of managerial perspectives (an elite), engaged in an ethics improvement process (McCurdy, 1993).

The ethics committee or forum (or perhaps, in the earliest stages, a smaller forerunner group) can serve a variety of functions. It may support ethical consciousness and decision-making in staff members' work with clients by providing educational resources, offering consultation to staff members who must make decisions in difficult cases, and developing policies and procedures to guide practice in recurring situations. The group's initial activities may receive helpful direction from a survey asking the organization's staff and leadership what ethical concerns or problems they see or simply—if the term "ethical" sounds ominous or seems to confine people's thinking unduly—what problems they find troubling or disturbing in their services to clients, in other aspects of their work, or in the organization's life generally. As a complement or alternative to a written survey, the group might also consider individual interviews, open meetings, or focus groups to identify and discuss ethical concerns.

On the basis of the information gathered by these means, the ethics group might proceed to draft a statement of its mission and purpose. Such a statement could serve not only to guide the ethics group's activities but also to inform the organization's leadership of the group's direction, elicit leaders' opinions, and engage them in the ethics effort. Early dissemination of the mission statement among staff members can serve both to alert staff to the group's existence and plans and to raise consciousness about the reality and importance of ethical concerns.

Also at this early stage, the ethics group might undertake a course of self-education in ethics and begin to plan and facilitate educational events for staff members, such as lunchtime ethics "brown-bags" (to discuss cases or particular ethical issues and concepts), inservices, and perhaps a half-day ethics seminar or conference (Hamel, 1997).

SITUATIONS AND CASES

Given a stated organizational commitment to becoming a more ethically aware and responsive organization, and the formation of a nascent ethics structure and process, what issues and situations might the organization and its newly established ethics forum choose to address? And how might the group and the organization address them? Here are a few possible examples.

Situation 1. A home care agency, CareMost, provides homemaking services to Mrs. Z, who is unable to walk. She has a grandson living with her to "take care of" her meals and other personal needs. A daughter (the grandson's mother) tends to Mrs. Z's finances. Mrs. Z has taken a liking to the homemaker. She talks freely to her about the inattentiveness of the grandson ("My house is just a place where he can stay for free") and her disagreement with her daughter's management of her money ("She wants to make sure there's plenty left for her after I'm gone").

Mrs. Z begins to do more than merely confide in the homemaker. She offers her gifts of jewelry and cash ("After all, I can't take it with me"). Citing agency policy, the homemaker declines the gifts. But she feels sorry for Mrs. Z, who obviously is lonely and derives little companionship or support from the inconsistent attentions of her family. She begins to visit Mrs. Z on her days off and occasionally on weekends. The daughter complains to the agency: "She's trying to steal my mother's affections. She's after her money. She's not a 'friend' and I don't want her in the house. I want the agency to send a different homemaker." The administrator who fielded the daughter's call brings the situation to the CareMost ethics forum.

It is most appropriate to bring cases like this one to an ethics group. Since the agency wants to support staff members in "doing the right thing," a mechanism that offers consultation and advice in particular cases is one means of such support. In this regard, the forum does well to make itself just as available to an alert administrator who recognizes an ethical problem as to line staff, such as the homemaker in this case, who might also have approached the committee. At the same time, attending to the particulars and subtleties of specific cases will help the forum to see the organization's "big picture" issues in a more nuanced way.

Several avenues of response to this situation are possible. The ethics forum might suggest a case management reassessment, with special attention to possible signs of abuse or neglect, while noting the legal obligation to report suspicious signs to the state's elder abuse agency. Such a response can be appropriate, but as a sole recommendation it might smack of retaliation against the family for daring to express displeasure with the homemaker. Such a recommendation would also beg the question of the agency's *ethical* responsibility, as distinct from its legal obligation (although the two may overlap). For example, what ethical obligations might exist alongside the legal duty to report possible abuse?

In any event, the group will need some ethical framework or perspective from which to assess the situation. As it begins its work, the ethics forum might formulate a list of values and virtues that it finds central to home care and to CareMost's mission. Candidates for such a list might include the following: *client self-determination, client safety and protection, client dignity and self-respect, compassion, professionalism, family integrity, caring attitudes and practices,* and *stewardship of agency resources.* The ethics forum will acknowledge that these values and virtues (and others that it might include in its distinctive list) are not always in harmony with each other, and that the organizational challenge in difficult situations is to find creative, acceptable ways to honor as many of them as possible.

In deliberating about the case of Mrs. Z, the forum may think not only about this case but about the wider ramifications for CareMost as an *organization* that aspires to grow ethically. This case, for example, is one manifestation of a wider range of concerns, often known as "boundary issues," in which the impulse or felt responsibility to provide care to someone perceived to be in need threatens to override the limits on one's action that other important values (such as client self-determination, family integrity, or professionalism) may suggest or require. Insofar as struggles with boundary issues are a common phenomenon among those who provide home care, the ethics forum might think about developing a policy or, perhaps better, guidelines for the management of various sorts of boundary situations in light of the organizational values it has identified. In addition, since the ethics forum's mission is not only to identify sound practices but to promote their actualization, it might suggest or sponsor a training session designed to identify the dynamics that draw or drive those in caregiving fields into boundary-issue conflicts, and to address those dynamics with reference both to psychological and social-scientific wisdom and to the values implicit in those conflicts.

> *Situation 2. A client has told a CareMost homemaker that she has been pushed, pinched, and sometimes hit about the chest and face by the son who cares for her (the son is never in the home when the homemaker is present). The client does not, however, want the homemaker to "tell the state" because she is dependent on her son and remains devoted to him. After some hesitation, the homemaker tells her supervisor. The supervisor informs the case manager designated by the agency to report suspected abuse to the state's Office of Elder Abuse.*
>
> *After about two weeks, the homemaker notices new bruises on the client's upper arms and neck. The homemaker reports these observations to her supervisor and asks what "Elder Abuse" has done after receiving the initial report. The supervisor answers that she does not know but "has to" believe that the state office has investigated the situation. She reminds the homemaker of the state office's "absolute confidentiality" policy regarding reported abuse. Since a reporting agency is never told whether or when the state investigator visits a home, both the homemaker and her supervisor wonder whether in fact "the state" has done anything or, if an investigation did take place, whether the investigator found anything and whether the client agreed to any protective measures. Moreover, the homemaker cannot know whether or when to be alert for some reaction from the son should he suspect her as the source of the report.*

The reporting case manager and the ethics forum might recognize this case as typifying a pattern that emerges when agency staff report elder abuse. The forum might, again, choose several avenues of response. On one hand, the group might interpret to all CareMost staff members the Elder Abuse policy that precludes "getting back to" those who report abuse and might reiterate the policy's ethical basis (probably respect for client "self-determination"). The forum might also summarize relevant regulations and laws (e.g., some states mandate reporting suspected abuse to criminal authorities, while others do not), suggest ways to support line staff who continue working in a home where they have reported abuse, or suggest joining with other agencies in asking the state office to review its confidentiality policy and perhaps ease some of its restrictions.

It is worth noting that advocacy in the bureaucratic and political arena is not necessarily off limits to a forum that seeks to enhance the ethical nature of its organization. Sometimes ethical conduct needs more external support than it currently is receiving; one task of an ethics group might be to call attention to that need, e.g., by bringing the issue and the need for advocacy to the attention of the agency's board (with the authorization and assistance of the administration). Moreover, if the options outlined here involve significant administrative or political dimensions, that fact does not preclude also seeing them as *ethical* interventions because they address an ethical problem. In such instances, perhaps an appropriate criterion for classifying a problem as "ethical" is whether "some of the arguments and some of the analyses are or would have been moral arguments, and thereby the ultimate decision that of an ethically responsible organization" (Goodpaster & Matthews, 1982).

> *Situation 3. CareMost has committed itself to providing services in neighborhoods and situations where other agencies normally decline to become involved—indeed, the organization prides itself on offering such services. However, both line staff and supervisors complain of the dilemmas this stance can create for them. Homemakers are sometimes asked to provide services in circumstances that can only be described as filthy, and long-time homemakers tell chilling "war stories" of occasions when cockroaches and other vermin have crawled over their purses, jackets, and other personal items. Supervisors feel guilty when they must send workers into situations that they themselves would avoid, and some add that it is doubly hard to "do this" to staff members who earn so little per hour for the privilege. (Agency policy that recognizes clients' "right" to choose their living conditions as part of their "self-determination" is, predictably, little consolation either to staff or to supervisors.) As a result, sometimes supervisors who are also case managers will actively look for reasons to deny services*

> to would-be clients whose dwellings would present an undesirable environment for line staff members. This problem has now been brought to the ethics forum's attention.

This situation is an example of the need for organizational attention not only to client and interagency issues but also to internal issues in the area of human resources, human relations, and what might be called "the [organization] as a just society" (Ewing, 1990). The fact that these distasteful duties are "given" to those who are paid the least and have little control over their assignments raises questions of fair and equitable treatment of staff members. Are there, for example, more equitable and creative ways to share the burdens of such unpleasant working conditions among staff members, possibly including the supervisors? Moreover, for those who ultimately "accept" (or even volunteer for) these assignments, is specific training in negotiating such situations provided? Can or should they receive bonus compensation, on the order of "hazardous duty pay"?

The fact that this problem arises repeatedly is, again, a reminder that the organizational issues extend beyond the treatment of particular people in particular cases. On one reading of the situation, the organizational challenge lies in figuring out how CareMost can honor its simultaneous commitments to clients and to staff members while retaining the priority of client service as the heart of its mission. However, this situation may present an opportunity to ask a prior question about the mission itself, or about the prevailing interpretation of the mission.

If resources to support client services in such distasteful circumstances are insufficient, or if meeting this commitment means questionably subjecting staff members to degrading conditions, is it time to reconsider the commitment? Is CareMost unwisely trying to be all things to all people? Must the organization accept clients whose living conditions so viscerally repel staff members (or even put them at physical risk)?

To some in the agency, such questions might be "unaskable." By raising the unaskable questions, however, the ethics forum would act consistently with a vision of organizational ethics as continual reflection on the organization's activities and commitments—even long-standing commitments that may have seemed beyond question. Such inquiry can do the organization a service by prodding it to peer more deeply into its sense of mission. Perhaps it is time for a change of perspective on what the mission requires, or should require. Alternatively, this reexamination might help CareMost affirm the existing interpretation of the mission, but to do so with a greater awareness of the real costs—financial, human, and indeed moral—that maintaining this commitment entails.

Situation 4. CareMost has been approached as a potential partner by a for-profit hospice. The hospice would like to outsource those aspects of its care and service that do not require specific training in health care, and has concluded that CareMost is the local agency best able to meet the need. The contract offered by the hospice appears generous, especially when its payment rates are compared with the fees the agency normally receives through its contracts with the state. Care-Most's board of directors is likely to approve the arrangement.

Some of the agency's managers are uneasy with the proposed partnership, however. They worry that working regularly with hospice clients will require a new level of training—and probably ongoing emotional support—for homemakers, case managers, and other staff members. There is also concern about the legal and ethical issues staff members would face if a client directed them not to call paramedics in the event the client took a turn for the worse or suffered a cardiac arrest.

Last, but not least, there is widespread unease in CareMost because the hospice is a publicly traded corporation with a reputation for aggressively soliciting clients to generate revenue for its bottom line. CareMost, on the other hand, is a not-for-profit agency with a solid reputation built on its commitment to serve its community. (That reputation, in fact, is no small factor in the hospice's choice of CareMost as a prospective partner.) Should CareMost enter into a significant partnership with "this sort of operation," as one manager puts it?

Not every partner, and not every partnership, is likely to be desirable when measured against an organization's mission and central values. On the other hand, the pot of gold at the end of the rainbow can be enticing for an agency that normally must struggle to make ends meet. Moreover, "not-for-profit" status does not mean that an agency must be *against* any legitimate "profit" or surplus that would help it fulfill its mission. In its initial self-education process, the ethics forum will have been wise to study and discuss financial issues as one aspect of organizational ethics, and to recognize that "making money" is one legitimate value under the overarching umbrella somewhat euphemistically labelled "stewardship of agency resources."

But the forum is now faced with a more specific question involving financial considerations: Should CareMost enter into *this* partnership arrangement, however lucrative it promises to be? The questions about the impact on agency operations and on staff members of caring for "dying" patients are worth pondering. Are staff members adequately trained and prepared to care for this new clientele? If providing home care to hospice patients truly means a significant change in practice, or in the emotional impact of client relationships, the agency must assess carefully whether it is (or can become) prepared to take on this new burden. Moreover, for its part, is the hospice prepared to help with such training and support issues if called upon to do so?

On the other hand, the ethics forum might ask just how "different" caring for hospice clients would actually be. Many of CareMost's existing clients are likely to be elders whose current life expectancy is not long, and some may in fact, or could, be hospice patients. These clients have already experienced a substantial deterioration in their health; otherwise, they would not be receiving home care. (It is quite possible that some agency workers have already been faced with client requests not to call 911 if a medical crisis arises.) The forum might help managers raising the hospice question to think through their own images of hospice patients and their care. Perhaps thinking of prospective hospice clients as more like than unlike clients they know, e.g., as persons seeking to make the most of their lives in limiting circumstances, is a helpful way of reframing this concern.

The perception that the hospice is (or is known as) an avaricious and marginally ethical "operation" deserves both sympathetic and critical consideration. Such perceptions of "outside" organizations often surface when partnerships or (especially) mergers are proposed. Often they carry a measure of truth; in any case, they must be taken seriously. They can, however, also signal anxiety about significant change, and a not uncommon tendency to "demonize" the unknown organizational other. In this case, the widespread apprehensions may also reflect a bias against a stereotypical "for-profit" mentality that is attributed to the hospice.

The ethics forum might suggest a careful, objective review of the hospice's publicly observable financial and marketing practices, and perhaps a spot-check of the hospice's reputation in the eyes of external observers whose judgment is considered reliable. The question of reputation is both important and inherently difficult to assess. At the least, the ethics forum should recognize that CareMost's reputation is part of its moral capital in its community and is itself a resource requiring stewardship. The agency's choice of partners inevitably affects that moral resource. There are legitimate questions about whether, and how, the hospice plans to capitalize on CareMost's stellar reputation. Might it, for example, tout its affiliation with CareMost in its advertising?

But suppose that thorough investigation demonstrates that the hospice's negative reputation is essentially unfounded, i.e., that its business and marketing practices raise no significant questions. As an organization that desires to be ethical in its own partnership decisions, CareMost must decide whether it will take the relative risk of affiliating with an agency that it believes to be ethical when some in the community believe otherwise. If the partnership possibility has become public knowledge, and if CareMost chooses not to affiliate on the basis of reputation rather than substance, the agency might contribute to the hospice's unfairly attributed reputation, and thus add, however unintentionally, to the injustice. Even so, if CareMost perceives that the reputational risk of affiliating with the hospice is simply inordinate, it is not obligated to jeopardize its own well-being by pursuing the partnership. As a matter of compensatory justice, it might nonetheless seek a way to signal publicly that rejection of the partnership offer does not reflect an unfavorable judgment about the character of the hospice.

Such organizational issues as the choice of partners and partnerships may not come before every home care or adult day care agency's ethics group. If and when such situations do arise, however, an organization and its ethics forum are wise to recall that these business questions are simultaneously ethical questions whenever the analysis of the issues involved includes moral judgments. The challenge is to make those judgments, and the analysis and reasoning behind them, explicit; meeting that challenge is one task of organizational ethics and of an organization's ethics mechanism, however it is constituted.

BAD NEWS AND GOOD NEWS

Those who earnestly desire to increase ethical consciousness and conduct in their organization will inevitably encounter frustrations in pursuing this aim. The "bad news" for those who have a sense of moral urgency is that creating an ethical organization takes time. Acknowledging this reality may, however, be "good news" in disguise if it eases an unrealistic pressure to "do it all now." Conducting ethical "benchmarking" with comparable organizations will likely confirm that every organization desiring to be more ethical has its growing pains; this knowledge may be a source of reassurance and comfort to those who wish that more would happen more quickly in their own organization. This acknowledgement should not, however, lessen the laudable moral zeal that drives the ethics improvement process; rather, it counsels the virtue of patience as a needed ingredient of any improvement effort that is "in it" for the long haul. The moral challenge here is that of blending firmness and flexibility, of firmly adhering to high expectations (Herman, 1997) while flexibly adjusting time frames and accepting the inconsistencies that plague any improvement process.

Further, it may enhance the morale of everyone involved in the organization's ethics improvement process if the administrative leadership and the ethics group recognize and publicly acknowledge that in important, identifiable respects the organization already *is* ethical. For one thing, any home care or adult day care agency is likely to be composed of leaders and staff members who already act ethically in the vast majority of their activities. This supposition is especially probable in an organization whose mission is to provide vulnerable people with services that they truly need, and whose staff members could often earn more money in other employment. Generally speaking, those who provide home care and adult day care not only want to be ethical in their practice but are motivated by a strong desire to care for persons and meet human need. Indeed, many caregivers connect this desire and motivation with their sense of religious calling (McCurdy, 1997). Staff members' motivations to care and to do the right thing should thus be recognized, celebrated, and enlisted in the organization's ethics efforts (Paine, 1994).

It should also be recognized that the ethics task is not solely, or even primarily, to help line staff, supervisors, and administrators deal with "hard cases" or moral dilemmas (Beauchamp & Childress, 2001) that confront them with difficult choices. The general ethical climate in the organization (its "moral ecology"), the day-to-day attitudes and actions of staff members in "routine" situations, and the characteristic ways in which the organization views and treats employees (perhaps especially those who are paid the least) all deserve significant ethical attention by organizational leadership and the designated ethics group. The responsible parties should identify and plan to address these ongoing concerns even as they recognize the need to help those who seek ethical counsel in the heat of pressing situations (Holstein, 1998).

Those—both organizations and individuals—who seek to provide home care and related services to elders are not only responding to a perceived need; they are also accepting a social responsibility. Perhaps unfairly, this is true even though all too often community-based care is underfunded and those who offer it receive far too little recognition for the genuine, indeed indispensable, service they provide. It is this very indispensability that, in our current societal climate, underscores organizations' social responsibility: "Those who undertake to perform critical social functions must accept stringent social obligations. If they have the means, they must use them; if they do not have the means, they must demand them" (Donabedian, 1986, p. 3). The ethical organization will both recognize the inescapability of its social responsibility and seek to flesh out the meaning and scope of that responsibility. As Donabedian implies, the obligation to use society's resources to meet society's needs, whether fully acknowledged or not, may well require political advocacy and public consciousness-raising efforts by those who must have the resources if they are to meet the needs. In the end, the ethical organization must be a socially and politically aware and active organization as well.

REFERENCES

Beauchamp, T. L., & Childress, J. F. (2001). *Principles of biomedical ethics* (5th ed.). New York: Oxford University Press.

Bioethics Consultation Group. (1992). *Forming a moral community: A resource for health care ethics committees.* Berkeley, CA: Author.

Boyle, P. J., DuBose, E. R., Ellingson, S. J., Guinn, D. E., & McCurdy, D. B. (2001). *Organizational ethics in health care: Principles, cases, and practical solutions.* San Francisco: Jossey-Bass.

Donabedian, A. (1986). Quality assurance: Corporate responsibility for multihospital systems. *Quality Review Bulletin, 12*(1), 3–7.

Ewing, D. W. (1990). The corporation as a just society. *Business Ethics,* (March-April), 20–23.

Forrow, L., Arnold, R. M., & Parker, L. S. (1993). Preventive ethics: Expanding the horizons of clinical ethics. *Journal of Clinical Ethics, 4*(4), 287–294.

Goodpaster, K. E. (1998). *Conscience and its counterfeits in organizational life.* Public lecture given at DePaul University, Chicago, IL., October 28.

Goodpaster, K. E., & Matthews, J. B., Jr. (1982). Can a corporation have a conscience? *Harvard Business Review, 60*(1), 132–141.

Guinn, D. E. (2000). Corporate compliance and integrity programs: The uneasy alliance between law and ethics. *HEC Forum, 12*(4), 292–302.

Hamel, R. (1997). A question of value. *Health Progress, 78*(3), 24–26, 32.

Herman, S. (1997). *Durable goods: A covenantal ethic for management and employees.* Notre Dame, IN: University of Notre Dame Press.

Holstein, M. (1998). Ethics and Alzheimer's disease: Widening the lens. *Journal of Clinical Ethics, 9*(1), 13–22.

McCurdy, D. B. (1993). Should expertise in bioethics be required for serving on a [sic] HEC? NO. *HEC Forum, 5*(6), 371–373.

McCurdy, D. B. (1997). Appreciating staff members as moral stakeholders. *Ethical Currents,* (48), 9–10.

Millspaugh, D. (1998). From anonymity to respect: Lessons in the establishment of a bioethics forum. In S. F. Spicker (Ed.), *The health care ethics experience: Selected readings from HEC forum.* Malabar, FL: Krieger Publishing.

O'Reilly, C. (1989). Corporations, culture, and commitment: Motivation and social control in organizations. *California Management Review, 31*(4), 9–25.

Paine, L. S. (1994). Managing for organizational integrity. *Harvard Business Review, 72*(2), 106–117.

Potter, V. R. (1996). Individuals bear responsibility. *Bioethics Forum, 12*(2), 27–28.

Schein, E. H. (1992). *Organizational culture and leadership* (2nd ed.). San Francisco: Jossey-Bass.

Schyve, P. M. (1996). Patient rights and organization ethics: The joint commission perspective. *Bioethics Forum, 12*(2), 13–20.

Tronto, J. (1993). *Moral boundaries: A political argument for an ethic of care.* New York: Routledge.

CHAPTER 8

Organizational Ethics in a Nonprofit Agency: Changing Practice, Enduring Values

Phyllis Mitzen

Can a nonprofit, community-service organization become more focused on the "bottom line" and still remain true to its ethical values? In 1997, staff of the Council for Jewish Elderly (CJE) in Chicago met to express concerns about the lack of an approach to integrate the agency's values into all organizational practices. Prompted by significant change over the past several years in the way CJE operates, the staff had two main ethics-related concerns: first, that CJE not lose sight of our mission as we change and, second, that as we establish new services and business practices, they embody the values of the organization.

The Council for Jewish Elderly in Chicago provides services to 20,000 older people and their families yearly in the northern metropolitan Chicago area. We serve many needs (related to transportation, independent housing, assisted living, home health, adult day care, in-home services, mental health services, and nursing home care) with a substantial budget from a number of funding sources (private fees, Medicare, Medicaid and Title III, foundation grants, private donors, the Jewish Federation, and others). We are accountable not only to the consumer of our services, the older person, but also to our funding sources, to our board of directors, and especially since we are a sectarian organization, to our community.

In recent years, we have undergone major organizational change as we respond to the marketplace. We have relied on the quality expert Edwards Demming's concepts of continuous quality improvement, process thinking, strategic planning, and market-driven programs as we shift from a social welfare model to a more market-driven model. A philosophy that focuses on the "bottom line" has been introduced, to coexist with our long-standing commitment to provide quality services, as we anticipate a growing need for services to the aging and in order to position ourselves to provide more services to more people.

CJE has had an ethics program since 1984. Two ethics committees were established, one dealing with nursing home issues and one dealing with community issues. Within a couple of years, the committees developed ethics guidelines for community-based practice and for the long-term-care facility. These guidelines are now used to orient new clinical staff and as a guide for practice and for the work of the ethics committees.

The CJE ethics program has been providing a number of services, including ethics training for our practitioners and occasional seminars on selected topics for clients, families, and other staff. In the community, where the clinicians seldom have "ethics emergencies," we created monthly ethics brown bag lunches to discuss cases. Over lunch, an ethicist joins our home care staff to discuss topics that could range from a moral conflict about their role in a case to questions about distribution of resources when at-risk clients refuse services to, most common, questions about a client's self-determination when the person's judgment is perceived to be impaired. These clinically focused mechanisms have served the needs of the agency and the professional to work out the often complex issues that arise in day-to-day service delivery to older people.

The recent changes in the CJE operations have been of real concern to the clinical practitioners. And, because of their sensitivity to ethical issues, they have framed some of their concerns in ethical terms, expressing worries about creation of a "two-tiered system" and "not throwing the baby out with the bath water." At a particularly heated ethics brown bag last year, one social worker raised her concern about an ad CJE was running in local papers for our new assisted living program. The ad cleverly made reference to forgetfulness in a way that could be taken in more than one way. The clinicians harshly challenged CJE's commitment to organizational values, stating that their colleagues outside of CJE expressed surprise at what could be interpreted as CJE's insensitivity and use of stereotypes. CJE's marketing staff responded that the ad was targeted to families and that it had generated many inquiries about the facility, fulfilling the purpose of the ad, which was to generate new clients for CJE, part of the organization's strategic plan. (Because the ad had fulfilled its purpose, it was discontinued.) This kind of issue, only a small matter, served to show that our values were being challenged in unforeseen ways, and it became clear that we needed to think of organizational ethics differently.

A team was assembled with the responsibility to plan an organizational ethics strategy for CJE. The team consisted of the two chairs of the agency's ethics committees, an assistant to the executive director, and another agency executive. Also serving were the ethicists from both committees and the ethicist from a nearby hospital that had gone through a similar process. The team started by making a distinction between the needs served by CJE's already existing clinical ethics program and CJE's need for attention to organizational ethics. The team agreed that the mechanisms CJE has in place are not sufficient to address the problems that lie ahead.

The process started with the group defining *values* and *ethics*, words that were confusing when we tried to discuss an organizational ethics program. These are the definitions we agreed to:

Values refers to strong and enduring beliefs that motivate and define behavior. Values inform the choices we make. They are a statement of what is "good" for individuals and for society. Between groups, values are often in conflict, which necessitates ethics discussions. Values constitute the practical pieces of our work—what we believe in, what is important in our work.

Ethics refers to a fleshing out and carrying out of our values. Ethics is the practice of values and the critique and assessment of values. An ethical dilemma is a clash of values or responsibilities or rights.

Several years ago CJE developed a core values statement that embodies our mission and values. This statement is included in all of the agency's official communication and is well known in the agency and throughout much of the community. The ethics team identified all the values expressed by this statement and were surprised to find that there is inherent potential for conflict within the statement itself. In other words, at our very core, there is the potential for ethical dilemmas, even when we do everything right. For example, the core value statement calls for "commitment to Jewish communal values" and "delivering quality programs and services for all older people and their families." The basis of conflicts arising from these two statements could be in the ways the board, the community, governmental bodies, and clinical workers interpret them. For example, if we serve everyone, what happens if an African-American client interprets "quality programs and services" to mean services available on Saturday when, because of our Jewish orientation, we cannot provide them? What happens if by attempting to serve all older people, we begin to serve fewer Jewish people?

We speculated that there are three major areas in which ethical problems could arise and where the enhancement of organizational ethics mechanisms would benefit CJE: in our business practices, with our employees, and in our relationships with the larger community.

As our business focus changes from a social welfare to a market-driven service-delivery system, there will be casualties. Some services that have been provided for many years and are perceived by many people as being important may be dropped or significantly modified. Long-standing relationships with other providers may change or end. CJE may be inviting relationships with new partners that include for-profit businesses and certainly with health care providers. CJE has a care ethic and is highly regarded in the community for that reason. We do not want to lose this quality and respect as the changes are being decided.

Ethical behavior of an organization begins with ethical behavior toward its own employees, which means communication and a supportive environment that supports even whistle blowing, with all its potential for conflict. Ethical behavior requires us to clearly articulate our values and how they are put into operation. We must be accountable for our commitments to our clients and to our employees.

In addition, influences from outside the organization will have great impact on our development of organizational ethics. The Joint Commission on Accreditation of Healthcare Organizations requires "business ethics mechanisms" for nursing home and home-health accreditation. We have a nursing home and have opened a home-health agency, both of which are subject to these provisions. In addition, in the future and as our organizational ethics program advances, we foresee the possibility of identifying and seeking to influence policy and legislation that may raise ethical questions and have unanticipated consequences for our clients and for the agency.

By initiating an organizational ethics mechanism, we want to enhance our clinical ethics program by educating people about ethics-related issues and look for ways to integrate this work into the existing organizational structure.

CHAPTER 9

Ethics in Clinical Practice With Older Adults: Recognizing Biases and Respecting Boundaries

Robyn L. Golden and Sallie Sonneborn

An elderly man wandered throughout the neighborhood, his clothes disheveled and usually out of season. He wore a heavy worn-out winter coat, knit hat, and scarf in the summer and went gloveless in the winter. The neighborhood merchants all knew him; they saw him wandering into the heavily-trafficked street, and when he went to their stores begging for money they often gave him a cup of coffee and some cookies.

The local social service agency for older adults received numerous phone calls from neighborhood residents and merchants who were concerned about this congenial man who was at risk of being beaten by local thugs, hit by a car, dying of hypo- or hyperthermia, or some other tragedy. They assumed the man was alone, had no family to care for him and was living off his meager social security income that was not enough to pay the monthly bills. The social service agency, of course, was concerned, and staff went into the street to find the old man. He immediately charmed the workers who learned he had three grown, professionally successful children, all of whom lived within 10 miles of his home. The elderly man said his children did not care about him; none of them ever called or visited. The workers were infuriated at his children for their neglect and lack of concern. How could they ignore the needs of this charming elderly man who obviously needed their help?

The agency made a home visit and was further incensed by the deplorable condition of the home, which the old man said he owned free and clear. The agency sent services to him: home-delivered meals, housekeeping, and case management. Feeling badly for him with Thanksgiving arriving at the end of the week, and believing that his family would not pay any attention to him, the worker decided to take him to and from a community dinner.

The case manager understood that she needed to talk with the man's family, and he finally gave permission to speak with the children. During these conversations, the worker learned that this "sweet and destitute gentleman" had been a violent and abusive father to his children when they were young and in their teen years. He had several hundred thousand dollars in the bank, and a like amount invested in the stock market. His children, all separately, spoke of him as being selfish, spiteful, and evil-hearted. The worker began to question her preconceptions and think differently about her interventions. She felt frustration at the realization that his dress, demeanor, and charm had deceived her.

"A boundary . . . is not the figurative line in the sand or any other kind of apparent demarcation, but a metaphor for the rules and limits—if not the unspoken rituals—that are supposed to govern the worker-client relations" (Goldstein, 1999).

INTRODUCTION

The literature on ethics in social work, case management, nursing, and other helping professions has largely focused on decision-making, rather than on the decision maker (Abramson, 1996). Most literature addressing ethical issues in work with the elderly focuses on client-driven situations. This chapter examines the question of ethics from the perspective of the worker. It explores a process by which practitioners—the decision makers—can evaluate their own perceptions and actions in relation to their elderly clients within a self-directed ethical framework. This process will increase their awareness and consequently improve their practice.

We argue that practitioners who skillfully identify and work through ethical dilemmas while comfortably and consistently exploring their own personal prejudices and biases will practice more effectively than those who do not. Powerful conscious and unconscious motivations, bias, and countertransference can influence how clinicians perceive and/or address ethical dilemmas; for these reasons they should be major areas of concern to clinicians working with older adults. Experience suggests that three common myths or misconceptions often hinder a practitioner's effective work with the elderly. By contributing to a faulty view of what is happening, these views subtly influence moral judgment and clinical practice. One perception is that older adults are helpless, rejected by family and society, and thus must be "rescued," perhaps the misconception under which our case manager labored in relation to our elderly gentleman. Another misperception is the conviction that because old age is "merely" a time of decline and loss, we should not bother with the elderly. A third misconception is that the elderly cannot significantly change because they are rigid and incapable of making adaptations. Beliefs in stereotypes and the ageism that often results may lead even a professionally educated clinician to be either unnecessarily resistant or unusually motivated to do something different from what is his or her "normal" practice.

In their research, Levkoff et al. (1994) found that health care providers who assess the needs of the elderly often make decisions based on their own preferences, attitudes, beliefs and other external factors of which they may be unaware. These preferences and inclinations may result in biases. All people have biases, many of which are not conscious. These unconscious processes can prejudice how the clinician determines the mode of practice with older clients; they can also blur the acceptable boundaries set forth in professionals' respective codes of ethics and standards of practice. Biases can also impede a central feature of moral practice—attentiveness to the particular needs of *this* client in *this* particular context. For these reasons, if practitioners are to make conscious decisions about their actions, awareness of their own biases and their origins is essential. We should be cautious not to automatically identify our biases as "bad" or "wrong," since doing so would tempt us to cover them up rather than consider how they may be influencing our practice.

Recognizing personal biases and respecting professional boundaries are closely intertwined. A boundary violation occurs when the practitioner's actions—shaped by his or her unexamined biases—are not checked by the rules of professional conduct. In our case example, the worker was troubled enough to think about how her own personal biases may have affected or motivated her decisions. If she had initially been more cognizant of her preconceptions, would she have developed a different care plan for this man? If she had asked the client about his plans for Thanksgiving, or how *he* felt about his children not attending to him, how might his answers have led to different decisions on her part? Even without the information she subsequently learned about his relationship with his children, she made plans for him for Thanksgiving without exploring how he felt about it or what it meant to him.

Recent efforts to explore the ethics of working with the elderly have paid little attention to the development of the clinician's knowledge of his or her own values. Values shape moral perceptions and judgments which, in turn, influence treatment of the client. Clinicians working with the elderly must be encouraged to explore their views about old age, aging, and the elderly, what they fear most about aging, what they look forward to in their own older years, and the rules and beliefs they have learned about aging and the elderly from their own families.

Countertransference and blurred boundaries are among the most important consequences of unexplored personal biases. Countertransference refers to conscious or unconscious phenomenon involving feelings that occur when the clinician reacts to a client based in large part on the clinician's own past experiences, preferences, preconceptions, fantasies, and fears. Very simply put, countertransference is the powerful linkage between helpers' personal feelings and their interventions and behaviors (Genevay & Katz, 1990). While Freud (1912) defined countertransference as "an unconscious process involving the arousal of the analysts' unresolved conflicts and problems which had to be eliminated in order to function effectively," the countertransference process is now regarded as an appropriate, natural emotional response. It may be conscious or unconscious, and, if it is understood, it can be an important therapeutic tool, serving as the basis for empathy and deeper understanding. Left unchecked, in contrast, countertransference may result in a professional's tendency to "over help" or "under help" based on his or her feelings, rather than on the client's situation and needs. Unchecked countertransference can lead the practitioner to unwittingly overstep a professional boundary. Boundaries are the often thin lines between what is therapeutically helpful and what is not. Generally, a professional relationship with a client remains, on the practitioner's part, professional. The clinician tries to keep the content of his visit with the client to the point and within the realms of acceptable practice. If a young practitioner unwittingly identifies elderly men with her grandfather, she may get off subject or assume the role of a granddaughter. Perhaps the worker in our case scenario identified the older man on the street with her grandfather, and rushed to help him prior to gathering the facts of the case.

Genevay and Katz (1990) identify frequently reported countertransference issues that occur in work with older adults. They include: denial, fear of growing older and being helpless, fear of dying, the unknown and contagion ("death is catching"), anger, need for control and professional omnipotence, and the need to be needed. When clinicians identify countertransference issues, we may respond to them appropriately. In doing so we can recognize elderly clients as individuals and avoid pitfalls such as overcompensation, paternalism, premature termination of the therapeutic relationship, the false need to "make everything better," and acting as if the client has no one else in his social/familial network upon whom to rely. These reactions can affect whether or not we ever engage with older adults, force unnecessary services on them, or over-address their underlying problems. Both overly positive and overly negative attitudes about the elderly can affect the intervention.

ETHICAL SELF-ASSESSMENTS

The American Heritage Dictionary (2000) defines ethics as "set principles of right conduct; the study of the general nature of morals and of specific moral choices." Since most aspects of work in the helping professions have ethical implications, it is important for all clinicians to develop a personal code of ethics. Personal ethics are our individual rules of conduct: They tell us what we believe is right and what is wrong. Our behaviors stem from the values we hold. The practitioner's personal rules of conduct will often decide the nature and quantity of care he or she provides. If we value independence, then we are more likely to do things *with* a client rather than *for* a client. If we value privacy, we are more likely to keep quiet about our client's personal business. In times of stress when we must make a judgment call, we act on our individual, frequently unspoken, and internalized values. But values alone cannot govern what we do in relationship to others. Reliance on personal ethics can be problematic if the client and others in the caregiving picture are not involved in thinking together about care.

Professional, organizational, and societal ethics also affect our behaviors and may conflict with our personal rules. The practitioner must be mindful of these other ethical stances, balancing them with their personal ethics and, as we shall discuss below, bring them into the open through conversation or more formal ethics mechanisms.

Abramson (1996) suggests a process of self-assessment to increase the clinician's moral self-awareness and, therefore, permit her or him to respond more empathically to clients' values and to ethical issues. Abramson's suggested framework for self-assessment consists of guidelines in eight areas:

Prejudgments—Challenge your understanding of your own world before deciding what to believe.

Character and Virtue—Know what makes you feel good about yourself. What do you love and from what do you gain personal satisfaction?

Principles—Ascertain how you use and prioritize your own ethical principles, such as autonomy, beneficence, nonmaleficence, justice.

Ethical Theories—Be aware of and recognize your own patterns of thinking in relation to the two most commonly discussed ethical theories: utilitarian or consequentialist ethics and deontological ethics. The former suggests that actions are right or wrong according to their outcomes; the latter holds that certain acts are intrinsically good or bad in themselves, irrespective of their consequences (Beauchamp & Childress, 1989).

Free Will and Determinism—Ask yourself whether you believe problems are within or outside the individual's own control.

Spirituality—Identify the ultimate concerns about identity, destiny, purpose and meaning that give force to your life.

Individual and Community—Examine your ideas about individual rights versus the good of the community (social responsibility).

Voice—Examine how you tend to approach moral problems. Is your approach from the perspective of rights, privacy, and noninterference, emphasizing individuation, separation, and autonomy, or from the perspective of relationships and connection, emphasizing intimacy and a view of the self as connected with others?

This self-assessment process should help practitioners become more conscious of the values, beliefs, and feelings that may underlie their decision-making and interventions. Then, when a decision must be made, the clinician will be more open to weighing the evidence that is there rather than defending her own position. Based on this assessment, practitioners learn to perceive moral problems from different perspectives, facilitating their ability to engage with the client and the clients' families. Others, for example, may think differently than the practitioner about privacy. Unless practitioners are aware, from the start, that such differences are possible, indeed probable, then they may not even think to ask certain questions. This self-knowledge can help practitioners make intervention decisions that are harmonious with the client's definition of the problem. In this way, it increases the chances of successfully engaging the client in a plan of action that best meets the client's needs.

Beyond these fundamental features of self-consciously and attentively caring for clients, practitioners also face specific ethical dilemmas that often arise when there are two or more conflicting values that demand self-awareness of biases and prejudices. Safety versus independence is one such key ethical conflict. For example, clinicians working with older people want to assure that clients remain both as safe and as independent as possible. A situation wherein a client lives alone in a neighborhood that the clinician feels is unsafe and therefore potentially dangerous to the client's well-being raises this question for the clinician: What role should he or she play in encouraging the client to move, even though the client has expressed satisfaction with his present living arrangements? Such an ethical dilemma can become even more complicated if the clinician is unaware of how his own personal values and biases may influence his thinking, and hence his decision-making process. The clinician, in trying to act self-consciously, must explore how fears of aging subtly prejudice how he thinks about safety and independence. Even more specifically, such self-understanding may lead to an awareness that neither safety nor independence are fully available to any of us and that some compromise is part of daily living.

We make value judgments and other kinds of judgments, for example, about how we think people should behave and what we think the outcomes of service for a client ought to be. One such value holds social activity to be desirable for all older adults. This value can lead a worker to be concerned about a situation that does not concern the client. If an older person has few social contacts, family members and the clinician may want to involve her in a program that includes socialization so she may make new acquaintances. The reality may be that she enjoys her time at home and feels quite satisfied.

Another set of conflicting value judgments occurs when the obligation to protect the client's welfare conflicts with the duty to protect his or her right to self-determination. While the National Association of Social Workers (NASW; 1996) supports the obligation to enhance clients' capacities and opportunities to address their own needs, the clinician's duty to protect the older person's safety, health and welfare may often conflict with this other obligation. For example, what happens to the right to self-determination when the clinician is confronted with an elderly client who is judgmentally impaired? What is the proper balance between a client's right to engage in self-destructive behavior and a practitioner's obligation to prevent it? How do we balance the rights of the community and the rights of the individual in forcing services and interventions? Do we view autonomy as appropriate only when clients are competent enough to exercise it? Is it ever acceptable to pass along seemingly inconsequential information to a concerned family member without the older adult's permission before competency or risk has been assessed?

Control, autonomy, and dependency continue to be core issues of late life, and as a result, conflicts related to the relative merits between dependence and independence often occur in professional relationships with older adults. According to Galambos (1997), autonomy has three specific components: autonomy of the person (acting according to a person's own choices without interference or restriction); autonomy of actions and choices (giving consent, raising objections, refusing to make choices); and respect for autonomy (recognizing an individual's capabilities, desires, and wishes). Clinicians who are supportive and respectful of autonomy enable people to think independently, make their own judgments, and pursue self-developed goals within the limits of their physical and mental capacities.

Some ethical problems may be rooted in an older person's judgment that needs and vulnerabilities are weaknesses. As a result, some older people are reluctant to engage in a therapeutic relationship because they fear it may exacerbate their sense of helplessness, they fear a loss of independence and dignity, or they may view the helping professional as an intruder. Increased dependency may lead to feelings of shame and, in turn, a resistance to intervention as a method to preserve a sense of self. Older adults represent a unique group of clients who may not ask for help directly, but who are persuaded, even coerced, into getting help by a well-meaning family member. Engaging such older people often requires a willingness to be flexible in one's professional role, that is, making a reasoned, planful decision to cross a boundary that in another situation might be considered a boundary violation.

UNIQUE ASPECTS OF CLINICAL WORK WITH OLDER ADULTS

As professionals, we must be willing to relinquish our own agenda and begin the therapeutic relationship on the client's terms. For example, when an elderly client with declining capabilities and increased need resents the need for professional intervention, it may be appropriate for the clinician to help with tasks of the client's choice (e.g., paying bills, balancing a bank book, filling out forms, shopping, cooking), rather than delving headfirst into issues of medical or emotional health and well-being. This may be a successful way to support the client's autonomy and need for independence while setting the tone for more therapeutic activities in the future. While "starting where the client is" is a hallmark of good practice, it is often tempting to jump-start the process when the practitioner identifies more serious problems. We must guard against this tendency. The professional's internal self may affect his or her ability to empathize with a reluctant client. If his or her values lead to compassion and understanding of what the client is experiencing, it will be possible to help the client without interfering with his or her sense of self-respect.

A FRAMEWORK FOR ETHICAL-CLINICAL ANALYSIS

When we experience a problem working with a specific client, it is often difficult to distinguish whether the issue at hand is one of ethics or of practice. That is, when a question arises about a given assessment, intervention or goal, it is not always clear where the locus of the conflict resides. Is it an ethical issue, a practice difficulty, or an interaction of the two? Often, in fact, there is an overlap between ethics and practice. Sometimes the problem is misinterpreted as an ethical conflict when in reality the practitioner has been unable to understand the underlying dynamics of the client's situation and has not attended to the clinical issues. This inability to deal with the clinical dynamics of the therapeutic relationship is sometimes related to not recognizing countertransference and biases. When a clinician is very attached to a client, he may neglect to notice the client's functional problems and limitations that could be due to memory loss. Mutual admiration between the client and practitioner may not allow for, or may cover up, the client's and practitioner's genuine feelings.

An ethical dilemma is a specific situation involving competing values. These conflicts may be between or among personal, professional, or societal values. If an ethical conflict causes the problem, the practitioner should try to identify the two or more competing values and determine how to resolve the conflict. If competing values cannot be identified, the practitioner needs to reexamine clinical issues. When there are questions about boundaries and limits, the practitioner's unrecognized feelings and beliefs are often the root cause and need attention.

Once a practitioner identifies an ethical dilemma, she faces the task of resolving it, if possible. Sometimes ethical conflicts cannot be resolved, but they can be mitigated so that all parties achieve relative comfort. Frequently the worker feels uncomfortable acknowledging conflicting values, particularly when the conflict is between personal values and those held by the client, agency, or profession. This reluctance is often due to shame or embarrassment or to a belief in the superiority of one's own values. At other times, the clinician may not acknowledge the legitimacy of these conflicts. In all of these cases, good clinical practice requires both recognizing the conflict and exploring the issue. When professionals are reluctant to engage in this examination and to discuss ethical matters as they arise in work, the integrity of their work is questionable and the client's best interests may be discounted.

Such ethical clashes may cause reactions or feelings on the practitioner's part. The clinician needs to consider the ethical problem based on criteria other than her own personal values. The clinician must remember that people have a right to make choices, even if in her view they're the "wrong" choices, and also must recognize that sometimes a client has no good choices. When a client is competent, the clinician must try to respect his or her autonomy and address the problems or behaviors directly. It is more difficult when the clinician's standards suggest the older person is unable to make autonomous decisions. How can the clinician be sure that he or she is correctly assessing the older person's competence? If a client wants to live in a roach-infested house with a drug-dealing grandson, does that mean that the client is exercising poor judgment and should be moved against her will? Since the client is living in a harmful and dangerous situation according to the clinician's standards, when should the clinician supersede a client's right to self-determination? What about concern for others who must enter the home? In these situations, practice and ethics blur. Usually our values tell us to intervene in order to protect, maybe even to an extent that otherwise would be considered outside our preconceived boundaries and role. Only when the practitioner acknowledges value clashes and identifies a process to examine them can she be more certain that the emotion that tells her to intervene against the client's wishes is coming from a place of consciously evaluated and chosen personal and professional values, and not from unexplored biases or countertransference.

ETHICS IN PRACTICE IN CLINICAL SETTINGS

We often struggle between what we feel is best for the client (e.g., nursing home care for a very frail and dependent individual) and the client's strong wish to maintain her dignity by remaining in her own home with assistance. When our own codes of ethics and good standards of practice are operating, and when we are aware of our biases and countertransference, we are more apt to make decisions based on rational facts rather than pure emotion. For example, a practitioner who is simply striving for client safety may advocate for premature institutionalization rather than explore the variety of in-home services and housing alternatives that may allow the client to remain in the community. The clinician is obligated to ask whether the plan is the least restrictive, least humiliating and least demeaning intervention that can be designed for the client while at the same time minimizing risk for the client or the practitioner. A benchmark in evaluating the plan of action is whether the intervention is just, appropriate, and respectful.

Practitioners cannot resolve these ethical and clinical issues in isolation. Organizations need to create learning and supervisory processes that allow them to explore feelings of uncertainty and professional vulnerability. Perhaps the educator/supervisor's greatest challenge is to train clinicians in the area of ethics. It is important for practitioners to feel free to identify "red flags" that indicate a need to think hard about a reaction to an issue, a gut feeling, countertransference, or bias. It is also helpful for clinicians to seek consultation with a supervisor or colleague when they feel that their values or preconceptions may be affecting how they intervene in a case. Supervisors must allow clinicians to be open about their countertransference issues, and encourage openness and self-evaluation in a non-judgmental atmosphere.

Larger home- and community-based organizations should also have a formalized volunteer ethics committee (see McCurdy, chapter 7, this volume), where practitioners can present vignettes of complicated cases. The committee might consist of various internal staff members and administrators, as well as community members. It is always helpful to have myriad perspectives represented, and members can include practitioners, supervisors, community members, physicians, psychiatrists, clergy, attorneys, philosophers, and, of course, a trained ethicist. Some organizations also have less formal "ethics brown bag sessions," which can be held during lunchtime, when workers can discuss ethical concerns with colleagues and an ethicist. Brown bag lunches usually occur more frequently than ethics committee meetings, so cases can be discussed with colleagues and trained ethicists in a timelier manner.

CONCLUSION

A therapeutic relationship is distinct from all other relationships. First, it is a fiduciary relationship: the client places his or her confidence in the practitioner who possesses special knowledge, expertise, and authority (Black, 1991). As the fiduciary, the practitioner is expected to be competent and trustworthy and to act in accordance with the standards of the profession and in the best interests of the client (Bayles,

1981). Like any fiduciary relationship, the therapeutic relationship results in unequal power and unequal responsibility. The practitioner has a duty not to abuse this power and to be honest, candid and loyal (Kutchins, 1991). In order to succeed in not abusing the power inherent in the relationship, it is incumbent on the responsible practitioner to be self-reflective vis-à-vis possible ethical conflicts and to understand their origins. In the case example, the case manager needs to understand why she made the judgments about the client's family without first making her own self-assessment. She needs to examine her values about filial responsibility and client self-determination. The client in this situation did not ask for help. In fact, there is no indication that he even expressed regret about being alone for the holiday. What are the case manager's beliefs about older persons' ability to take care of themselves, physically as well as emotionally? Had she engaged in the kind of self-reflective exercise we advocate here, she might have been better able to look more objectively at the client's strengths as well as weaknesses; she might have gained a better understanding of his relationships with others, not only his family; and she might have learned how her own biases prevented her from knowing her client.

Social services can be crucial for the well-being and continued adaptation to the challenges of old age for older people and their families. Any bias that might influence the clinician's decisions in serving a client represents a barrier to appropriate service delivery. Countertransference, biases, and value conflicts can all lead to consequent boundary problems. These must be identified and addressed by clinicians in the field of aging in order to eliminate or temper potential barriers to effective service delivery for our clients. An open and examined practice is an ethical practice.

REFERENCES

Abramson, M. (1996). Reflections on knowing oneself ethically: Toward a working framework for social work practice. *The Journal of Contemporary Human Services*, CEU Article No. 61, 195–201.

Bayles, M. D. (1981). *Professional ethics*. Belmont, CA: Wadsworth.

Beauchamp, T., & Childress, J. F. (1989). *Principles of biomedical ethics*. New York: Oxford University Press

Black, H. C. (1991). *Black's law dictionary*. St. Paul, MN: West.

Freud, S. (1912). Recommendations for physicians on the psychoanalysis method of treatment. In E. Jones (Ed.), *Collected papers of Sigmund Freud*, Vol. 2. New York: Basic Books, 1959, pp. 323–333.

Galambos, C. M. (1997). Quality of life for the elder: A reality or an illusion? In C. Corley-Saltz (Ed.), *Social work response to the White House Conference on Aging.* New York: Hawthorn Press, Inc.

Genevay, B., & Katz, R. (1990). *Countertransference and older clients.* Belmont, CA: Sage Publications.

Goldstein, H. (1999). On boundaries. *Families in Society, 80*(5), 435–438.

Houghton Mifflin Co. (2000). *The American Heritage Dictionary.* Boston, p. 471.

Kutchins, H. (1991). The fiduciary relationship: The legal basis for social workers' responsibilities to clients. *Social Work, 36,* 106–113.

Levkoff et al. (1994). Progression and resolution of delirium in elderly patients hospitalized for acute care. *American Journal of Geriatric Psychiatry, 2,* 230–238.

Murray, A. M., Levkoff, S. E., Wetle, T. T., Beckett, L., Cleary, P. D., Schor, J. D., Lipsitz, L. A., Rowe, J. W., & Evans, D. A. (1993). Acute delirium and functional decline in the hospitalized elderly patient. *Journal of Gerontology, 48*(5), 181–186.

National Association of Social Workers (1996). *NASW code of ethics.* NASW, Washington, D.C.

CHAPTER 10

Ethics and the Frontline Long-Term-Care Worker: A Challenge for the 21st Century

Robyn I. Stone and Yoshiko Yamada

The U.S. health care and long-term-care systems are experiencing major shifts in the way that care is financed and delivered for people with chronic disabilities. Managed care and integrated care systems are changing the way that older people and others with chronic care needs get services, and financial incentives are pushing people with acute care needs out of hospitals as quickly as possible into nursing homes and their own homes. Indeed, while the nursing home is still the dominant care setting for people with long-term-care needs, recent developments include an aggressive move to keep individuals in the community, in their own homes, or in alternative residential care environments.

At the center of this health care chaos are the frontline long-term-care workers—the nursing home and home care aides providing the bulk of formal, paid personal care and instrumental assistance to elderly and younger disabled people. New ethical issues are emerging in relation to how paraprofessionals do their jobs as terms such as *choice, autonomy, privacy,* and *managed risk* become part of the long-term-care vernacular. In this article, we identify some of the key ethical concerns and highlight several major trends that heighten the need to address these issues from the worker perspective.

THE ETHICAL CONTEXT: AN OVERVIEW

A number of frameworks may be applied in addressing the ethical concerns surrounding the paraprofessional nursing home and home care worker. A look at the elements of medical ethics is an obvious first step in examining the role of the long-term-care worker and her or his relationship to the care recipient (Hayley, Assel, Snyder, & Rudberg, 1996). These elements include (1) the degree to which the worker respects the autonomy of the care recipient (e.g., as related to such concerns as self-determination, privacy, respect for the individual); (2) beneficence (or doing what is best for the care recipient); (3) fidelity (i.e., establishing trust and maintaining confidentiality); and (4) justice, that is, the extent to which the worker applies equitable treatment and distribution of resources to all care recipients. The professional ethical code for nursing assistants includes respect for client autonomy but also emphasizes the need to choose the greatest good for the least harm, knowing one's own limits, and applying a fairness test to all actions.

Discussions about ethics in long-term care tend to address these issues from the perspective of the care recipient, focusing on the moral and ethical concerns of caring for the elderly or younger disabled client. But Kane (1994) has argued that the discussion needs to be broader. An examination of ethics, she says, must include not only the responsibilities of the worker (the worker's behavior toward the client and family and decision making about the care), but also responsibilities *to* the worker (policies regarding the deployment and working conditions of these frontline caregivers). These frontline workers have rights as well as responsibilities, and the ethical concerns regarding their status and treatment in the workplace and in society must be recognized. What is more, Kane says, nursing home and home care aides are moral agents, and the ethical soul-searching should not be left to the workers' superiors, as some have argued (e.g., Kjervik, 1990).

Given the very close and often intimate relationship between frontline workers and their clients, Aroskar and colleagues (1990) argue that to address special and perhaps difficult situations it is not sufficient to simply have a formal code of ethics. Rather, there is a need for "everyday ethics," defined by Kane (1994) as "an ethic of intimacy, one that recognizes human need for affiliation and responds to the myriad of issues that arise from day to day, not a set of ethics procedures that are trotted out for large life and death decisions." In ethical decision-making, where, for example, does a worker draw the line between petty theft and "keeping the change"; what should she do about accepting small gifts from family members for special services rendered? One home care aide might choose to visit a needy client outside the formal work schedule; another may falsify the number of visits to one client in order to spend more time with a needier individual. These decisions are very difficult for the workers, who are closest to the care recipients and who are trying to balance good physical and emotional caregiving with their own needs for respect and dignity.

SPECIFIC ETHICAL CONCERNS

A number of specific ethical concerns are particularly relevant to the situation of frontline workers.

Lack of Authority and Autonomy

Like many of the elderly or younger disabled people for whom they care, paraprofessionals in long-term care have little power. Frontline workers typically have great responsibilities without much authority (Aroskar, Urv-Wong, & Kane, 1990; Eustis, Fischer, & Kane, 1994). Care plans are established by others (e.g., nurses, care coordinators) and client information is often not shared with the aides. At the same time, workers are often alone with their clients, facing great responsibilities without clear authority and channels of accountability. Nurse aides in the nursing home, residential care and home care settings are at the bottom of the nursing pecking order, which significantly limits their autonomy. In many cases, simply challenging a supervisor may threaten the worker's job security. Care recipients are affected in many ways by this situation—both directly and indirectly. As was articulated so eloquently by William Thomas (1994), founder of the Eden Alternative long-term-care organization, nursing home residents and community-dwelling care recipients can never be more empowered than the staff who care for them.

Clement (1996), a feminist analyst who has examined the theory and practice of care, autonomy, and justice, emphasizes the importance of autonomy for the caregiver. She claims that an autonomous caregiver is more likely to give ideal care than a nonautonomous one. A problem arises when the requirements of the work undermine the individual's autonomy. The worker's own definition of good care may be overridden by the "experts" for whom the caregiver works or by the care recipient, who is expressing his or her own desire for autonomy.

"Caught in the Middle"

The frontline worker in any long-term-care setting is most often the person caught between at least two masters (Aroskar, Urv-Wong, & Kane, 1990; Foner, 1994; Clement, 1996). For nursing home aides and home care workers employed by an agency, the frontline caregiver must respond to the demands of the employer (as represented by the administrator, the supervising nurse, and sometimes other personnel) as well as the client. Frequently, family members of the care recipient become additional masters, in institutional as well as home care settings. In many cases, the definition of care subscribed to by the frontline worker may conflict with that of the employing agency, the family, and even the care recipient.

Because of the unique, intimate relationship of the worker to the client, aides tend to focus on personal dynamics between them and their care recipients, while organizations and sometimes relatives are more interested in the quantifiable aspects of the "production" of services—for example, viewing care for the client's psychological and social needs as secondary or even irrelevant compared with the personal care and instrumental tasks required. The worker is often caught between the formal rules and performance requirements, on the one hand, and the personal, often informal relationship with the client, on the other. Such a situation can create uncertainty and confusion. For example, informality between the worker and the client can be positive, but it can also lead to ambiguity about the worker's tasks and the possibility of exploitation of the worker and to worker "burnout" (Eustis, Fischer, & Kane, 1994).

Compensation and Working Conditions

Nursing home and home care aides have the lowest status of any workers in health care and long-term care, which their pay levels, access to benefits, and job security reflect. Their remuneration and benefits tend to be poor; in fact, many have no access to health care benefits, sick leave, or annual vacation. This situation is particularly true for independent providers—those individuals who are not working for an agency but are hired directly by the client or family.

It is clear that many of these workers are not doing this type of work for financial compensation alone. Research has suggested that for many, the altruistic returns of caring for a needy individual are important motivating factors (Bayer, Stone, & Friedland, 1993; Feldman, 1993). Studies have also demonstrated that these individuals do respond to nonmonetary rewards including formal recognition of a job well done and opportunities for climbing a career ladder. The extent to which such opportunities arise is somewhat dependent on the local economy. In areas where unemployment is low and where it is difficult to recruit workers, providers are more likely to offer incentives to attract and retain nursing home and home care aides. How frontline workers can be provided with adequate compensation is a central ethical and practical concern that the health care system must address.

Working conditions are also a major issue. One of the most serious work environment concerns that frontline workers face is the potential for verbal and physical abuse by their clients. The academic literature and popular media are replete with stories about elder abuse. Less attention has been paid to the workers who are the victims of care recipients. Yet, though such abuse goes largely unrecognized, it does exist (Mercer, Heacock, & Beck, 1993; Foner, 1994; Aroskar, Urv-Wong, & Kane, 1994). When client-worker struggles over power and control occur, the nursing home or home care aide may become the recipient of client violence and abuse. This is especially true for those caring for individuals with dementia, where belligerent behavior is frequently a manifestation of the disease. In her recent qualitative study of ethics in dementia day care, Hasselkus (1997) explored situations where the client or the worker was said to be "crossing the ethical line." She noted the dilemma of a female worker caring for a demented male daycare participant who continually made sexual advances toward her. The worker was torn between the desire to give good care, in light of her understanding of his condition, and her fear of sexual abuse. In another instance, family members falsely accused workers of unethical behavior ranging from tying up someone's husband to completely ignoring another care recipient.

Ethnic and racial differences between the worker and the client may exacerbate the potential for abusive behavior. Most long-term-care recipients are white, and most workers are people of color, often immigrants, sometimes without legal status (Kane, 1994). These workers are often targets for exploitation by the client and the client's family. In addition, because long-term-care administrators and supervisors tend to be white, in institutions where racial tensions exist, the worker may be vulnerable to the employer as well as to the care recipient.

EMERGING TRENDS

The ethical issues related to the frontline worker are becoming more critical in light of several emerging trends: the expansion of client-directed care, the movement toward more delegation of what were formerly nurses' duties to less skilled workers in both acute and long-term care, and the development of a number of options for paying family caregivers.

Client-Directed Care

While wealthy individuals have long been hiring private care workers, the concept of client-directed care as a formal long-term-care option has been aggressively promoted only over the past decade, mainly by the physically disabled community's independent living movement. This philosophy of allowing and encouraging individuals with long-term-care needs, particularly nonmedical needs, to manage their own care has now permeated long-term-care programs for the elderly as well as the younger disabled. In many instances, frontline workers are selected, trained, supervised, and fired by the clients themselves (Flanagan, 1994). For example, in several European countries (including Germany and Austria) and some state programs in the United States, long-term-care consumers are given cash payments in lieu of services, with varying levels of discretion in how they use the funds.

While the notion of empowering consumers with enhanced choice and autonomy is intuitively appealing, serious ethical issues arise for the frontline worker when the concept is actually put into effect. As noted in the previous section, the benefits and working conditions of the long-term-care workforce are frequently not adequate; workers suffer from low wages, lack of benefits, and less than optimal working environments. With the growth in client-directed care comes the potential for these workers to be even more exploited by clients who fail to pay the minimum wage, who choose to offer no benefits, and who also have the option of hiring and firing at will. The Department of Health and Human Services and the Robert Wood Johnson Foundation have jointly funded a four-state demonstration project for "cashing out" long-term-care services—that is, providing funds directly to clients, who then hire and pay their own long-term-care workers. The project has received significant criticism from those who are concerned about the ability of disabled clients to manage cash wisely and the potential abuse of clients and workers. Traditional home care agency staff argue that many disabled people, and especially the elderly, are not prepared to be an employer and will be at the mercy of untrained, unsupervised workers. Advocates for the workers, including the Service Employees Industrial Union and others, have strongly opposed client-directed care on the grounds that there are no mechanisms for protecting the rights of the worker. The demonstration project includes some elements designed to mitigate these employer-employee problems, particularly the development of state-level counseling programs that would provide technical assistance to clients in hiring and managing workers as well as the more technical aspects of paying Social Security, workman's compensation, and other benefits. These counseling programs, however, are voluntary and cannot provide the full range of protections for either the client or the worker.

The goal of client-directed care is, in fact, to provide more choice and autonomy for the long-term-care recipient, but if this goal is realized, will it be at the expense of the worker? Asch (1993) has identified many ethical dilemmas in agency-directed home care, including the lack of oversight and accountability that may result in workers being treated unfairly by the client and the client's family or by the agency. These ethical concerns will undoubtedly escalate as client-directed care becomes more prevalent. Policy makers and providers involved in developing such programs need to understand these tradeoffs and face them squarely as they design new options to enhance client empowerment. Formal and informal strategies for minimizing abuse of the worker as well as the client must be implemented, and mechanisms for protecting the rights of both parties should be explored.

Nurse Delegation

Recently, health care providers in both acute and chronic care have been utilizing increasing numbers of paraprofessional aides in the provision of direct care. Those aides often replace licensed nurses, and they perform more and more complex tasks. The delegation of nursing care to aides, if carried out appropriately, can enhance the efficiency and quality of the nursing care (Simpkins, 1997). Furthermore, nurse delegation has been critical, if not essential, to the development of new long-term-care options like assisted living that allow significantly disabled people to remain in community settings. For example, allowing an aide to administer oral medication to an elderly resident with long-term-care needs may make the difference between that person having to move into a nursing home or remaining in her own home or an assisted living residence. In states like Oregon, where the philosophy of autonomy, choice, and deinstitutionalization has motivated the expansion of residential care alternatives, nurse delegation legislation allows elderly and younger disabled people who are eligible for nursing home care to be cared for in assisted living and adult foster care at a much lower cost, with more freedom and privacy, and with no discernible evidence of lesser quality care (Kane, 1997).

However, when nursing tasks are delegated to aides, several issues need to be considered in order to assure quality of care for patients as well as to clarify each staff person's job and point of accountability. As aides provide more complex care for their patients under nurse delegation, a question arises as to the skills and experience levels required to perform those tasks. Under the Omnibus Budget Reconciliation Act of 1987 (OBRA '87), nurse aides in nursing homes or home care agencies that receive Medicare or Medicaid funds are required to receive a minimum of 75 hours of training within four months of employment and to pass a competency evaluation program. Yet, as the complexity of aides' tasks increases, the adequacy of these training requirements becomes questionable. Moreover, since OBRA '87 does not specify contents of the training, a great discrepancy exists between the training itself and the aides' actual skill levels. Utilizing aides in nursing activities may produce cost savings, but without quality assurance and sufficient training for aides, delegation may cause tremendous harm to patients and ultimately increase costs.

In addition, improper nurse delegation can have negative effects not only on patients but also on aides themselves and on higher-level health care workers, where role ambiguity and lack of accountability can cause major problems. Erlen and colleagues (1996) highlight role conflicts that can ensue when the rules and boundaries of nurse delegation are not clear. In one example, the authors identify problems arising from a discrepancy in the documentation of a nursing home resident's status prepared by the aide on the night shift and the nurse on the following day shift. Without clear direction and mutual understanding about delegation of tasks (who should do what under which circumstances, who can delegate to whom for which tasks), role confusion is inevitable, resulting in a lack of respect for, mistrust in, and perhaps even outright hostility toward other staff members (Erlen, Mellors, & Koren, 1996). The issue of accountability in the event of a serious error is paramount. If, for example, inaccurate documentation by the night aide leads to a deterioration in the resident's condition, who bears the responsibility—the aide or the nurse who delegated the task to the aide?

In response to those concerns, states have increased efforts to provide standards by which licensed nurses delegate tasks to unlicensed aides (American Nurses Association, 1997). Several states, including Colorado, Oregon, Kansas, and Texas, have nurse-delegation provisions in their nurse practice acts (Kane, 1997), and others like Hawaii, Arizona, and Pennsylvania have introduced legislation on nurse delegation in 1997 (American Nurses Association, 1997). These states are motivated by the desire to reduce expenditures for health care and long-term care, an interest in promoting more autonomy for consumers and workers, and the need to ensure quality without jeopardizing the safety and well-being of the care recipient. As nurse delegation continues to expand across the country, it is essential that policy makers, providers, and consumers understand and address the ethical concerns that result from the tensions among these competing interests.

Paying Family Caregivers

While family caregivers informally provide the bulk of long-term care to disabled elderly and younger relatives, an increasing number of state programs in the United States and long-term-care programs in other countries pay family members for their assistance (Keigher & Stone, 1992; Stone, 1997). Most of the industrialized countries that pay family caregivers (usually women) view this financial assistance as wage compensation for work (Glendenning & McLaughlin, 1993). According to a study of home care in California by Benjamin and colleagues (2000), clients tend to prefer paid family care providers to other, unrelated caregivers. From a client perspective, having a paid family provider meets certain security, choice, and satisfaction needs when compared to receiving assistance from a nonrelative. They argue that to the extent that permitting paid family caregiving makes the client feel safer as a care recipient, a sense of security becomes a highly desirable benefit of this service arrangement.

Although compensation for family caregivers may be preferable for many people, the transformation of an informal caregiver to a paid frontline worker raises some important ethical questions. Kane (1994) has identified several concerns including the following: (1) whether consumers and payers have the right to demand a certain level of quality from paid caregivers and, if so, how to measure and monitor it; (2) whether the consumer should accept a family member as a paid caregiver; and (3) how the consumer resolves dissatisfaction with the paid family caregiver. In addition, Stone (1997) also notes policy makers' reluctance to introduce the idea of financial compensation for services that they believe should inherently be the responsibility of family members and others in the informal network. The preoccupation of policy makers in the United States with the question of potential abuse of cash payments by family members has not dominated the European debate, where many countries do pay family members for long-term-care assistance. At the same time, anecdotal reports of abuse by family members in the long-term-care program that has relatively recently become a part of the German social-insurance system, including families getting cash but not spending it on care, highlight the ethical issues emerging from the transformation of informal caregivers into paid workers (personal communication with J. Wilburs, 1998).

As we approach the twenty-first century and the graying of America, the ethical issues related to providing care must be addressed from the worker perspective as well as the consumer perspective. Codes of ethics are important, but they must be bolstered by ethical practice, which means consideration of ethical issues in treatment plans and treatment care conferences, the development of in-service education programs on ethics for frontline workers, and the expansion of policies that empower aides as well as care recipients. We need to promote and practice "everyday ethics" to ensure that all the parties involved in long-term care are treated with respect and human dignity.

REFERENCES

American Nurses Association. (1997). Unlicensed assistive personnel legislation: 1997 [on-line]. Available: http://www.nursingworld.org/gova/hod97/uap.htm.

Aroskar, M. A., Urv-Wong, E. K., & Kane, R. A. (1990). Building an effective caregiving staff: Transforming the nursing services. In R. A. Kane & A. L. Caplan (Eds.), *Everyday ethics: Resolving dilemmas in nursing home life.* New York: Springer Publishing.

Asch, A. (1993). Free to be a bigot. In R. A. Kane & A. L. Caplan (Eds.), *Ethical conflict in the management of home care: The case manager's dilemma.* New York: Springer Publishing.

Bayer, E. J., Stone, R. I., & Friedland, R. B. (1993). *Developing a caring and effective long-term care workforce.* Bethesda, MD: Project HOPE Center for Health Affairs.

Benjamin, A. E., Matthias, R., & Franke, T. M. (2000, April). Comparing consumer-directed and agency models for providing supportive services at home. *Health Services Research, 35*(1), part II, 351–366.

Benjamin A. E., Matthias, R. E., & Franke, T. M. (1998, September). Comparing Client-Directed and Agency Models for Providing Supportive Services at Home. Final report to the U.S. Dept. of Health and Human Services.

Clement, G. (1996). *Care, autonomy, and justice: Feminism and the ethic of care.* Boulder, CO: Westview Press.

Erlen, J. A., Mellors, M. P., & Koren, A. M. (1996). Ethical issues and the new staff mix. *Orthopaedic Nursing, 15*(2), 73–77.

Eustis, N. N., Fischer, L. R., & Kane, R. A. (1994). The homecare worker: On the frontline of quality. *Generations, 18*(3), 43–49.

Feldman, P. (1993). Work life improvements for the home aide workforce. *Gerontologist, 33*(1), 47–54.

Flanagan, S. (1994). *Consumer-directed attendant services: How states address tax, legal, and quality assurance issues.* Cambridge, MA: SysteMetrics.

Foner, N. (1994). *The caregiving dilemma: Work in an American nursing home.* Berkeley, CA: University of California Press.

Glendenning, C., & McLaughlin, E. (1993). *Paying for care: Lessons from Europe*. Social Security Advisory Committee Research Paper No. 5. London, England: Her Majesty's Stationery Office.

Hasselkus, B. R. (1997). Everyday ethics in dementia day care: Narratives of crossing the line. *Gerontologist, 37*(5), 640–649.

Hayley, D. C., Assel, C. K., Snyder, L., & Rudberg, M. A. (1996). Ethical and legal issues in nursing home care. *Archives of Internal Medicine, 156*, 249–256.

Kane, R. A. (1997). Boundaries of home care: Can a home-care approach transform LTC institutions? In D. M. Fox & C. Raphael (Eds.), *Home-based care for a new century*. Malden, MA: Blackwell.

Kane, R. A. (1994). Ethics and the frontline care worker: Mapping the subject. *Generations, 18*(3), 71–74.

Keigher, S., & Stone, R. I. (1992). *Payment for care in the US: A very mixed policy bag*. Paper presented at the International Meeting on Payment for Dependent Care. Vienna, Austria, July.

Kjervik, D. K. (1990). Beyond the call of duty: A nurse's aide uses her judgement. In R. A. Kane & A. L. Caplan (Eds.), *Everyday ethics: Resolving dilemmas in nursing home life*. New York: Springer Publishing.

Mercer, S. O., Heacock, P., & Beck, C. (1993). Nurse's aides in nursing homes: Perceptions of training, work loads, racism, and abuse issues. *Journal of Gerontological Social Work, 21*(1/2), 95–112.

Simpkins, R. W. (1997). Using task lists with unlicensed assistive personnel. *Insight, 6*(2). Available on the Internet: http://www.ncsbn.org/files/insight/vol62/tasklist.html.

Stone, R. I. (1997). Integration of home- and community-based services: Issues for the 1990s. In D. M. Fox & C. Raphael (Eds.), *Home-based care for a new century*. Malden, MA: Blackwell.

Thomas, W. (1994). *The Eden alternative: A new paradigm for long-term care*. Presented at a symposium of the Lester E. Cox Medical Center, Springfield, Missouri, April.

CHAPTER 11

When the Helper Needs Help: A Social Worker's Experiences in Receiving Home Care

Nan G. O'Connor

As I drove to a gathering of former high school classmates, I wondered if it was a good idea to go at all. Increasing pain in my left hip had forced me to resign my position as a social work supervisor in the spring of 1997. I was weak and fatigued from the constant battle with the pain in my hip. Still, I felt it would be uplifting to be out, so I made the long trek to the western suburbs where the gathering was to be held. Toward the end of the evening, one of my classmates approached me to express his concern over my medical problems. I confided that I had consulted two top orthopedic surgeons in Chicago. The first felt my complicated medical history ruled out surgery to unfuse my left hip. The hip had been fused after high school graduation in 1970 and was now creating the pain and strain I was experiencing. The second surgeon said he could perform the operation but had only operated on three patients. My friend told me his neighbor was an orthopedic surgeon, and suggested I consult him. A week later, I went to see the physician my friend recommended and, after a thorough review of my history and a lengthy physical exam, he quietly told me that my situation was beyond his purview. He then told me about Dr. Henry Finn, a surgeon at Weiss Hospital in Chicago who had performed hip fusion takedowns, a rare and complicated procedure, on several patients with great success. A few weeks later I met with Dr. Finn, who listened attentively as I gave him an overview of my medical history. (At the age of nine, I had fallen through a hole in the first floor of an unfinished house I was exploring, landing many feet below on both hips. That trauma triggered a congenital degenerative joint disease, resulting in a total of seventeen major surgeries dating back to 1962.) At this point, I was no longer able to work, and was barely functioning. After hearing my history, Dr. Finn gently responded: "I think I can help you get your life back." Although unfusing a hip posed many risks, which included the possibility of infection, he felt there was a 90% chance for complete success. After a few more months of questioning and soul-searching, and two additional consultations with Dr. Finn, I decided to have the surgery.

As I prepared for what I felt would be the most major of my 17 surgeries, I knew I would need help once I returned home. I did not want to make the same mistake I had made after my right hip replacement 4 years earlier, when I had no help except for a nurse's aide who assisted me in the shower three times a week. It was such a struggle then to make meals, clean up, and even make my bed, that I felt my healing was delayed from lack of proper help. Dr. Finn had told me there was a good possibility I would be in a body cast for several weeks after this surgery in order to hold the new hip in place, and did not feel I could be alone at home afterwards. I commenced my search for home care resources by calling community agencies as well as the state Office of Rehabilitation Services (ORS), who informed me that arrangements for care could be made by the hospital social worker just before my discharge.

I had lived alone for several years, and had recently moved to a different community. The Department of Human Services could only arrange home-delivered meals on a temporary basis since I was under 65. Several months previous, I had become eligible for Medicare, and I knew Medicare would provide home physical therapy and a nurse's aide to assist with bathing. I had started to receive income from Social Security disability as well as benefits from my employer, which equaled about half of my previous income. Having had many surgeries and costly medical bills over the years, I had depleted my savings and knew I could not afford private-duty care.

On November 11, 1997, I entered Weiss Memorial Hospital in Chicago to undergo the procedure to unfuse my hip. As Dr. Finn came into the surgical holding area to see me before the operation, he asked, "Are you ready?" I hesitated, but knew deep inside that if I did not have this surgery I would continue the downward spiral of the physical decline I was in. I answered, "Yes."

Coming out of the anesthetic a few hours later, I felt there was something terribly wrong. I didn't verbalize my fear to anyone, but it persisted. Dr. Finn had discovered during surgery that the gluteus medius, the large muscle that holds the hip in place, was only 25% intact, the rest having been surgically removed during the hip fusion in 1970. In order to keep the hip from dislocating while it was healing, I was put into a body cast that extended from above my waist down to where it encased my toes. After a few days in the hospital, I was transferred to an extended care facility, where I was to stay for several weeks. I was depressed over being in a nursing home environment, and dreaded the endless days. The care was adequate at best, and the staff seemed frustrated and overwhelmed with the unfamiliar scenario of a younger woman in a body cast who needed to be frequently repositioned and turned.

I started to experience pressure inside the cast, and within a week I was taken to the emergency room to have the cast split at the heel. My left hip and leg continued to swell, and the decision was made to change the cast under general anesthetic. As I woke up in the Recovery Room, the orthopedic resident came to my side and said: "Ms. O'Connor, I'm afraid I have some bad news: your hip dislocated when we were transferring you off the operating table, and we have to take you back into surgery." In my mental fog, I struggled to understand. Dr. Finn appeared and confirmed the news, saying he would put the hip back into place under general anesthetic, and hoped he wouldn't have to open me back up to do so. With mercifully little time to react, I went into the Operating Room once again. They were able to move the hip back into place without surgery, and a new body cast was applied.

I was transferred back to the nursing home. A few days later, the Director of Nursing at the extended care facility attempted to position my bed to relieve the swelling that persisted in my hip. She allowed the electrically controlled bed to go so high it hit the overhead light fixture, and the bed crashed to the ground. Immediately, I was in excruciating hip pain. I knew she had been trying to help me, but I was furious over her inattention, and in shock from the trauma. Although portable X-rays taken at the nursing home showed the hip was still in place, the pain worsened. I was finally taken to the emergency room the next day, where X-rays there showed that the hip had indeed dislocated again.

Since the hip was slipping in and out of place too easily, Dr. Finn decided I would need a new, constrained hip, which had a ring-like device around the ball of the prosthesis to hold it in place. On December 7th I woke up with pain from what I thought was a pulled muscle in my calf. A scan showed that I had a blood clot traveling up my right leg. I had a history of blood clots, including one that caused my heart to stop while recovering from the hip fusion 27 years previous. A filter was put through my chest wall into my abdomen to prevent any future clots from traveling to my heart. On December 9th I was operated on and the constrained hip was put in. Immediately after this surgery, I was fitted with a special brace to stabilize the joint.

I had been bedridden for over a month, so I entered the rehabilitation unit at Weiss Hospital, where I had intensive physical and occupational therapy. At first, I was placed on a tilt table that helped my body get gradually used to being upright. I then learned to walk a few steps using a walker, and was only able to stand for less than one minute. A custom reclining wheelchair was ordered, since the muscles in my hip were not healed enough to sit fully upright and I did not have a chair at home that was high enough and had arms. The insertion of the filter for my blood clot had injured the muscle in my chest wall that controlled my right arm, and the occupational therapist gave me exercises to regain its use. Arrangements were made for home-health services to begin immediately upon my discharge. These services included physical and occupational therapy. The ORS approved 20 hours of home care per week to assist me with bathing, laundry, cleaning, and meal preparation, and a personal care assistant was lined up through one of ORS's contract agencies. The brace was removed, and I returned home January 13th, two months to the day since I had entered the hospital.

The morning after I returned home, I received a call from the home care agency informing me that the personal care assistant had changed her mind and would not be able to come. They could not locate another worker, but promised to continue working on it. A friend who had offered to stay with me for two weeks came the next day, and until she came, I stayed in bed as much as possible. I did not have the strength to fix myself any meals, so I was grateful when my friend arrived. The panic I felt over the worker not showing up slowly dissipated. I called the agency every day, and was informed they were having trouble finding someone with a car who was willing to come out to the suburbs.

On January 22nd, a young woman who lived in Chicago came to meet me and begin services. The next day, I was informed by the agency that the woman felt it was too far to drive. Fortunately, I had a nurse's aide through the home-health agency who helped bathe me twice a week. Since ORS was having no luck in finding help for me, my friend offered to commute from her home to mine a few times a week for a short period of time. Two other friends who lived nearby came every week to do laundry and cleaning, and drove me to doctor's appointments. My family members provide enormous financial and emotional support, but they do not live in close proximity and are unable to provide immediate care.

In the next few weeks, I started to receive short-term home-delivered meals five days per week through the human services program in my community. Through their office, I was matched up with a young mother who volunteered to shop for groceries twice a month. There were some days that no one was able to be with me. I found myself trying to prepare meals and pick up after myself, which expended the little energy I had on household tasks. This left me feeling very frustrated trying to cope with my limitations. I was also filled with anger at the "system" that could not provide me with basic care. At times, I was too weak to even walk down the hall with my walker to the kitchen and back, and worried about whether I was safe. Fatigued and emotionally spent, I became withdrawn, and some people started to withdraw from me. I became unreasonably resentful of others who had mobility and who could get out, and felt hurt by those who did not or could not call. I did not want to burden others by asking for help, and because I had grown weary of hearing that no one was available, I stopped calling the agency.

On March 2nd, almost 7 weeks after coming home, the private home care agency finally found a Certified Nurse's Assistant (CNA) who lived in Chicago but who was willing to make the drive to my house. During her first visit, the home care worker, whom I will call Marian, made it very clear that she would come only if I would sign her time sheet for more hours than she would actually work. Marian felt justified because "everyone does this" and because she lived an hour from my home, received no mileage reimbursement, and was paid only $6.50 an hour. She put great pressure on me for a decision that week by calling me several times from her home. Although I sympathized with her plight, I was still not feeling strong physically or emotionally and was worn down by her calls. After much struggle and soul searching—desperate for assistance—I reluctantly agreed to her request. I felt as if I was being blackmailed and was upset over violating my strong ethical principles, but necessity seemed to demand capitulation.

Even though Marian expressed being uneasy with this arrangement, I felt that she was taking advantage of me and that she had the upper hand, since she only agreed to care for me on her terms. This sense became all too real when she began calling the night before her designated work day to say something had come up, and that she would have to come another time. Such late notice meant I could not make other arrangements even if it were possible, and I was left alone on those days. She also started to come late and leave early, saying she wanted to avoid heavy traffic for her drive home. I began to exert my own subtle form of control by being uncommunicative some days, or by not telling her what needed to be done until she was about to leave—hoping, I suppose, that she would stay. I slowly realized I resented needing help, and that underneath the resentment was deep sadness over the change and loss that had occurred.

Marian came from a country near India, but life in the United States did not meet her expectations. She lived in a one-bedroom apartment with her two teenage children, and because her husband had recently left her for another woman, she often arrived at my door in tears over the hurt and betrayal she felt. She did her work distractedly and incompletely, leaving me to finish tasks that caused me both pain and physical setbacks.

During this time, I became Marian's confidante and companion as she struggled with emotional problems caused by her children and husband. I began to feel resentful: *she* was supposed to be helping *me!* Torn between anger and compassion, I suggested that Marian seek counseling. She replied that her beliefs would not permit her to do so, and out of the need for physical privacy and emotional protection, I started to withdraw. I was afraid to tell her how I felt, fearful she would leave if I did not listen to her woes. I became testy and irritable, especially on the mornings Marian would have to bathe me. I felt humiliated by having someone else perform this intimate act, and hated feeling helpless and vulnerable, emotions that were exacerbated when Marian made personal remarks about my scars or appearance. I really don't think she meant to be unkind, but her comments added to my deep and overwhelming shame.

I had lived alone for several years, and having someone in my home who was not of my choosing was a great strain. I was constantly accommodating myself to Marian's schedule, which often meant getting up quite early after an exhausting session of physical therapy the day before. There were also cultural and racial conflicts: Marian asked me constant questions about the value of my furnishings and whether I had money, always remarking, "In our country we do not have such things." One of Marian's tasks was to shop for me, but she would not always pick up the items I asked for, instead buying the brand that was on sale. After a while, I stopped asking her to go to the store for me. It was often hard to find things after she had moved them while cleaning, and, although I didn't worry about her stealing from me, I could understand the fear and confusion many homebound people experience over this issue. Sometimes when preparing my meals, Marian would have to be instructed in the use of what seemed to be unfamiliar ingredients: when I asked for an egg salad sandwich, she did not know how to make one. There were also occasions when I would find the mirrors wiped with furniture polish, or the floor mopped with a bathroom cleanser that contained bleach, which left the tiles permanently discolored. We did not have the same standards of cleanliness, and Marian's lack of regard for my personal belongings by flinging them to another spot while she cleaned culminated in an extremely upsetting incident.

While dusting a table in my living room, she carelessly shoved a handpainted vase to the side, where it rolled off the edge and onto the floor, breaking into several large pieces. It was a treasured gift given to me by a friend many years before, and one of the few possessions I felt attached to. I was distraught. As I explained why I was so upset, Marian said, "You shouldn't have left it out." With no offer made to fix the vase or buy something in its place, I realized that not only did we not share the same values, but she did not value my things. I wondered if Marian was jealous of my nice surroundings, and also wondered if, on some unconscious level, she deliberately broke a vase that she possibly saw as frivolous. This entire incident seemed to magnify and crystallize all the losses of privacy and independence I had suffered.

The next week I talked with Marian again, telling her how upset I was over the vase incident. I told her she needed to work more hours, and that I could not tolerate the way she constantly changed her schedule. I also told her I was paying the price for her actions through the pain and fatigue that would result when she didn't come. This conversation did not change anything. In weary resignation, I became quieter and often withdrew to my room.

As the months went by, Marian and I developed a guarded yet comfortable interdependence. Her personal and financial problems escalated, however, and Marian began to spend fewer hours in my home. I was reluctant to report her to the agency, out of a strong sense of loyalty and my own need for the few hours Marian showed up. I did, however, finally tell Marian that I could no longer sign her time sheets for hours she did not work. I also requested that she work the hours that had been approved, since my friends were bearing the burden of performing tasks she was being paid to do.

Physical therapy was progressing slowly. I could see some improvement in my ability to walk with the walker, and was able to sit up in my wheelchair in the evening, which the pain in my hip had prevented until then. I still fatigued easily, however, especially after any extra activity. In the meantime, in desperate need of a change of scenery, I decided to fly to Colorado for a 10-day visit with four of my brothers. I left for Denver the last week in September, knowing it would be physically taxing but mentally uplifting to go. While there, one morning as I was getting out of bed, my right knee suddenly gave way. I was in such severe pain I could not move my leg or walk. An ambulance took me to the local hospital, where emergency room and orthopedic physicians concurred that I needed to get back to Chicago to see my own doctor. Since it was the end of my trip, I flew back home as scheduled and went to see Dr. Finn. His exam revealed an unstable knee joint, and X-rays showed that the plastic part of the prosthesis, which had been put in 10 years earlier, had worn away. Hesitantly, Dr. Finn decided that I would need either a partial or total knee revision, and was worried that since this was my "good" leg, the healing of my other hip as well as this knee may be compromised. Surgery was scheduled for October 29th, and I was fitted for a knee brace to help minimize the pain.

This chain of events devastated me and as I tried to prepare for this, my twentieth surgery, I was filled with anger and fear. What if something went wrong? What if, after all I had been through to rehabilitate my other hip, I couldn't walk? I depend on my right leg greatly, and realized I would actually need more help at home after this procedure because my hip had not healed and could not support my injured knee.

The surgery to replace the prosthesis went as planned. I returned to the rehab unit, where I progressed slowly because I was in constant, severe pain. I was discharged from the hospital in 11 days, almost 1 year to the day after my hip surgery. When I returned home, Marian told me she had taken another job, and would not be able to give me the hours I needed. Since I could barely get myself out of bed, let alone maneuver with my walker or wheelchair, I was panic-stricken. What would I do? Who could come to be with me? The agency tried to find another worker but to no avail. Since I was weak and not able to make many phone calls, a friend intervened for me and called the hospital social worker, who gave her the name of a private agency she thought could help. My family paid for a private CNA who came five days a week for four hours. She was a wonderful, upbeat person, and her presence gave me a sense of peace and security that I had not experienced after any of my other surgeries. I looked forward to her visits; she was very nurturing, and brought me delicious food she had made at home, and did little extras as well, like combing and fixing my hair after my shower, which was quite lovely and soothing. I liked giving her little treats to take home to her family as a way of thanking her—and maybe keeping her. However, she too was having personal and financial problems. Three weeks after she started she called to say that her car had broken down and was in the shop. Then she stopped coming at all. I was stunned, and felt bereft. When I called the agency that she worked for, they were equally puzzled, and could not reach her. I felt that she was probably embarrassed to come back after missing so much time, and also began to wonder: Was it me? Did I do something to make her leave?

A few weeks later, the agency called me to say they had found a woman who lived close by and who was eager and willing to begin work. She was delightful and we hit it off immediately. She told me a little about her personal life, saying that they lived in subsidized housing, and that she felt the neighbors treated her family differently. She then cried as she told me about their financial problems, and the shame she felt her children suffered. She was hardworking, and in the second visit was already talking about being with me "next Christmas" as she helped me put my decorations away. The next day, I received a phone call from the agency that her husband had called them to say, "My wife had to go out of town and is not coming back to work for you—ever." This disturbed both the supervisor of the agency and myself as we wondered if she was being abused. We never heard from her again, and I was left feeling shaken by her sudden departure. I felt abandoned.

In December I started to receive physical therapy at home five days a week because I could not endure the ride to the outpatient clinic. The pain in my knee prevented much progress, and in January and again in February I was admitted to the hospital for knee manipulations performed under a general anesthetic to break through scar tissue formation.

During this time I was on the phone constantly with my ORS caseworker, who admitted to me the chances were slim to none that a worker could be found for me. The home-health social worker called the ORS administrator in Springfield, who admitted there are "terrible" problems getting workers for clients in the Chicago area. He had no solutions.

Last spring, I tried to hire someone on my own who would be paid directly by the state. A woman at our church gave me several names, and one woman came to meet me who seemed well suited for the job. In the course of the interview, she broke down and started sobbing: her son was in prison and the hearing was scheduled for that week. She also confessed she was receiving Social Security disability for severe depression. Since I had been without formal help for 3 months, I tried to quell the concern and doubt I felt, and asked if she could start immediately. She agreed, but was concerned that income from the state would jeopardize her Social Security benefits. I called Social Security, who confirmed what she had told me: that the money she would receive for assisting me was over the amount allowed. I could not pay her in cash, so we parted ways. A few weeks later, I was put in touch with a college student who was looking for extra income. She knew I had seen many people come and go, and promised she would not be one of them. She was very enthusiastic and grateful for the job. After coming to my house three times, she disappeared as suddenly as she had come. She did not return my phone calls, and I found out later she had abruptly and inexplicably quit a long-standing job at a nearby restaurant.

Tired of riding an emotional roller coaster between hope and despair, I gave up looking for help completely. As a result, I paid the price of pain, fatigue, and setbacks in my progress.

I am, perhaps, the epitome of the wounded healer. As a social worker for almost 2 decades, I have cared for elderly clients, advocated on their behalf to receive the help they needed, heard the panic in their voices when the person who was supposed to help them was late again. Now I know how my clients feel as I experience the multiple losses of dignity, mobility, independence, privacy, and self-respect. Despite an extensive personal and professional support system, I cannot rally the formal help I need. What options does someone frailer than myself have? Is it a right or a privilege to have good health care—to have care at all? Does our society, our country, value those who are in need . . . even when the need is physical? And do we value the very necessary and important work of home care workers? We pay them such low wages and provide little agency supervision or support. The frustrations and personal problems the workers face are brought into the client's home, and, as I can attest to, affect the quality of care provided.

It has been almost a year since my knee surgery. I have had many complications and setbacks, but am making slow progress. I still use a walker and wheelchair, and am gaining strength and endurance in weekly physical therapy. I do have two wonderful friends who come every week to help me with laundry, cleaning and transportation to various appointments, while other friends and my family continue to provide tremendous financial and emotional support.

As I struggle with the loneliness, isolation, and physical and emotional pain that accompany a long recovery, I do find comfort in faith, family, and friends. Time set aside for prayer each day alleviates the despair I sometimes feel, and brings me a peace that is greatly comforting. I have learned to appreciate the virtues of patience and humility, knowing that in accepting care from another, the gift of grace is given to us both. I have overcome some of the pride that perhaps blocks the help I seek, and in the process have forged a new and more honest relationship with my family, my friends, and myself. My compassion for others and for the struggles of home care workers has increased. I have a new understanding of what suffering really means.

In many ways, receiving—and not receiving—home care has tested and strengthened my faith, and increased my capacity to endure. Now, not knowing what shape or form my future will take, I wonder if my experiences are meant to help others.

CHAPTER 12

Care at Home: Virtue in Multigenerational Households

Hilde Lindemann Nelson and James Lindemann Nelson

Mrs. Morse, shriveled and bent from osteoporosis, is 76 years old. She broke her hip in a fall five years ago, at which time she moved in with her daughter and son-in-law, Carolyn and Matthew Broome. A second fall three years later left her bedridden, and now she is back in the hospital with a long list of problems. Among other things, she has developed serious pressure sores—some bad enough that bone tissue shows through—from being bedridden for so long. She needs regular changes of dressings on these sores, and while this is quite a painful procedure, medication has kept the pain at manageable levels. Her daughter (and to a lesser extent, her son-in-law) is deeply involved in her care.

When the physicians ask Mrs. Morse for permission to do a procedure, she invariably responds, "I don't know. You'll have to ask my daughter." Carolyn Broome, who is an attorney, keeps explaining to her mother that she must make these decisions for herself, but Mrs. Morse just shakes her head and says, "You decide." Carolyn's decisions have been reasonable ones, but recently she has become very concerned about the amount of pain medication her mother is getting. She had a long phone conversation with her aunt Bessie, Mrs. Morse's sister, about this and has been demanding ever since that the analgesics be administered much more sparingly. She says they make it hard for her mother to visit with her, and she wants her mother to be alert.

In the opinion of the treatment team, Carolyn Broome is becoming overinvolved in her mother's illness, letting her own psychological needs push her into making decisions that are increasingly inappropriate. The team learned that the sister has not even visited Mrs. Morse in a number of years. The call goes out to the hospital's ethics committee in hopes that some strategy for changing Carolyn Broome's mind about reducing the pain medication can be worked out. Failing that, perhaps there is a way of getting her out of the decision-making loop. As one nurse puts it, "I feel as though I'm being forced to participate in the abuse of a vulnerable patient." [1]

This is obviously a story about ethical conflict between a patient's professional caregivers and a member of her family. Less obviously, though, it is also a story about the care that is given by one generation of a family to a member of an older generation. In what follows, we explore a moral challenge common to multigenerational family life, particularly as it involves generational differences in household roles and responsibilities. We will argue that unless professional providers of health care are aware of this challenge and respectful of the demands that it places on family caregivers, providers can inadvertently exacerbate the difficulties the family faces when an elderly person requires medical care. Mrs. Morse's treatment team is on the very brink of doing just that. So first we will identify the challenge, then we will offer ways to respond to it, and finally we will consider what the professionals involved in Mrs. Morse's care are doing to hurt this family.

We conceptualize the challenge in a particular way, as a version of the general social problem of dealing with diversity—in this case, differences related to gender and generation. We identify three linked factors that make it difficult to deal well with intergenerational diversity within households-change, identity, and death. In reflecting on the virtues that are needed for coming to terms with these factors, we find the resources that can keep Mrs. Morse's treatment team from standing in the way of the daughter's attempts to care admirably for her mother.

THE MULTIGENERATIONAL FAMILY AS A 'MULTICULTURAL' FAMILY

Consider two prominent features of many contemporary families, especially middle-class American ones. The first feature is their role in

---

[1]This story is adapted from "Mrs. Shalev and Her Daughter," in H. L. Nelson and J. L. Nelson, 1995, *The Patient in the Family*. New York: Routledge.

providing fairly comprehensive care for their members, particularly those who are very young and those who are very old. The second is the pride of place given to homogeneity in our perception of families. Families share traditions, memories, and hopes, as well as genes. Their members very often take special pride in each other's accomplishments and feel particular shame at each other's failures. Love them or hate them, how we feel about the people who are members of our family is different from how we feel about the people who are not.

What makes it seem natural and right for family members to provide special care for each other is the perception of homogeneity; they all share in common something very important. But a second look at the supposed homogeneity of families reveals that things are rather more complicated. There are differences among family members too, some of them enormous. A piece of advice that feminist mothers sometimes pass on to their daughters is that every marriage is a "mixed marriage," in the sense that husbands and wives are culturally very differently situated. Should the daughter be inclined not to take this piece of maternal wisdom seriously—after all, she might think, women work outside the home just as men do, and wives have all the same privileges and responsibilities as their husbands—she might reflect on a "complication" in the ways families discharge their care-providing roles. Women still provide the vast majority of the hands-on caregiving that flows across generations, whether it be directed to a couple's children or to their frail elderly parents.

Families are actually remarkably diverse places. In one household, living in close proximity, one will find people distinguished not only by different temperaments, abilities, interests, and the like, but by some of the general marks of human difference through which we identify ourselves—differences that interact in complicated ways with powerful systems of social meaning and practice. Gender identity, of course, is one of these marks. Generational identity is another.

Gender identity has received immense attention in the last thirty years or so. Thanks to feminist theorists and activists, we now have a better sense of how gender shapes our ideas of ourselves and each other, and we have some strategies for how to resist the still prevalent and powerful ideologies of gender that unfairly restrict human lives.[2] One of the most powerful of those strategies is to let gender lie more lightly on us. If, for example, we do not mark everything in our lives

---

[2]The relevant literature is extensive. For a few examples of how feminist analysis has been useful in helping us think about intergenerational analysis, see M. Pearsall, ed., 1997, *The Other Within Us* (Boulder, CO: Westview), and M. U. Walker, ed., 1999, *Women and Aging* (Lanham, MD: Rowman and Littlefield).

in strongly gender-related terms—this is what men do, this is what "not-men" do—injustices against women will be less common, and people who happen to be female and people who happen to be male can live more harmoniously and comfortably with each other.

Is there the start of a lesson here for dealing with generational differences? Steven Sabbat and Rom Harré (1992), Tom Kitwood and his associates at the University of Bradford (Kitwood & Bredin, 1992), Margaret Morganroth Gullette (1997), and many other writers have, either explicitly or by implication, argued that being marked "elderly" is in many ways similar to being marked "female": You are taken less seriously than people who are not so marked, and your agency is more restricted. You are disempowered, not as a matter of your body, but as a function of your culture. Your place in your society gives you a different perspective from that of people who are regarded as essentially unmarked by gender or age, but those "paradigmatic people" tend to discount your special perspective if they acknowledge it at all.

Like sexism, whose ill effects in the larger society are mirrored and reproduced within families, ageism too finds its way into the home. Consider the household of a middle-aged, single mom, her elderly father, and her two teenage sons. Mom has a demanding job and the boys are busy with after-school sports, so dinner is usually a casual affair—people graze from the refrigerator or snack in front of the TV. Grandpa was brought up in the tradition of the family dinner table, where people gather for an evening meal and discuss the day's activities. When he suggests to his daughter that he might cook such meals at least a few times a week "so we can be a family," she replies, "Oh, Pop—we *are* a family. That's not how people live now." Grandpa feels dismissed and useless, knowing that his generation's view of how family members ought to interact simply does not count. Because his daughter and grandsons see family dinner as quaint and foreign, he is cut off from a custom that is important to him.

It might be useful to ask how we could resist the ideologies of age that disrespectfully restrict family members' lives. More specifically, it might be useful to wonder whether we could let membership in our own age cohort lie more lightly upon us. What virtues do we need to develop in ourselves if we are to live well in intergenerational households and, not incidentally, to grow old gracefully in the bargain?

THREE CHALLENGES: CHANGE, IDENTITY, DEATH

Virtues, as we will think of them here, are habits developed to protect or promote things that are valuable but somehow at risk, or difficult to achieve, or rare. Compassion, for example, is a virtue because the feelings of others are important in themselves, as well as being important guides to what we should think about the world and how we ought to act in it. Being in good touch with the feelings of other people is not always easy, however. It takes imagination and a willingness to be engrossed by something other than oneself. Taking "virtue" in that sense, then, we want to rough out some virtues particularly appropriate to living in a multigenerational household. To do so, however, we first need to get a sense of the three factors we mentioned earlier that make it difficult to deal well with intergenerational diversity at home.

Change

When one of us was 10, he clearly remembers being told, by someone in authority, that the human race's store of scientific and technological knowledge was doubling every seven years, and that soon it would double in six years, and then five. Whether this is or was true we do not know, but he remembers being both exhilarated and frightened by the pronouncement. How could he keep up with such a rate of change? How could he continue to be a vital part of a world moving so fast? At 10, he was already starting to fear his own obsolescence.

While these concerns (like, perhaps, his source) were overblown, they don't seem to have been altogether misplaced, or completely idiosyncratic. Consider how commonly people respond to social change by mooring themselves to some particular time that they see as the golden age. The stories they tell of that definitive time become the referents by which all other periods of their lives are measured. So common a mechanism must have many advantages, but it also can make it harder for people of different ages to be fully in sympathy with each other. It also buffers people from developments that might make their lives easier if they could but welcome them.

We would do well to look for better kinds of responses to the vertigo induced by social change. Rather than think of the stories of our past as anchoring us to the golden age, we might consider the ways such stories hold us captive, imprisoning us in one era of our lives and thereby estranging us from other eras that have also contributed to our lives in important ways. Such stories should be resisted. But they are powerful; they can become part of our very identities. Which brings us to the next theme.

Identity

We mean by "identity" the actions, experiences, and characteristics that people describe in answer to the question, Who am I? (Schechtman,

1996). Such answers take a narrative form, as we arrange the events of our lives in ways that allow us to make sense of them. The idea here is that as we reflect on the course of our life, we give it a narrative shape. The content of the stories of ourselves will include particular people, places, and times as well as particular actions we have taken and refrained from taking. These are among the things that we can hold on to in staking our claim to an identity. Being of our own generation and, by implication, not being of other generations, will often be an important part of these stories.

We want to draw attention, though, to a feature of identity that is problematic for living well in multigenerational intimacy—namely, that the narrative forms by which we make sense of our identities are, as a rule, taken from a cultural warehouse stocked with such forms, not all of which are harmless. For example, many of us take up the stock plot according to which it is a great thing to be young, but then one must inevitably fall from that original grace into a regrettable, decrepit old age (see Gullette, 1997).

This "aging as a fall from grace" plot is problematic for a number of reasons. In the first place, if you see your own aging as a story of decline and fall, it is hard to imagine how you could stop yourself from seeing other people, now in old age, as anything other than characters who have already declined and fallen according to the specifications of that plot. Second, if you make sense of old age by using this particular narrative, you will experience a kind of cognitive dissonance. On reflection, you will find it hard to think of your own life as having been in every important respect much superior when you were in your teens or early twenties. For many of us, it is just the reverse. And despite the commonly shared intuition that extreme old age really does involve a decline, there is another commonly shared intuition that says that death is a greater harm to a young person than to one who is very old. The reason for that intuition is surely that very old people have the advantage of having enjoyed many more years in which to experience the good things of life, and so are better off. And there is a dissonance in thinking of the old as both better off and yet fallen from grace.

A positive response to the challenge of living in diverse households comprising identities affected by stories of gender and generation is to meet the question, Who am I? with some others. How firmly am I that thing? How firmly *should* I be that thing? How strongly ought I to identify with stories whose plots and characters are supplied by forces not always friendly to the best ideals and aspirations? Perhaps we can find ways of answering these questions that will make generational differences seem less significant, ways that will make family members who were middle-aged when we were born seem less foreign. Perhaps the kind of identity we ought to encourage in ourselves, our elders, and our juniors is more fluid than fixed. To return to the story of the family dinner, for example, it might have been helpful if the single mother had not supposed that a very casual lifestyle was an unalterable feature of her and her sons' identity. Her father seemed willing to meet her halfway: He was not insisting that the family gather around the table every evening, and he was willing to do the cooking himself. Perhaps his daughter could learn a little more flexibility and teach it to her sons as well.

In addition to asking questions about our identities, we can also learn how to tell, and hear, counterstories. A counterstory is a narrative that resists sexist, ageist, or other oppressive identities that have been imposed on people through their own or others' narrative activity. Counterstories challenge or offer alternatives to the master narratives that identify us unjustly and thereby restrict our roles, relationships, and agency. The "fall from grace" narrative, for example, is a master narrative that identifies elderly people as being past it, no longer capable of exercising certain roles even if these constitute their identity. The counterstory that is needed here is one that resists the idea that the elderly person has "fallen from grace," affirming instead the grace that is now present in the person's life and so freeing the person from arbitrary restrictions. Counterstories can help break up the ways in which we think of ourselves or others as fixed against a template of generational meanings (see Nelson, 1995).

Death

Now it is time to examine a final master narrative, the "old age is about death" story.

Daniel Callahan (1987) has observed that people who are young can become middle-aged and then old; people who are middle-aged can become old. But people who are old have nowhere to go. If they don't stay old, they die.

It seems to us that this observation is too simple to provide much guidance as we try to respond to the diversity of real lives. But it is a way of articulating something that is widely believed about people in their eighth or ninth decade of life: The important thing about them is that they are going to die. Now this belief is odd, when you stop to think about it. Why pick out that age group as having a special connection to death? Up until this century, for instance, women were much more likely to die in childbirth than to live out the biblical life span, yet we have never strongly correlated being in one's twenties with dying. Our guess as to why we do correlate being old with dying is that people who are very old no longer center their lives around large projects, and people without such projects, we are tempted to think, are just marking time. They have nothing to do but wait for death.[3]

One interesting response to this problematic way of thinking about the very old—a counterstory, if you will—has been to try to see old age as indefinitely extended middle age. Callahan has criticized this strategy, in part on the ground that if old people see themselves in this way, they will typically pursue only the pleasures of middle age without being disciplined by its responsibilities. The strategy would conceptualize old age as a time of continual self-gratification, but since death cannot be integrated into such a conceptualization, death must be feared. Callahan proposes what amounts to a different counterstory. He has suggested that a project be fashioned, specific to the estate of being old, that involves self-effacement and a willingness to promote the projects and interests of younger generations. Such a course, Callahan argues, would make both death and old age more meaningful and easier to take.

We want to suggest another sort of counterstory altogether. Ours is one that resists the idea that the value and significance in human lives come mostly from having projects—either of the kind Callahan has in mind or the project of self-gratification. There are sources of meaning outside our endeavors, and these sources may be of special importance to the very old. To have lived at all, and have thereby contributed to shaping the history and the future of the world, is surely one of these sources of meaning. That our life stories have become part of the life stories of many other people, some of whom will survive us, is surely another. Many of us care deeply about certain people who will live after us, and their continuing experience can provide us with a sense of meaning that is not a function of our having current projects, or indeed, our being in the picture at all. Families connect one not only to a past, one's heritage—they connect one to a future, one's legacy. Our counterstory, then, has a "hands across the generations" plot to it.

FLEXIBILITY AND STORY TELLING AS VIRTUES

We have roughed out here the outline of some rather nontraditional virtues that allow us to meet the challenges of living in a multigenerational household. One such virtue is a kind of imaginative fluidity with respect to the shifts in one's cultural and social surroundings, with

---

[3]See the discussion of "career selves" in M. Walker, 1998, *Moral Understandings*. New York: Routledge.

respect to one's own identity, and with respect to how society presents death as a harm. The virtue of fluidity requires that one not be dominated by destructive narratives of change, identity, age, or death, and thus is much abetted by another virtue—the virtue of narrative competence. Such competence involves knowing how the stories we have told ourselves over our lives, and the stories others have told to and about us, shape us for good and ill. Such competence also involves knowing better how to undermine the stories and narrative fragments that are bad for people, and to resist them with more compelling, more admirable, more respectful stories.

We have been working out the idea that intergenerational households should be seen as multicultural households and that living well in this multicultural setting requires a set of habits, of ways of seeing and acting, that allow all family members to move more freely among the different cultures. This, we might argue, is what Carolyn Broome was doing when she phoned her aunt. She was taking seriously the differences between her generation and her mother's, and trying to honor those differences in the treatment decisions she made on her mother's behalf.

Carolyn's own golden age is the 1960s. In protesting U.S. military involvement in Vietnam, she and many other students were also demanding autonomy over their own lives. Her passionate commitment to self-determination is one reason she went to law school; it is why she wanted her mother to make her own decisions regarding her health care. The story of Carolyn's golden age held her captive until she started reflecting on the difference between her generation and her mother's. It was then that she turned to her mother's sister, who gave her a short tutorial in the rather different values that the older generation held dear. Theirs was the World War II generation, to whom solidarity in the face of a common threat was more important than individual freedom; interdependence prized above independence. Carolyn came to see that her mother was less interested in asserting her own preferences than in having her daughter make them for her. She valued the loving trust that existed between them.

Carolyn also came to see that she had been imposing on her mother the stock plot of decline in old age and, along with it, the story that what is important about old age—especially infirm old age—is that the person is going to die. Her talk with Aunt Bessie convinced her that her mother has something better to do than to lie there obtunded by morphine until death catches up with her. There is still grace in her life, but she cannot experience it when she is in an analgesic stupor. The visits from her daughter and son-in-law are a source of joy for her, worth the pain they cost her.

Carolyn Broome is thus trying to practice the virtues of flexibility and narrative competence as she enacts a counterstory to the narrative the treatment team is inadvertently telling about her mother. If the professional caregivers succeed in getting her out of the decision-making loop, they will be diminishing Mrs. Morse's old age and disrupting the bond between mother and daughter. That would be seriously wrong.

Are we advocating, then, that Mrs. Morse be left out of the loop? Not at all. If the treatment team can elicit from her a clear sense of what she wants, so much the better. It is likely, though, that she will say again what she has said before: "Ask my daughter." We are not suggesting that the staff exclude Mrs. Morse from the decision-making process. Our point is merely that patient autonomy is not the only value here. Equally important, it seems to us, are the values of love and connection across familial generations. These are worth preserving even if doing so makes of medical decision-making a messier business than the professional staff would like.

The virtues of flexibility and narrative competence do not by themselves suffice to perform well the many and difficult tasks of multigenerational living and caregiving. They cannot take the place of adequate social resources to allow decent care for frail elderly, very young, or ill family members who need it. But the challenges of dealing with different generations under one roof are not all, and perhaps not even primarily, financial. Whether the growing percentage of people who are old in our society will have good relationships, be honored, respected, loved, and, when necessary, cared for, is not only a question of what we have. It is also a matter of who we are.

REFERENCES

Callahan, D. (1987). *Setting limits.* New York: Simon and Schuster.
Gullette, M. M. (1997). *Declining to decline: Cultural combat and the politics of the midlife.* Charlottesville, VA: University of Virginia Press.
Kitwood, T., & Bredin, K. (1992). Toward a theory of dementia care: Personhood and well-being. *Ageing and Society, 12,* 269–287.
Nelson, H. L. (1995). Resistance and insubordination. *Hypatia, 10*(2), 23–40.
Sabbat, S., & Harré, R. (1992). The construction and deconstruction of self in Alzheimer's disease. *Ageing and Society, 12,* 443–461.
Schechtman, M. (1996). *The constitution of selves.* Ithaca, NY: Cornell University Press.

IV

Practice

CHAPTER 13

Mapping the Jungle: A Proposed Method for Ethical Decision Making in Geriatric Social Work

David Fireman, Sharon Dornberg-Lee, and Lisa Moss

INTRODUCTION

On some days when we, as geriatric social workers, head out to see our clients in the community, we may feel as if we are entering a jungle, where we never know what we might encounter around the next bend. Thus, when we have the opportunity to pause and reflect upon our practice, it is a welcome one. Attending "brown bag" ethics discussions at the Council for Jewish Elderly (CJE) has been an informative and thought-provoking way to explore, in a relaxed setting, serious ethical questions arising in geriatric social work. Yet a recent discussion at such a brown bag forum about expanding traditional ethical formulas left many of us social workers curious about where the rubber really meets the road. For example, academically speaking, it is worthwhile to uncover the philosophical meaning(s) of such concepts as autonomy or self-determination. But in real-life case work, such discussions rarely provide useful means for moving forward in the tough and wrenching dilemmas we face with our elderly clients and their significant others. So when we were approached about contributing to this project, we immediately began considering practical guidelines to be used when ethical dilemmas impinge upon our work. In this effort, we decided to marry two instruments produced by CJE and to illustrate the use of these instruments through case material.

CJE has developed two practice-based instruments aimed at clarifying assessment and decision-making processes associated with geriatric casework in home- and community-based settings. First, the *Ethics at CJE Community Programs: A Guide for Staff to Assist in Their Thinking of Ethical Situations*, hereafter referred to as *CJE Ethics Guide* (Council for Jewish Elderly, 1993), has proved to be helpful in organizing practitioners' thinking when working through ethical dilemmas. It succinctly identifies general ideas and principles in expanding thinking about issues on a case-by-case basis. It does not purport to offer answers, but rather helps pinpoint issues and conflicts at stake by identifying pertinent questions relating to ambiguous concepts, such as rights, values, competence, and incompetence. We intend to illustrate usage of this guide by way of presenting case material in the body of this chapter.

Second, the "risk chart" (see Figure 13.1) assists practitioners to examine the key risk factors in a given case. The assessment tool utilizes a chart format to place clients either at no, low, moderate, or high risk. Though the tool suggests these are discrete categories, in fact risk occurs along a continuum. Nonetheless, the assessment tool can be very helpful in placing clients along that continuum in each of five domains: cognitive, psychological, physiological, environmental, and social. This risk assessment tool will be used in the three case discussions that follow as a means of quantifying the level of risk. Our aim in this chapter is to use case material to illustrate the benefits of the risk chart in struggling with intervention considerations and actions on behalf of older persons.

Our main goal in all three cases is to counteract what we have perceived as a lack of method in making some of the hardest choices with which we are faced in geriatric social work. One such example centers on quality of life in a context of potential danger. Here, philosophical and academic discussions are generative only insofar as they produce practicable steps in real-life case work. By marrying the aforementioned tools, sticking to an actual method, and considering its bearing upon specific cases, we hope to point out the gaps in practice and suggest ways to constructively fill them. Yet, experience has taught all of us that often ambiguity is the rule. As a Zen poet once remarked, "The map is not the territory." For various reasons we all struggle to work in situations which are, by their very human nature, unpredictable and difficult to control. The superimposition of charts, graphs—essentially

	Minimal Risk	Low Risk	Moderate Risk	High Risk
Cognitive	• Intact memory • Memory loss with adequate supervision ADLs*: Yes IADLs**: Yes	• Some memory loss (Oriented x 3)*** ie: loses keys, forgets to shave ADLs: Yes IADLs: Yes	• Moderate-high memory loss (Oriented x 1 or 2) ie: burnt pans, eating properly?, forgets to take medication ADLs: Yes IADLs: No	• Severe memory loss (Oriented x 0 or 1) ie: wandering, confusion, explosive behavior, auto accidents ADLs: No IADLs: No
Psychological	• Psychological needs being met	• Mild to moderate impairment ie: depressed mood, sad, anxiety, bereavement ADLs: Yes IADLs: Yes	• Major impairment ie: depressed mood, anxiety, delusional, paranoia, psychotic, substance abuse ADLs: Yes IADLs: ?	• Severe impairment (danger to self or others) ie: suicidal, homicidal, unable to meet basic needs ADLs: ? IADLs: ?
Physiological	• 1 or 2 treated chronic diseases ie: diabetes, hypertension, heart disease	• Multiple treated chronic disorders • An untreated, less severe chronic disorder ADLs: Yes IADLs: Yes	• Multiple untreated chronic diseases • 1 or more untreated severe chronic diseases • Lice, scabies • Medication non-compliance • Significant weight loss ADLs: Yes IADLs: ?	• Life threatening health condition ie: major infection, gangrene, frequent falls, internal bleeding ADLs: ? IADLs: ?
Environmental	• Well maintained • Safe and secure	• Not maintained ie: unkept, roaches, mice, things in need of repair	• Potential danger ie: extreme clutter, no locks, stacked garbage, major appliances out of order	• Dangerous situation ie: no heat, water or electricity, no refrigeration for food that requires it, fire hazard
Interpersonal	• Closes contacts • Socializes	• No close contacts • No socialization • Unsafe neighborhood	• No/minimal contacts • Unintentional neglect by caregiver • Verbal abuse • Exploitation	• Total isolation • Intentional withholding of basic needs • Physical abuse • Danger due to others' behavior (psychotic family member, substance abuser)

*ADL = Activities of Daily Living (i.e., feeding, grooming, bathing, dressing, transferring, continence, toileting, mobility).
**IADLs = Instrumental Activities of Daily Living (i.e., housekeeping, preparing food, using telephone, doing laundry, taking medicine, handling finances, shopping).
***Oriented x 3 = Oriented to time, place, and person

Developed by Council for Jewish Elderly.

FIGURE 13.1 Risk chart.

the practice of putting things into boxes—goes only so far. Therefore, while we wish to point out the virtues of using a method to help unpack ethical dilemmas in geriatric home- and community-based social work, we also acknowledge its limits. Indeed, all methods eventually self-destruct in the face of reality, that is our dynamic and constantly changing world.

As geriatric social workers, we see clients both in their own homes and in assisted living facilities. Both of these settings create unique challenges and ethical dilemmas. Thus, two cases will explore home care ethical issues for social workers. The final case will elaborate some of the ethical issues inherent in assisted living for older persons. In addition to selecting cases that spotlight ethical decision-making across settings, we have selected cases that underscore another key challenge: deciding whether, how, and when to intervene in situations where a client's competence is in question. Thus, before moving to the cases, we elaborate further some of the key considerations that occur in home and assisted living settings, especially with clients who have impaired decision-making capacities.

ETHICAL CONSIDERATIONS IN HOME AND ASSISTED LIVING SETTINGS

Visiting clients in their own homes is often rewarding for geriatric social workers, as it affords an opportunity to see clients in their natural social milieu, and to assess their functioning in that environment. However, working with older adults in the home setting can present ethical dilemmas, particularly when a client is isolated. Ideally, other team members such as a nurse, the client's physician, and members of the client's social support system (such as family and neighbors), can join the social worker and client in establishing and implementing a treatment plan. But what of the all-too-common scenario in which a client is completely isolated and refuses outside intervention by anyone other than a social worker who has, over time, gained the client's tenuous trust?

When ethical dilemmas arise in these cases, the worker may feel isolated in his/her decision making, giving rise to a host of countertransference issues. As Golden and Sonneborn (1998, p. 83) point out, "[l]eft unchecked ... countertransference may result in a tendency for the clinician to 'overhelp' or 'underhelp' based on his or her own feelings, rather than on the client's situation and needs." For example, the worker's anxiety may cause her to intervene too aggressively, rather than to bear alone the moral responsibility of taking no action when a client appears at risk. Conversely, when a social worker is the only one in contact with a client, she may become complacent, lacking the "reality check" that professionals in other disciplines can provide as they question one another's assumptions and inform one another's practices. Certainly, in these situations, ongoing supervision and consultation are essential.

Another dilemma in home-based social work arises when a client's living environment presents potential health threats, such as the presence of rodents or risks posed by a client's hoarding behavior. Unlike more structured settings, such as assisted living, the client's environment is potentially a greater threat and the client's behavior is relatively unmonitored on a day-to-day basis. Certainly, as social workers, we have all felt relieved when clients who had lived in their own homes made the change to assisted living and the greater protection and structure we perceive it provides.

However, assisted living settings create a host of other ethical concerns. Practitioners, as well as consumers, have a perception that there is greater protection and structure in assisted living. Yet, at the same time, assisted living promotes an ethic of independence for older adults. As Bianculli and Wilson (1996, p. 13) have pointed out, "We talk historically about assisted living being a shift in paradigm with philosophical underpinnings of autonomy as opposed to safety." This shift seems to create ethical concerns that beg the same questions as those raised in a community setting, but with a different twist. In assisted living, the term negotiated risk has become a frequently used concept. The negotiated risk process has been described as a "process of identifying risks and trying to accommodate them" (p. 5) and "a process of negotiating the way that services required by a resident are going to be provided by either a facility or a service provider" (p. 7) (Bianculli & Wilson, 1996).

A common scenario in assisted living plays itself out around decisions regarding discharge from the facility. Residents age in place and their care needs begin to exceed the service package provided by the facility. This puts the residents at risk because their needs cannot be met with the level of staffing provided. In an effort to avoid nursing home placement, many residents or families want to "negotiate the risk" and say that they will assume the risk. A common discussion follows, with promises that the family won't sue if anything happens and the resident/family fully understand the risk associated with their choice to continue living in the facility. Often this discussion focuses on two issues: the risks of falling or wandering. This puts the practitioner in the position of having to wrestle with questions of autonomy versus safety, as well as the responsibilities and the risks involved for both the facility and the client. The fact that a negotiated risk process has taken place does not, in and of itself, free the practitioner from stopping to think about the ethical issues at hand.

What are the rights of the client? Who is making the decisions? And, the question that seems to come up often: Is the client's situation such that he or she really is not best served in an assisted living facility? Quality-of-life issues arise similar to those in the community. Often in assisted living, the resident is in a more structured environment and physical safety is not imminently compromised. Basic needs are met. However, in the case of a person with significant cognitive deficits who cannot participate in activities or direct him/herself within the setting, are there other factors to consider, such as psychosocial and spiritual sources of meaning? Is this individual best served in assisted living with no dementia care component just because she or he is not at risk in the physical domain? Those working in assisted living must struggle with these questions. The use of a planned method for identifying risk and asking questions to guide practice is essential to providing care that is not simply adequate, but based in an ethical framework.

ETHICAL CONSIDERATIONS CONCERNING DECISIONAL CAPACITY

The *NASW Code of Ethics* (National Association of Social Workers, 1996, p. 7) states, "social workers respect and promote the right of clients to self-determination and assist clients in their efforts to identify and clarify their goals."

We all believe that a competent elderly client has the right to decide how and where she or he lives and whether she or he receives health and social services. Yet the ethical principle of beneficence—to do good—may supersede the principle of client self-determination when the client lacks decisional capacity. However, in practice, decisional capacity—the ability to make meaningful and informed choices—is not easily gauged, nor is it a one-time determination. A cognitively impaired client's capacity to make decisions may vary from decision to decision, and even from day to day. Thus, concerns surrounding the assessment of decisional capacity can and often do create moral dilemmas for practitioners (Egan & Kadushin, 1998). Further, lack of adequate training in the assessment of decisional capacity can exacerbate these concerns (Healy, 1998).

As the *CJE Ethics Guide* explains, on a scale from lowest to highest ability a competent individual has the ability to demonstrate:

1. Communication of a choice;
2. Factual understanding of the issues;
3. Appreciation of the situation and its consequences;
4. Rational manipulation of information.

Conversely, an individual is deemed incompetent, and therefore lacking in decisional capacity, when he/she:

1. Is unable to understand the risks of compliance/noncompliance;
2. Is unable to explain the rationale for his/her decision; and/or
3. Is unable to determine possible ramifications of his or her decision and/or behaviors that are inappropriate to the situation.

(Council for Jewish Elderly, 1993, p. 9)

Even when a client appears to lack decisional capacity, the right to self-determination should prevail if the client is able to communicate a choice *and the assessed risk of abiding by that choice is low.* For this reason, assessment of the level of risk for any given client is intimately tied to the resolution of ethical dilemmas when self-determination and beneficence are the competing values.

Often our duties to protect the older person's safety, health, and welfare come into conflict with the ideal, indeed the duty, to respect his or her autonomy and self determination. We believe that it is wrong to leave clients with the impression that their interests' will—without exception—be considered primary. And yet, it is also essential to attempt at all costs to refrain from forced interventions just to make practitioners feel better. Here the concept of "welfare" comes into question. It seems "welfare" is chiefly defined in terms of physical safety. But, must physical safety considerations always be primary? Is quality of life strictly defined in terms of safety? Can one maintain quality of life in the context of potential danger? Put another way, how much credence is really given to psychosocial and spiritual sources of meaning in our definition of quality of life? Cases involving older persons with cognitive impairments invariably give rise to such considerations.

The case discussions that follow illustrate the complex web of factors that come into play in working with older adults in home- and community-based settings. Three diverse cases will be presented, the level of risk in each case will be assessed, and a discussion of relevant ethical considerations will follow.

The following case illustrates a central ethical dilemma, namely, that of the conflicting duties to protect the older person's welfare and rights simultaneously. The method utilized begins with the risk chart, plugging in relevant assessment data and thereby identifying the level of risk: no risk, low risk, moderate risk, or high risk. Then, relevant ethical questions arising from the *CJE Ethics Guide* are applied.

THE CASE OF MR. B

Psychosocial History

Mr. B is an 86-year-old Jewish man born in Hungary. He is the oldest in a family of four children. He has one daughter with whom he lives. He is a widower. Mr. B is a published author, clinical psychologist, and lawyer. He has led a life of considerable social and political activity. He is described by himself and family members as a radical thinker who has always wished to save the world with his ideas.

Physical, Cognitive and Emotional Status

Mr. B is diagnosed with probable Alzheimer's disease. Behaviors and personality changes suggest he is at the beginning of mid-stage. His physical health is stable after a quadruple bypass surgery 2 years ago. However, due to his cognitive decline he is unable to perform most activities of daily living (ADLs) and instrumental activities of daily living (IADLs) independently. Historically, he had others (e.g., a wife, maids) manage these tasks for him while he attended to his writing and practices. With prompting and cueing from his 24-hour live-in caregiver, he manages to do certain personal care tasks such as dressing and bathing. He is able to walk and negotiate stairs independently. Mr. B's emotional state is predominated by feelings of worthlessness and frustration. He had determined that his only hope is to resume his active social and political life. Although he is aware of his cognitive "slipping," he often does not acknowledge some of the real and potential limits it imposes upon his mobility. As his physical health is sound, he continues to have energy to be active outside of his home. However, without supervision he may be at risk for wandering, and getting lost and/or injured.

Social Support and In-Home Services

Mr. B currently lives with his daughter and live-in caregiver. His daughter is away most of the day. She manages household tasks such as bill paying and repairs, but is psychologically and emotionally estranged from her father. In fact, the two have had conflicted, often ruptured relations with each other for years. Consequently, Mr. B spends most of his time alone or with his live-in caregiver. He does not have access to and from his home without this individual.

Areas of Potential Risk

Mr. B is desperately trying to find a way to get his house key back from his daughter. She has confiscated it on grounds that he would get lost or hurt if he were to leave the house. Despite the fact that he has cognitive impairments, there is no past evidence that Mr. B could not find his way home, and when asked how he would manage in an emergency situation he responds appropriately. Moreover, Mr. B denies that there is a problem of risk and asserts that his rights are being violated. He argues this point quite lucidly and vehemently. Perhaps as a result of this forced intervention, Mr. B is becoming increasingly angry and at times agitated. His mental world is characterized by suspiciousness, violent images, even suicidal/homicidal ideation. In addition, depressive symptoms such as pervasive sadness, feelings of worthlessness, and changes in sleep and appetite have increased.

Assessing the Level of Risk

Mr. B's level of risk will now be explored in each of the five domains on the risk chart.

Cognitively, Mr. B appears to be at high risk. His mid-stage, probable Alzheimer's is affecting all aspects of normal mental functioning. Without assistance he appears unable to manage his ADLs/IADLs. His judgment and rational thought processes are declining in quality. He is at high risk, mitigated, however, by the fact that he employs a live-in caregiver. Yet, as is the case with many such afflicted individuals, Mr. B frequently has lucid, meaningful episodes in which he is both understood and understanding.

Psychologically, Mr. B appears to be at high risk. He has been increasingly delusional, suspicious, and angry. His suicidal/homicidal ideation in response to feeling imprisoned in his own home predominates and infects his psychological well-being. Again, even with the live-in caregiver he remains at high risk in the psychological domain.

Physiologically, Mr. B appears to be at low risk. His basic physical needs are being adequately addressed.

Environmentally, Mr. B appears to be at low risk. The immediate home and neighborhood environment are relatively safe and adequately maintained.

Finally, on the social contact domain, Mr. B is at low risk.

Questions/Issues Regarding the Case of Mr. B

We intend to show that, despite low risk in the important domains of physiological, environmental, and social contacts, Mr. B's entire world seems precariously balanced due to cognitive and psychological reasons. The following is a consideration of our own internal questioning process, to be followed by the major questions identified in the ethical guidebook at CJE.

Practice and ethical questions can become blurred, perhaps inevitably so. For example, there may be realistic ways for Mr. B to have a key to his home. Various possibilities within a problem-solving context have been generated. Perhaps having a key in his hand is what is most important to him. Perhaps it would meet a profound psychological need. Perhaps having it would lead to a reduction in his agitated state. Perhaps he would never use it. And what if he did? These are practice questions, yet it remains an ethical question as to what the proper balance is between a client's right to engage in (potentially) self-destructive behavior and a social worker's obligation to prevent that behavior. This question is particularly relevant since Mr. B has yet to be judged "incompetent" (adjudicated disabled) in a court of law, even though his daughter has so judged him.

An ethical dilemma involves two competing values. So, which of the values takes precedence? Physical safety or psychological well-being? Quality of life or quantity of life? No matter the answers, Mr. B perceives his own life to be increasingly bereft of meaning. To the extent that he is not allowed free access into and out of his own home, his right to self-determination is being diminished, stripped away.

Perhaps there are elements in Mr. B's case which give rise to possible elder abuse/neglect issues. Given the longstanding, conflicted relationship, could it be that his daughter is exacting a certain kind of vengeance by refusing to give him a key? Why has she not been willing even to consider some of the alternate possibilities? Does not the key to his house also represent a key to his happiness? What happens to considerations of Mr. B's happiness within the swirl of concerns about his physical safety? Is the no house key policy really for the client's protection or is it primarily in place to allay his daughter's potential concerns for his well-being, for that matter his estate? As the client has said himself, "My daughter perceives her action as helpful in order to satisfy her own thoughts and needs." In this sense, "protection" can be seen as an excuse. The client's wishes are being ignored. Consequently, he feels as though he does not matter. If he does not matter, then neither does his daughter, hence the suicidal/homicidal ideation. Surely, the fact of his mental deterioration contributes to this state of being (non-being), but what measures could be taken now to counteract the negative spiral into which he is falling? The suggestion is that, when there is a family member assuming a primary caregiving role whose behaviors may be directly or indirectly damaging to the older person, ethical dilemmas abound. Indeed, social workers in the aging field are often inundated with feelings about entering what may be a surrogate decision-making role on behalf of their vulnerable elderly clients. This case begs certain questions revolving around possible elder abuse/neglect that this chapter does not address specifically. Suffice it say that these possibilities only serve to further complicate smooth and easy decision-making.

Next, given the cognitive and psychological high-risk nature of Mr. B's case (as identified on the risk chart), the ethical guidebook leads to two essential areas of ethical exploration. The questions are provided to help the social worker determine when, and to what degree, a certain kind of intervention is justified: (1) family, support system, and community dynamics and (2) client self-determination and paternalism.

As home- and community-based geriatric social workers, we must attempt to understand the dynamics and quality of the client's relationships with family members, friends, neighbors, religious organizations, or community agencies. In this effort, it is essential to determine who the client(s) is/are. If the client has a support system, who are they? What are their capabilities and limitations? If the family is involved and caring, is the social worker advocating for the client's needs and acting as an advisor, rather than an executor? Does the client have family/other support system members that empower and advocate for him or her? How do these members of the support system affect the well-being of the client? How can the worker help to balance the interests of the older person with those of the family? Is the worker clear about the differences between the responsibilities of the agency (CJE) and the responsibilities of the family, and does the worker remember that it is not his/her role to take the place of the family, even if there is none or it is dysfunctional?

While client self-determination is a central social work tenet, geriatric social workers are keenly aware of its limits. Indeed, the right to self-determination is not absolute. Yet, the force of self-determination (as a value, a tenet, ethical principle) is not necessarily diminished as a justified claim even in cases when it is clearly on shaky ground. Thus, the question of whether to act paternalistically on behalf of the client becomes central. What exactly are the wishes of the client? What are the capabilities and limitations of the client (client system)? Is the client "competent"? To what extent has the risk been evaluated *and how? Is there a valid reason to override the stated desires of the client? Are there circumstances involving imminent harm? Does the social worker respect and encourage the autonomy of the client? Is the social worker fulfilling his/her responsibility to assist and/or bolster the client's ability to live and act autonomously? Is a paternalistic attitude appropriate?*

In sum, the method used to identify where Mr. B falls on the risk chart and what related ethical questions are generated, provides a kind of "map" of the territory. As controversial a practice decision as it might be, the social worker might lean toward attending to the need for Mr. B to have a key for himself. The decision to give him a real key, coupled with the stipulation that he be supervised in the beginning stages of his travels to and from the home, would be the most ethical action to take. It is not good enough to merely address the physical safety aspects of his situation. After all, his life—like all of ours—is multidimensional and complex. Though physical safety is important, we must ask pointed questions about who it is we are really trying to protect. At this stage, not having been adjudicated incompetent, not showing any compelling evidence that he would get lost or hurt—in some way physically damaged—he should be given the benefit of the doubt. His psychological well-being is suffering gravely, putting him and others at risk for the deeper, perhaps more permanent wounding of lost hope and dashed personal dignity.

As in Mr. B's case, the following case details the complex and often ambiguous nature of home- and community-based social work, forcing the professional to refine assessment and ethical decision-making skills on an ongoing basis.

THE CASE OF MRS. M

Psychosocial History

Mrs. M is an 82-year-old Catholic woman of Czechoslovakian descent. She has suffered numerous and severe traumas throughout her life. The older of two siblings, she reports a history of severe emotional and physical abuse by her mother. Mrs. M's brother died in childhood of a heart condition, a profound loss for Mrs. M. Mrs. M was married four times. Her first husband, a Jewish professional, was killed by the Nazis on his way home from the synagogue. Her second husband, a businessman, was killed during a bombing, also during World War

II. She describes her last two marriages as severely abusive. Mrs. M has had ten pregnancies, but only one surviving child. All of her other pregnancies ended in miscarriage or stillbirth. She has long been estranged from her son, citing his alcoholism and cruelty toward her. Mrs. M emigrated to the United States in 1952, shortly after her third marriage.

Physical, Cognitive and Emotional Status

Mrs. M now lives alone in a subsidized studio apartment in the low-income Uptown neighborhood. She has a history of coronary artery disease, osteoarthritis, and asthma. Her arthritis often presents functional difficulty for Mrs. M during flareups. Mrs. M has symptoms of dementia, with some short-term memory loss, difficulty learning skills and retaining new information, and impairment of executive functioning. She frequently loses valued items. She is unable to initiate phone calls and hangs up on unknown callers. She has marked paranoid ideation. She believes misplaced items have been stolen from her, that her former housekeeper and the building janitor are breaking into her apartment, and that others are attempting to defame her. Her apartment is cluttered as she hoards items including bags of clothing and fast-food containers. She typically presents with a labile mood and pressured speech. At times she is charming, cooperative and engaging. At other times, she is agitated and irate, only to become suddenly tearful. Given the lack of any third party source of information on the client's psychosocial and psychiatric history, it is difficult to determine if the client's persecutory delusions are the result of long-term mental illness or related solely to her dementia. She takes no psychotropic medications and refuses psychiatric intervention and/or geriatric assessment. Regardless of Mrs. M's psychiatric history, it is clear that what she experiences as the assaults of aging have triggered past traumas, at times overwhelming her capacity to cope with either the past or the present.

Despite these challenges, Mrs. M has many strengths. She is resourceful; able to articulate clearly her feelings, values, and desires; and surprisingly resilient. She is able to perform most activities of daily living without assistance. With cueing, she can also perform most instrumental activities of daily living.

Social Support and In-Home Services

Currently, Mrs. M accepts a weekly visit from her care manager as well as home-delivered meals. She refuses other services such as a personal care worker and has developed paranoid reactions to such workers in the past. Mrs. M has developed a close and trusting relationship with her care manager. She has only one other social contact, a middle-aged business owner whom she befriended and sees infrequently.

Areas of Potential Risk

Mrs. M often demonstrates poor judgment, for example going out for bread during the height of a blizzard. On this occasion, she fell in a snowbank and was not rescued by passersby for nearly an hour. At times she has demonstrated poor food safety skills, such as leaving cooked meat on the counter overnight. She is generally compliant with her medication regimen, but on occasion suddenly will discontinue use of a medication as she misattributes symptoms of illness, such as arthritis pain, to medication side effects. She has difficulty understanding how to regulate the heat and air-conditioning in her apartment. Her level of agitation may also pose a risk to her physical health. In many instances she has yelled and pounded her fists on the table, only to virtually collapse into her chair in exhaustion, sometimes experiencing chest pains. Further, Mrs. M frequently lives in a state of anxiety and fear secondary to her paranoid ideation. Though care management visits consistently provide her with practical assistance and supportive counseling that bring her relief, these visits are limited to once a week. By continuing to live alone and remain socially isolated, Mrs. M must tolerate a fairly consistent level of psychic pain with which she must cope alone.

Assessing the Level of Risk

Mrs. M's level of risk is explored in each of five domains (see Figure 13.1).

Cognitively, Mrs. M appears to be at moderate risk. She is oriented to person, place, and time, and functions relatively well despite minor cognitive impairment. Though she loses items frequently, such as keys, eyeglasses and her bankbook, this behavior does not place her at serious risk, particularly given her resourcefulness in problem-solving when items are lost. Her questionable attention to food safety and her spotty compliance with medication pose a somewhat more substantial, i.e., moderate, risk.

Psychologically, she is at moderate risk due to her anxiety and paranoia.

Physiologically, she is at low risk as she has multiple chronic disorders but is receiving treatment for them and receives regular medical care.

Environmentally, she is at low risk as her apartment, though cluttered due to Mrs. M's hoarding behaviors, is free of debris and pests and does not pose a safety threat.

Finally, in the social domain, Mrs. M is at moderate risk. With the exception of contact with her care manager and one friend whom she sees infrequently, she is completely socially isolated. She spends most of her time alone. She is estranged from family, has difficulty forming and sustaining relationships, and rejects most supportive services due to paranoid ideation.

Discussion of the Case of Mrs. M

The key dilemma here for the social worker is whether to intervene to place this client in a facility that would maximize her safety or to abide by the client's wish to remain in her own home. Thus, the competing values in this case concern self-determination versus beneficence. Given the lack of assisted living options for a client with a very low income and mental illness, the only alternative setting for this client would be a nursing home. The very lack of appropriate placement options poses a moral dilemma for the care manager who must decide whether the client should continue to live independently in her current environment where she is at risk, or be placed in a nursing home, which exceeds her care needs and restricts her freedoms.

The CJE Ethics Guide *is useful in identifying the relevant ethical questions to consider in this case. First: Is the client competent? Mrs. M is able to articulate clearly her preference to continue living independently. Mrs. M has a factual understanding of most of the issues involved in this decision, though her perception of what an alternative setting such as a nursing home would be like is grossly distorted. For example, she believes that food might be withheld in a nursing home and minimal standards of cleanliness would not be maintained. She does understand that continuing to live alone has the consequence of her being lonely, lacking an optimal level of assistance and support, and leaving her vulnerable, for example in the event of a health crisis. Her ability to rationally manipulate information varies considerably from day to day, based on her level of agitation and paranoid ideation. When she is not agitated, she is able to discuss rationally various options for her future.*

Second: Is the person's bad judgment severe enough to put him or her at imminent risk? *Mrs. M is at moderate risk in the cognitive, psychological, and social domains. However, the risk in each of these domains does not place her at imminent risk, a central consideration. Though it is possible that the client's impairment and isolation can lead to harm, the risk remains just that, a possibility. The client's ability to function without coming to serious harm in the year and a half that her care manager has worked with her, and her demonstrated ability to mitigate harm through her own perseverance and resourcefulness, are testament to the fact that the risk of harm is not imminent.*

Finally, Has the worker thought about the harm, as well as the benefits, that his/her intervention will have on the client and on the client/professional relationship? *If the worker were to act paternalistically and attempt to have Mrs. M placed in a long-term-care facility, that action would have the benefit of markedly reducing the level of risk to this client. It would have the potential of additional benefits to Mrs. M, such as 24-hour access to staff that could provide support, reassurance and practical assistance as needed. Ideally, Mrs. M might also develop relationships with other residents in a more structured setting, thereby increasing her social support and diminishing her isolation and the anxiety this triggers.*

However, significant harms would equally be likely to occur. First, this type of paternalistic intervention, so at odds with the client's own goals for herself, would almost certainly bring about the end of the client/professional relationship. This would be experienced as a traumatic loss for the client in what has been a life marked by traumas. Further, the client would experience a very real loss of freedoms. She would no longer be able to walk around a familiar neighborhood, feeding the pigeons and running errands, or know the simple pleasure of making herself a cup of coffee in her own home. There is also a very real risk that the client might decompensate psychologically in a nursing home, removed from familiar surroundings and not permitted to engage in behaviors she finds soothing, such as hoarding certain items. In this scenario, her paranoia would likely increase.

At present, the care manager continues to see the client weekly to provide support and monitor the level of risk over time. While she has chosen in favor of self-determination at this time and against a paternalistic intervention to reduce the level of risk, the process of assessment—like Mrs. M herself—remains dynamic, changing over time and demanding continual reexamination.

Next, the equally subtle and complex ethical issues inherent in the area of assisted living social work will be explored. Here, the notion of "negotiated risk" is examined more thoroughly.

THE CASE OF MRS. J

Psychosocial History

Mrs. J is an 89-year-old widow. She lived in a group living building and moved to a more supportive assisted living facility a year ago when she needed more assistance. She has two daughters who both live in close proximity. Her daughters are very involved with their mother's care and, between the two of them, visit daily. They make all decisions for her. She has one sister whom she sees regularly. Mrs. J was a homemaker. She is a social woman who forms significant friendships with others and who makes new friends with ease. Mrs. J is depressed. She is often teary, expressing sadness about her situation.

Social Support and Services

Mrs. J receives assistance with bathing, dressing, and medication reminders. Staff provides these services as part of the package offered and included in the monthly rent. There is staff available to residents in the building 24 hours a day.

Areas of Potential Risk/Negotiated Risk

Mrs. J meets the criterion for discharge from the assisted living facility because of her frequent falls and episodes of incontinence. Staff has met with family and advised them of this. Her daughters respond that they value autonomy over safety and they are adamant that they do not want their mother to move to a nursing home. They feel that living in assisted living promotes their mother's quality of life and sense of dignity. They have been involved in continuous discussions of negotiated risk with staff and are comfortable living with the risks that have been identified. The two major areas of risk that have been discussed are: the possibility of a fall that would result in injury and the possibility of wandering from the building unnoticed and getting injured or lost. The daughters and the client's physician maintain that the client could fall in any setting she lives in and that the possibility of her wandering is remote, as the staff check on her frequently. They state that they are willing to accept the fact that the facility cannot provide services that will prevent these potential risks from occurring, and that they will accept the risk. The facility does not have a formal process for negotiating risk, nor a written negotiated risk agreement.

Assessing the Level of Risk

Mrs. J's level of risk may be explored using the five domains identified in the risk chart (see Figure 13.1).

Cognitively, Mrs. J would fall in the high-risk category because she exhibits general confusion and has wandered. She is disoriented to time and place. She is able to identify her family members and staff who are consistent and familiar to her. In the assisted living setting, an argument could be made that, because she lives in a structured environment that provides 24-hour supervision, this risk is mitigated.

Psychologically, she is at low risk. She does exhibit a depressed mood and expresses feeling sad about her failing health, however, she has close relationships with her family and actively participates in building activities. Her depression does not impinge on her functional abilities.

Physiologically, she is at low risk. The brain tumor was diagnosed many years ago and, though inoperable, it is not malignant or fast-growing. She receives regular medical attention.

In the area of environment, Mrs. J is at low risk. The building is not locked at night when Mrs. J is prone to wandering, but there is a staff person who is awake at all times.

In the area of contacts, Mrs. J has no risk.

In assisted living there are considerations other than those outlined above that must be taken into account when assessing risk. Bianculli and Wilson (1996) identify six questions as "a measuring stick for high risk":

Will behavior result in:

- *Severe or immediate negative consequences to resident and/or others?*
- *Imminent or very probable near-term physical or psychological harm?*
- *Physical harm to another resident, staff or visitor?*
- *Severe disregard for the dignity and/or security of others?*
- *Probable ridicule and/or isolation?*
- *Severe property damage?*

The last four of these six questions would not be factors in a home-based setting. There has been consideration of the ethical dilemmas faced by care managers who work in home health care, long-term care, and in the community (Healy, 1998), however, the dilemmas faced by those working in assisted living are emerging as the industry grows. It seems that with negotiated risk come a new set of ethical dilemmas. Negotiated risk is a concept that has come out of the assisted living industry. The case of Mrs. J illustrates some of the dilemmas that arise. Mrs. J is a compromised individual whose family is making choices for her. This family is very capable of negotiating systems to get their needs met. Giving them the option to accept the risks associated with staying in this facility enabled them to make a choice that respected their mother's autonomy. The social worker in this setting has obligations to both the client and the setting. The decision this family has made to keep the client in assisted living rather than a more restrictive environment does not pose harm to other residents, staff, or visitors and does not present severe disregard for the dignity and/or security of others. The episodes of incontinence could result in ridicule and/or isolation, but this risk is possible rather than probable. There is no risk of severe property damage. When looked at using these questions, the worker may conclude that Mrs. J could stay in this facility. If one were to examine this particular case using physical safety as the prevailing value, one might reach a different conclusion.

Ethical considerations in the case of Mrs. J touch upon the capabilities and limitations of the facility's staff and whether or not the client is really best served by staying in this setting. Does her family's wish to respect her dignity and autonomy override other values such as safety? Are there any obvious differences between the worker's values, those of the facility, and those of the client that may affect the worker's thinking and his or her ultimate decision-making ability? The latter is an interesting question in assisted living, as the value of autonomy is very strong. In this worker's experience, staff feels invested in "keeping" residents in the assisted living setting and out of the nursing home. They measure their worth by the ability to provide care that keeps an individual out of institutional long-term care. Using tools such as the risk chart and the CJE Ethics Guide can help staff identify the ethical concerns and ensure that they do not get buried in the language of negotiated risk.

CONCLUSION

All three cases chosen show the complicated nature of geriatric social work in home- and community-based, as well as assisted living, settings. We have explored some of the many ethical implications stemming from dilemmas such as physical safety versus psychosocial and spiritual well-being. Although crystal clear answers remain hard to come by, a method that aims to maintain the client's self-determination and dignity should be attempted. It has been said that if an artist did not have a frame she or he would have to paint the whole world. While it is impossible to capture the whole picture, it is important to proceed by way of a useful method as we strive to identify the most ethical intervention(s). First identifying the level of risk involved, and then proceeding to identify the most pertinent ethical questions concerning these risks, seems to provide a relatively clear and instructional way to do so. As client situations change, so do workers' assessments and therefore, so too would the outcomes of this same method. Though academic discussions partly fuel our work with expansive ideas and propositions, it is the on-the-ground, sometimes jungle-like environment of rights, values, and ethics that challenges us most to become methodical about the ways we intervene in concert with and on behalf of our elderly clients.

ACKNOWLEDGMENTS

The authors wish to thank Dennis Beauchamp, LCSW, and Carol Harris, RN, who developed the CJE risk assessment chart, as well our other colleagues at CJE from whom we have learned much as we struggle together to practice ethically-driven social work.

REFERENCES

Bianculli, J. L., & Wilson, K. B. (1996, October). *Negotiated risk in assisted living.* Paper presented at the American Association of Homes and Services for the Aging's 34th Annual Meeting and Exposition, San Antonio, Texas.

Council for Jewish Elderly. (1993). *Ethics at CJE community programs: A guide for staff to assist in their thinking of ethical situations.* Unpublished manuscript.

Egan, M., & Kadushin, G. (1998). The social worker in the emerging field of home care: Professional activities and ethical concerns. *Health and Social Work, 24*(1), 45.

Golden, R., & Sonneborn, S. (1998). Ethics in clinical practice with older adults: Recognizing biases and respecting boundaries. *Generations, Journal of the American Society of Aging, Fall* (Supplement: Ethics and Aging: Bringing the Issues Home), 83.

Healy, T. C. (1998). The complexity of everyday ethics in home health care: An analysis of social workers' decisions regarding frail elders' autonomy. *Social Work in Health Care, 27*(4), 34.

Loewenberg, F. M., & Dolgoff, R. (1985). *Ethical decisions for social work practice* (2nd ed.). Itasca, IL: F. E. Peacock Publishers, Inc.

National Association of Social Workers. (1996). *NASW code of ethics*. Washington, DC: Author.

CHAPTER 14

Adult Day Services: Ethics and Daily Life

Pat Stacy Cohen

Adult day service programs have been available to older adults and their caregivers in the United States since the late 1970s. These programs are designed for people who need supervision and/or assistance with activities of daily living (ADLs) and for their families who are committed to keeping them at home or in the community. Unique in the constellation of home care services, all the clients come to a center for socialization and services, then go home to families at the end of the day. A recent survey conducted by the National Adult Day Service Association (NADSA) demonstrates the vulnerability of the typical day service participant: Most are women with an average age of 76, and while some live alone, they most often live with a spouse, adult child, or other family members. Cognitive impairments are found in at least 50%, most require nursing services at least weekly and need help with at least two activities of daily living just to manage at home. The profile of this population is similar of that of nursing home residents. Family and adult day services make it possible for them to remain part of their community.

People involved in adult day services understand the special nature of the program. Families refer to it as "a lifesaver," participants call it "the club," and staff marvel at the twists and turns of a typical day at the center. Because participants go to the home of a relative or are dependent on others for some help when they are not at the center, relationships and intimacy are inevitable between families and staff. For example, in our Center we share techniques with families about how to best offer personal care to a participant; we know when the family car is in the shop; we intervene in health related situations; we hear about personal problems that affect attendance at the center; we are notified about job changes and moves; and we listen as the clients tell us stories from home.

At the Center, each of us brings our own values and sense of "right" and "wrong" to bear on day-to-day occurrences. Because of the intimacy of the setting, we are often called upon to expose our personal values and to have painfully honest discussions with each other before interacting with families about incidents that occur before, during, or after a day at day services. This chapter will describe some typical scenarios we have experienced over many years at the Center and will provide reflections on the moral terrain of this unique setting.

THE DECISION-MAKING PROCESS: SAM AND MARTHA

Sam and his wife Martha lived on the first floor of a two-flat apartment building; his daughter and her family lived upstairs. Sam was in frail health following several heart attacks but he got around with a walker and had no cognitive impairments. His wife ran the household, did all of the driving and managed Sam's life in a way that worked for both of them. He had carried many responsibilities as a bank vice president and was glad to relax in retirement. Sam started coming to adult day service when his wife's health began to deteriorate. He was well liked by everyone at the center. Sam's family drove him to day care everyday so other clients and staff got to know the family well over the years. His daughter ran a small catering business so it was not unusual for her to bring "treats" to the center.

Sam was 89 years old when he got the news that his leg needed to be amputated below the knee due to problems with his circulation. His family and doctor warned him that he might never walk again, and that he would not be the same again after the surgery and recuperation process. The news devastated Sam. He worried that his immobility would limit his chances of remaining active in the community, curtail his attendance at the center or even necessitate moving out of his lifelong home. He became visibly depressed as he resigned himself to spending the rest of his days in a wheelchair.

Sam's friends in adult day care encouraged him to talk about his situation and through a series of conversations with the nurse and his family, and encouragement from his peers, he decided he wanted to work toward a prosthetic device following the surgery. His doctor was skeptical . . . after all Sam was almost 90 years old and he didn't know anyone that age who had chosen the artificial limb instead of a wheelchair. The surgery went well and Sam's rehabilitation was remarkable. Several months later, Sam walked back into the center amidst the cheers of everyone.

The process that led to this happy ending involved a number of questions that merit consideration.

- Is it appropriate for staff to become involved in this type of decision since it has nothing specifically to do with adult day care? There are, no doubt, readers who think that staff became too involved with Sam and his medical situation. Sam trusted the nurse at the center; she was the first to learn that he wanted to do more than spend the rest of his life in a wheelchair. She encouraged him to speak to his family, his doctor and his peers at the center. She helped him explore all the possibilities and did some of the leg work for him. She spoke to other orthopedic professionals, educated Sam about what to expect and painted a realistic picture of what the recuperation could entail. The nurse treated Sam as a person with a right to know the facts and to decide his own future.

  At the same time, it was important to involve the family early in the discussion since this course of action, which included a prosthetic device and subsequent hours of rehabilitation, introduced added burdens for the family caregivers.

  Health care professionals tend to forget that people like Sam have held positions of power and carried responsibility and that they should be included in discussions of this nature. Such inclusion, however, does not depend on one's past position. It is something we owe to everyone. Morally, a trusting relationship is at the heart of caring practices. Day service staff and Sam's peers had such a relationship with him, and he benefited from it.

- The support Sam received from the day care staff and his peers could have created conflict between Sam and his family. When do the wishes of the family caregiver take priority over that of the client? The entire outcome of this situation would have been different if the family caregivers had been unwilling or unable to give Sam the opportunity to rehabilitate maximally. Imagine the discord if Sam's family had met his first conversation with negativism. The longstanding relationship between the family and staff at day care could have been jeopardized or lost forever. Think too of the impact on Sam if he were put in a position of having to stop trusting and sharing his thoughts, hopes, and aspirations with the nurse for fear of the negative repercussions with his family.

- It is not easy for staff to keep a balance between client wishes, family needs, and what seems to be the right thing to do. In a dramatic instance, such as when a client experiences a heart attack at the center, calling 911 is the "right" response. The "right" thing to do is less clear when the nurse discovers a client whose blood pressure is too high, phones the family, and is informed that the physician is "ok with that," and that the family intends to do nothing about it right now. The staff can attempt to educate, cajole, and advise the family about a situation but securing family involvement is never a guarantee that a perfect response will occur. The staff may feel powerless to influence a situation directly and must constantly come to terms with their feelings and still be ready and willing to offer information and advice when the next incident arises.

  A major dilemma for staff is how to emphasize the opinion of the client without discounting the family caregiver who in most instances must implement any decision. What happens when these are diametrically opposed? Should the dependent older adult always be expected to defer to the decisions of others? Should the family always defer to the autonomy of the dependent older adult? There will be times when staff at the center will be expected to support a plan or decision that is not what they would have chosen in the same situation. It may be difficult for staff to come to terms with these inner conflicts.

- In this case the nurse exercised good judgment. She got the facts, gave Sam information and facilitated conversations with everyone before any decision was made. What if that were not the case? It is possible for staff to offer "bad advice" or an opinion grounded in personal biases (see Golden and Sonneborn, chapter 9, this volume). Well-intentioned suggestions offered without enough background or knowledge can do more harm than good.

- Sam's peers and friends at the center confirmed and validated the direction he wanted to take. Should other clients at the center be able to hear about and discuss these things or is it a breach of confidentiality? What do you mean when you use the word confidentiality? How would it apply in this situation? In this example, Sam talked freely about his personal conflicts and his feelings. If staff believed that this free expression was inappropriate and asked him to stop, would that not be depriving him of an opportunity for peer support in the name of confidentiality? Should Sam's peers be encouraged to support Sam and give their opinions or should they be asked to stay out of his business since it just complicates an already difficult time for Sam? Some staff may think that protecting Sam and other clients from talking about certain subjects is their role and that hushing up certain discussions is good for the group. They may believe that it is in the best interests of their clients to squelch negative discussions in difficult situations, for example, when a participant dies, enters a nursing home, or makes a comment such as "I'm tired and sick and wish I could just die peacefully." Staff members need to come to terms with their own feelings and fears so that they can facilitate such conversations among clients. This may be the only opportunity for the older adults to receive peer support. Clients need a safe place to express "end-of-life" and other difficult thoughts, but if staff members are not attentive to the older adults' viewpoint, or are afraid of their own feelings about these issues, they may feel compelled to "cheer up" clients rather than listen. The fact that this level of support and interaction were available to Sam at the adult day care center indicates the nonjudgmental atmosphere that exists in that setting, and in most adult day services programs.

- Consider the comfort level that existed between staff, family, and client that enabled them to discuss options for Sam other than the permanent use of a wheelchair. When honest and open communication is nurtured at all levels and routinely applied, staff will respond in this manner when major events occur. In addition, they consider acknowledging and honoring the opinions of adult day service enrollees and providing them with opportunities to voice them to be a moral imperative. Consider what would have happened if the family or the personal physician were totally opposed to Sam's plan for wearing a prosthesis. Sam, in his wheelchair, would have needed his friends at the center to provide consolation and support. In that situation, staff would have grappled with the question of whether they did a disservice to Sam by giving him hope for another outcome or whether their sincere efforts during his personal crisis gave him a sense of belonging to a group who cared about his well-being. Consider the intrinsic moral value in the very action of working through this experience with Sam.

- Adult day centers usually employ a small number of people; the team approach to serving the clients often results in an overlapping of duties. Administrators and staff in adult day service wear a number of "hats." They are case manager, friend, helper, confidante, advocate, adversary, professional, and member of the family all in one day. These various roles and the staffing structure in adult day service centers can create a number of "moral dilemmas" or conflicts during the course of providing service. For example, does speaking the truth as a friend run counter to the advice a "professional" would give to someone like Sam? Staff would certainly have felt conflicted if Sam had come to them in their role as confidantes and disclosed that he was very upset about how things were going at home related to his medical condition and then requested that they not share these concerns with his family. It is difficult to honor confidential information offered by clients when the information is vitally important to their well-being and of a "need to know" nature to primary caregivers. The moral complexities linked to confidential sharing by a client can be exacerbated even further when staff fears that there could be negative consequences for the client if they reveal information to family members. The consequences may range from physical abuse to reprimands, punitive actions, or disparaging remarks. Staff, in their role as client advocate, must weigh each situation and opt for the course of action that either offers the greatest benefit or sometimes causes the least harm. Obviously having to make a decision that causes the least harm weighs heavily on staffs' moral sensibilities.

Sam's successful outcome was possible because staff believed that Sam's wishes were realistic and that his ideas had value. They made an investment in his personal decision that demonstrated a mind-set that is vital when clinicians practice ethically.

STAFF/FAMILY PARTNERSHIP

Staff members at the center and family members of the participants function as partners in the caregiving process. Families who drop parents off on the way to work share useful information with a staff member, "S/he was up most of the night, so s/he may be sleepy today," or, "S/he didn't really want to wake up this morning so s/he may be a little crabby." Staff may express concerns about the caregiver who looks very tired because she hasn't slept well or for the spouse who just isn't psychologically ready for a nursing home placement even if it may be time for that level of care. The next case explores some of the complexities in this partnership.

Clara, who is now in the later stages of dementia, has been coming to adult day care for about 6 years. She lives with her daughter, Alice, who is committed to keeping her at home even though Clara's other children think it's time for nursing home placement. Clara's functional ability is severely impaired. She often needs coaxing and hands-on assistance just to move about the center and staff members take turns

> feeding her at lunch. She has recently become bowel incontinent and because she is no longer able to follow directions, changing her has dramatically increased the ratio of one-to-one time with Clara.
>
> Clara is very gracious. Even with her limited abilities, she still intuitively knows when to sit next to an anxious client and calm her by putting a hand on her knee and offering a "word" of encouragement. Staff knows it is time to begin discharge planning with Alice but their love for Clara and their admiration for Alice's dedication makes it difficult to begin the process.

This case study illustrates the bonds that evolve between staff, participants and families at the center. It also illustrates that feelings of love and admiration can be a source of conflict and discomfort. Before taking action, the staff will need to discuss some of the following issues that have important ethical dimensions.

- There are service limitations in adult day service. Belief in the goal to keep Clara in her home just isn't enough to eliminate the frustrations staff feel when they provide care to her in the day service setting no matter how much they "want" to do it. Each center needs to develop discharge policies that it shares with family members before and during the discharge process. These policies serve as a framework for deciding about the appropriateness of clients to continue participation in the program. They can then be used as an objective tool in extremely personal and emotional discussions, while staff continues to empathize with Clara and Alice.

All staff involved in caregiving must have opportunities to deal with their own feelings when someone is about to leave the program. When making or implementing policies, managers should not discount the affections or frustrations of nurses and personal care aides who provide direct care. Discharge should be an interactive process within the center that allows staff to discuss options. Staff members who care for Clara must know their opinions count. Managers and staff must be able to communicate throughout the process so that everyone is comfortable, not only with the decisions, but with how decisions are made.

- Discharge from the program should include time for clients and family to make the transition to another type of service. Informal conversations about the status of the client should precede formal notices about a planned discharge. Specific time frames need to

be established and shared with family members so that alternative arrangements can be made. In some cases, family may even welcome the recommendation of the center because it removes the burden of deciding about the next level of care from them.
- The population in adult day service includes a variety of clients with different levels of need. Do higher functioning clients with fewer personal care needs than a person like Clara automatically receive less staff time? Is this situation ethically acceptable? A participant at the center who has a history of mental health problems such as depression could benefit from daily one-to-one contact of about an hour (the amount of time spent providing bathroom assistance to Clara) but that rarely happens. How can staff fairly balance the amount of time spent with clients in general? Since making choices are regular components of day service life, staff need to feel comfortable with the center's approach to care.
- Clara is a pleasant, easy-going person, and the staff admires Alice. The relationship of kindness that exists between this mother and daughter is a praiseworthy quality that the staff silently recognizes each time they interact with Alice or care for Clara. Do Clara and Alice receive preferential treatment because they are nice? Probably. Even though we know that all clients should be treated equally, staff care providers have an easier time helping people who are kind. There is also a risk that staff may interact more with clients who can offer feedback to them and unwittingly ignore clients with limited language or social skills. Self-monitoring and honest reflection by the staff group can help to insure that biases don't enter into how care is offered at the center.

It is probably true that staff members feel a sense of special commitment to Clara because she has been in the program for 6 years. Such staff loyalty to Clara and her family can generate internal conflicts among the staff. A new aide who has only known Clara for a short time will not have bonded with Clara in the same way as staff who have known her for a number of years. The staff feels admiration for the efforts of Alice on Clara's behalf. Are they seeing the situation clearly or do their emotions color what they see? Emotions and feelings are deeply important in this process of making ethical decisions. They strengthen our moral perception and give depth to our understanding of each situation and person. Can staff have feelings for clients and still be "professional" and ethical in their responses? Of course they can. Community-based programs such as adult day service do not rely on high-tech devices or state-of-the-art equipment but rather on the high-touch interactions of staff. Staff must feel the connection to families and clients in order to be effective professionals in this setting.

- Some participants in adult day service settings attend the center 5 days a week for up to 10 hours per day for several years. It is understandable that bonding takes place under these circumstances. These emotional attachments are the catalyst that motivates staff to treat clients as individuals who have a rich past and are worthy of respect. Knowing participants is an important feature of caring practices. Adult day service staff gets to know clients and families at an intimate level because they are partners with family members in caring for the clients. Workers are invited to their birthday parties, hear their secrets and many times learn about their home life in great detail. Day service employees frequently do "extra" things for participants. It is sometimes difficult for them to understand why other agencies or service providers don't have the same level of investment in the well-being of the client. This can lead to intolerance of other providers or unrealistic expectations when clients with complex needs are served by multiple agencies.

LEAVING THE ADULT DAY CENTER

Clients leave adult day service for a number of different reasons. In some instances the decision seems logical and is even encouraged by staff. In other instances the staff may have a hard time understanding the family's motivation. In those situations being supportive of a family and acknowledging things from their perspective can produce ethical quandaries for staff.

Harry is a retired attorney who lives with his children. He was diagnosed with dementia about 6 months ago but still attended board meetings and special events at his former law firm. His children were skeptical about whether Harry will "fit in" at the center but during the initial assessment interview, Harry agreed to give it a try. The plan was for Harry to attend two days a week, which still left him time to pursue his other interests. Within a week, Harry became one of the center's leaders. He announced to his family that he wanted to come to the center every day and he gave up most of his visits to the law firm. Harry's daughter-in-law was amazed and confessed to staff that the visits to the law office were getting pretty uncomfortable anyway.

After one year of attendance, Harry's family called to notify staff that he would be moving to a retirement home. All the clients and staff loved him. He was one of the higher functioning people at the center and everyone was shocked by the news. Harry really didn't like the idea but he told the social worker that he has resigned himself to the situation. Harry knows that he can't live alone anymore and has decided that his kids should not have to sacrifice their career goals to be with him. He has been out to visit the retirement village and he says it is "the best money can buy." The staff is having a very hard time dealing with this news. They think someone should talk to the family and try to change their minds. At a staff meeting they suggested that maybe Harry should be counseled to resist the idea and use his money for in-home companions and other options.

- The ability and capacity to care for an elder family member is unique to each family. Some family members seek advice, ask for options and talk to staff about their concerns, while others announce changes. Measuring and judging one caregiver's coping skills compared to other families or some ideal can create conflict. Family dynamics and past experiences affect present actions and decisions. It is critical for staff to acknowledge the perspectives of all concerned parties. Harry has come to terms with the arrangement. Are staff members listening to his opinion?
- What mechanisms are in place for staff to discuss their concerns? Maybe staff has a need to grieve and acknowledge the loss they will feel once Harry leaves. Working with low functioning clients can be a draining experience. Perhaps Harry's ability to interact with staff at a higher level was a type of reward for their efforts. Could something else be done to recognize staff? In a number of service settings, the needs of staff are not considered. What are the practical and ethical ramifications for the organization if staff needs are neglected?
- Staff rarely know about events that happen in the home. It is conceivable that Harry is more demanding at home or that he disrupts the household by wandering around all night. It may be difficult for staff to recognize that Harry's *persona* at the center could be quite different from his home self. Are the lifestyle needs of the rest of the family less worthy of consideration than Harry's? Grown children who are providing care are often filled with guilt when they choose placement outside the home. They want to do what's best for their parent, their own children, their spouses; pleasing everyone in this situation is highly unlikely. They just want someone to recognize and acknowledge that they are in a difficult

spot. Maybe adult day care staff should be expected to see that perspective.

DECISION MAKING WHEN COMMUNICATION SKILLS ARE LIMITED

There are a number of clients with limited verbal skills who still have opinions. These individuals present another challenge when decisions need to be made. Caregivers (family and staff) may be less attuned to non-verbal communication and may assume that lack of words is synonymous with a lack of ideas, desires, or preferences. It is a struggle for many of us to address the preferences of a person with dementia. The following case example repeats some of the discharge issues previously discussed but adds the dilemmas that family and staff face when providing care to someone with short-term memory loss.

> *Ellen is 75 years old and has a diagnosis of Alzheimer's Disease. She has been living with her son, Jeff, for the past 2 years. Her physical health had been deteriorating and Jeff informed the nurse at day services that the family was seriously considering nursing home placement for her.*
>
> *Despite the fact that Ellen has been attending the center for about 16 months, she still appears anxious, worries about everything, and needs constant reassurance. Recently, she began acting more anxious and asked staff questions (in her limited way) about nursing home placement because she overheard her family talking about it. Staff put her off temporarily by saying that they would check it out and talk to her about it later.*
>
> *Jeff is adamant about not telling his mother anything about the impending move. He knows Ellen will just start worrying about it and he is convinced that since her memory is bad she won't remember anyway. The social worker tried to explain to Jeff that Ellen knew a change was coming and that he should prepare her for it, even if it meant repeating the explanation over and over, but he cut her off, and said he wants to do it his way.*
>
> *Staff respects Jeff's wishes so they try to reassure Ellen that everything will be okay. They speak in generalities with her about the idea of moving, making new friends, etc. Then one Friday, Jeff picked his mother up early and told the staff that Ellen would not be back because she is moving on Monday.*
>
> *The next Monday, the participants missed Ellen and asked about her. They wished there had been an opportunity to say good-bye to*

Ellen and even began to talk about how terrible it was of her family not to say anything since the center usually has a little going away party. Staff made no comment in support of her family and suggested that the group make some cards to send to her. For about an hour during the morning activity the group reminisced about Ellen and other people who have left the center.

- Ellen knew something was going on, as demonstrated by her higher than usual anxiety level. Ellen has very limited language skills so it is virtually impossible to understand what she is trying to say. It is a real challenge to offer clients with dementia opportunities to process changes and talk about their feelings. The more staff knows about Ellen, the more they will be able to respond to her appropriately. Tuning in to behaviors, non-verbal communication, and listening to people like Ellen requires a high level of attentiveness. Physical comfort and assistance with ADLs is only one aspect of service to clients. Finding a private space and setting aside time for Ellen to "talk" about how she feels even when you cannot understand a word she is saying exhibits not only respect for her feelings but reflects staffs' belief that people with dementia face moral dilemmas that they long to express.
- Staff felt angry with Jeff for not preparing Ellen for the move. They totally disagreed with the way he handled the situation. They were visibly cool toward him when he appeared at the center. Is this righteous indignation cause for a formal reprimand from a supervisor? How ought supervisors handle feelings of staff? This scenario recalls the importance of frequent "reality checks" (what we would like to happen in an ideal situation rarely happens in the "real" world) and internal reminders that in everyday ethics all perspectives should be considered, not only in client relationships, but in managing staff.
- Other clients at the center also need to process changes. They had a chance to cope when staff responded to their comments and changed the plan for the day so that they could remember Ellen and others who left the center. The coping skills and common sense wisdom of the older adults at the center can be a learning tool for staff, too.

INTIMACY, BALANCE AND MORAL PREDICAMENTS

Adult day service is, by design, provided in a small group setting. The small group and the frequency of contact between staff and clients fosters a degree of intimacy that may not be duplicated by providers in other care settings. This individual approach is not without its own moral predicaments.

> Justine has been coming to the adult day center for about one year. Justine has been living with dementia for approximately 4 years. She has significant word finding and language deficits but she is still able to make her needs known. Usually Justine is cooperative and enjoys the activities offered at the center but she sometimes becomes very agitated for no apparent reason. One Tuesday, as soon as her daughter left, Justine became very upset. She went to the door and on the verge of tears started yelling, "Let me out of here; I want to go home." Peggy, one of the program assistants, reassured her that her daughter would return later in the day to take her home. She led Justine to the dining area for a cup of morning coffee. Justine joined the group for a while but left again to try to go home. The staff knew that the electronic lock on the door prevented Justine from wandering off, so Justine tried the door, looked out the window, and eventually returned to her coffee. Justine's morning was pretty typical, she joined the exercise group and the morning art project with some encouragement from staff but she left each session at least two or three times to check the door and look for her daughter.
>
> Justine's anxiety slowly escalated all day but increased dramatically after lunch. Peggy noticed her sitting alone; crying in the front lounge area while the rest of the group finished their desserts. Peggy brought Justine's brownie over to her and they "talked" for a few minutes. Peggy put on a tape, which seemed to have a calming effect on Justine and went back to finish her own lunch.
>
> Before long, even the other clients began to notice Justine's distress. They informed staff that there was a problem up front and this time the site manager left her lunch to check on Justine. Now, Justine was inconsolable; she was shouting in incoherent sentences about her husband (who had been deceased for many years), the babies, and various other memories.
>
> It was time to begin afternoon programming and because of the facility design, the only way into the activity room was to walk past Justine. Some clients tried to console her and others became anxious themselves when they saw and heard her. Normally, staff would "take turns" sitting with Justine to get through these episodes, but due to an unexpected staff absence and her high level of anxiety, the site manager decided to call Justine's family for an early pick-up (she usually stayed until closing time). Her daughter was in a meeting and none of the other emergency contacts were reachable. Staff modified afternoon

plans to include a sing-a-long, one of Justine's favorite activities. She stayed at the periphery of the group until her daughter arrived about 90 minutes after the original call.

- The amount of one-to-one time spent with Justine can affect the service provided to other clients. Some participants may feel ignored when they see how much time the staff spends with them compared to time spent with Justine. Staff may feel stress when heavy care for one client means having less time for other clients. Anxiety levels can increase dramatically among the client population if staff anxiety levels are high. It can be extremely difficult for staff to attend to individual client needs while maintaining a supportive atmosphere at the center when their own stress levels are high
- It is not uncommon for staff/managers to focus on clients first without realizing that staff also needs attention. Since clients are always present, staff in adult day service seldom get totally uninterrupted lunch breaks. On days when tensions are high, it is crucial for the staff group to remind each other to slow down and take a break from the clients. While Peggy's approach to Justine indicates empathy and an awareness of her preferences, this example also illustrates the staff's dedication to the program and their concern for each other since they willingly respond to Justine's behavior and to one another.
- Value conflicts arise when other program participants begin to complain about Justine and the staff time that she requires. It is difficult for young staff members to challenge statements older adults make even when those comments cause pain to others. Confounding ideas such as respecting one's elders, letting people express their opinions, avoiding conflict, giving in to strong personalities for the sake of peace, and blaming memory loss may prevent staff from having honest conversations with clients about the clients' tolerance levels or empathy for others with greater needs than their own. Prejudice against the less capable has no place in the day care community.
- Some people think that participants like Justine should be excluded from day care. Conflicts among staff members may exist about how to handle days like the one just described. Staff could easily feel that a call to the family in a situation like this is a sign of failure. After all, families who use the services of the center expect staff to handle problems don't they? Once staff decides to call the family, they must prepare for the responses. Family members are not always in a position to "drop everything" and get to

the center within minutes. Care must be taken not to equate being unable to respond immediately with a lack of concern on the family's part. Staff may also make value judgments about families who are "just home" compared to families who are at work while participants are at the center.

FROM THE PERSPECTIVE OF THE FAMILY

Family caregivers are an integral part of the adult day care equation. Their day-to-day routines include a commitment to maintaining their family member in the community. When things go smoothly, they receive accolades for their actions. When things do not go well it is easy to lose sight of their perspective. Professionals walk a fine line when evaluating what actions to take in a problem situation.

Angela has been attending adult day care for about 18 months. She suffered a stroke a few years ago and as a result, has physical disabilities. From a functional perspective, she is legally blind; unable to get around the center independently; she has very limited body/spatial awareness and she is unable to carry out directions (her body cannot seem to act upon her brain's directives).

Angela needs stand-by assistance with all ambulation and ADLs at the center. Her cognitive skills are largely intact so she participates during current events, word games, sing-a-longs and discussion groups. Angela tends to be a bit negative. She complains that it is always cold in the center, she hates to do arts and crafts, dislikes almost everything served at lunch, etc. She has told the case manager that she hates coming to day care and that what we do here is "just too childish for her," even though she is unable to follow any directions to complete even the most simple task. Angela lives in a garden apartment in a building owned by her nephew and his family. Angela's nephew and his wife both work and Angela rides the center's bus. There have been numerous times when Angela has forgotten her key and therefore can't get into the house. The bus driver brings Angela back to the center when this happens because the bus service believes it is not their problem. They are on the verge of denying her further service because the problem happens so frequently. The family members are unreachable when these "emergencies" occur and Angela has, on more than one occasion, remained at the center past closing time because family members work far away. They just beep the horn when they arrive and expect staff to walk Angela out to the car. They never say, "I'm sorry for being late," or, "Thanks for waiting," or in any way acknowledge the problem.

The family is not willing to leave a key at the center and they giggle about their hectic morning routine as an explanation of why Angela forgets her key so often. Suggestions have been made to involve the neighbors or other close-by family members, but the family is unwilling to work out any type of plan to avert future problems. They promised it wouldn't happen again but it does.

- The immediate resolution for this problem is for staff to stay at the center with Angela until her family arrives. Staff wants to consider everyone's perspective here and they realize that Angela cannot do anything to resolve the problem. They do not want her to be held accountable, but they are running out of ideas. Angela suggests that staff make an extra key and that it be "their little secret." This is totally against the family's wishes but staff is becoming frustrated. Since Angela does not have dementia, they are tempted to get the key. The staff has talked about this and they are worried about what might happen if and when the family finds out, a likely possibility since staff will need to go to the hardware store for the key. How far should staff be expected to go? It's hard for them to come to terms with doing something that they know is against the family's wishes. If the family finds out about the key it could create another set of problems. They also wonder if Angela will start asking them for other favors if they do this one thing for her.
- If families take advantage of you, or are uncooperative does that affect how you treat them or the clients? Maybe not intentionally, but if staff thinks that this family has no regard for them, they may care "differently." Staff does not expect to hear words of gratitude at every turn but they have a right to receive basic respect and appreciation.
- Staff begins to question whether this unwillingness to give the center a key indicates other neglect in the home. It is difficult to know what goes on in the home and staff is hesitant to overreact. To gather information, they contact the case manager who is responsible for an annual face-to-face with state-supported clients. Unfortunately a home visit has not been conducted for several years because Angela's family is never home during the day. Staff is now in a quandary about whether or not to delve deeper into Angela's home situation. Should they give the family the benefit of the doubt? Are they reading too much into the situation or is Angela potentially the victim of neglect?
- Even though Angela is not to blame for the problem, when does the only option for the center become excluding her? This is a

dilemma for staff because exclusion from the center is such a drastic measure. Yet, Angela hates coming to the center. Should such clients be expected to continue? Everyone involved knows that Angela really can't be left home alone but it is hard for staff to listen to complaints every time they interact with Angela. They, on occasion, make remarks to her about how much other people enjoy things around the center but that doesn't deter Angela from saying what's on her mind. Little by little, staff allows Angela to sit alone and listen to music while other activities are occurring at the center just so they and other clients don't have to listen to her crabby remarks. She says that she prefers to do that but staff still feels guilty that she is sitting alone.

BLENDING HOMOGENEOUS ATTITUDES

No age cohort is totally homogeneous. It is no small wonder then, that there are differences of opinion in the adult day services setting. People bring their personality traits, biases, and styles of interacting with others with them when they arrive at the center each day. The next two cases show how blending multiple preferences into a cohesive group consciousness is a goal but in most programs, it is definitely a "work in progress."

> *Agnes and Marty, two clients at the center, started flirting with each other. They go out of their way to sit next to each other during the day and often hold hands. They have even changed their days of attendance so they could be at the center at the same time. Agnes is younger than most of the other participants. She is smart, friendly, and plays the piano. She lives in a group home for people with chronic mental illness. Marty, who is blind, is the type of guy who has something to say about everything and has a ready joke for every occasion. He is married and one reason that he comes to the center is to give him and his wife time away from each other. Both Agnes and Marty are considered "high functioning" clients.*
>
> *Staff noticed what was occurring but it seemed harmless so they decide to "ignore it." Before long though, other clients began to point at them, whispering and laughing about their behavior. After a month's time, Dora, one of the other clients, told a volunteer that something needs to be done because what they are doing is very offensive and wrong. The volunteer agreed that things are getting out of hand between Marty and Agnes (though they are still only holding hands).*

She tells Dora to speak to the "boss." Dora speaks to the Director but after a week nothing happens. The following week Dora decided to talk to Marty and Agnes herself. She cornered Marty and Agnes one morning; their confrontation turned into a shouting match. All the clients joined in the conflict, expressing opinions on both sides. The site manager stopped the argument and the day went on as usual with no further mention of the problem.

- The first consideration is whether or not the type of behavior displayed by Marty and Agnes is harmless. They are just holding hands. What happens if their behavior escalates? There is considerable literature that suggests that physical contact is a good thing. Being noticed by Marty has heightened Agnes's self-esteem. She puts on make-up now and even looks happier. As long as it goes no further, how can this hand-holding be a bad thing?
- Obviously all observers do not agree about whether or not this behavior is appropriate. Dora knows that Marty is married and that may explain her strong reaction to their behavior. Some staff members feel that Agnes's mental health diagnosis must be considered. Would the situation be different if neither of them was married or if Agnes did not have the mental health diagnosis? There is a chance that two clients with dementia could act this way. Does that alter how one should handle the situation? It is critical that different perceptions be considered and discussed so that everyone is at least reasonably comfortable with the outcome and the processes used to arrive at the outcomes. It is also possible that total agreement may never be reached related to this subject. Perhaps the only solution will be an uncomfortable compromise.
- The staff also disagrees about the process of responding to this situation. Should all staff be expected/allowed to talk to clients about this type of behavior or only to the manager? There are managers who believe that their preference becomes the policy of the center. This type of rigid mind-set can be a source of considerable conflict for other staff. In this example, taking no action is itself a decision. A straightforward discussion about this actual event and plans for handling future dilemmas is necessary and beneficial in any setting. There are settings where honest discussions never take place. What moral responsibility does staff have to address the silence around these questions? Suppose all staff agreed that the behavior was "no big deal" but other clients had a different opinion. What obligation does staff have to honor the beliefs and perceptions of the older adults?
- Questions may arise about who to contact and how to document such an incident. Is formal documentation necessary? Should fam-

ily members be notified? What about Agnes's case manager since she is, in essence, Agnes's surrogate family? Staff wants to support Agnes but they are conflicted about how to respond when Agnes begs them to keep it a secret from her case manager. Marty's wife could learn of the situation, a possibility that makes staff very uncomfortable and even makes them feel a bit conspiratorial. This illustrates too, the dilemma of a manager who may always be in a position of making someone unhappy no matter what action is or isn't taken. What if Agnes and Marty keep holding hands even after someone tells them not to do it? There is always a danger of pushing too hard or making things worse when ultimatums are issued leaving open the question: What recourse do we have to resolve a situation like this?

Francis has attended the center for about 3 years. She has a history of depression and came to the center as an alternative to being alone and isolated at home during the day. Her peers viewed her as a natural leader and deferred to her judgment and wishes many times during an ordinary day. Francis had an opinion about everything that occurred at the center. She made comments about how people dress, which clients she likes, which participants take too long in the bathroom, and grumbled when people with dementia couldn't remember things. Recently, she started whispering about people to Teresa, another client. They said things just loudly enough to be heard by staff and other clients. Staff spoke to both of them and asked that they keep their comments to themselves but they persisted in their actions. Gradually people who were the brunt of their comments steered clear of them.

Francis liked to sit at the same place every day during lunch and there are a few other people who regularly sat with her at the table. One day when Francis was in the activity room finishing her project, Virginia, a new client, sat in Francis's seat by mistake. The other people at "Francis's table" started eating their salads and ignored Virginia. When Francis walked into the dining room and saw Virginia in her spot, she was very angry. She knocked over Virginia's salad, yelled at her for taking her chair, and was about to push her out of the way when staff intervened. By this time, Virginia was in tears and the other people at the table took Francis's side against Virginia. Staff and other participants try to reassure Virginia and apologize for Francis's behavior while they found her another place to sit.

After lunch, the Director took Francis aside to talk about what happened. Francis insisted that she didn't do anything wrong and that she was tired of having to give in to all these other "stupid" old people. She told the Director that she wouldn't coming back ever again and stormed out of the office.

The following day, both Virginia and Francis were absent. Both families called the center. Virginia's family wanted to know more about what happened and felt that with encouragement Virginia would be back the next day. Francis's family, on the other hand, expressed concern that Francis was misunderstood, she always was a bit outspoken, and she just needed a bit more attention. The staff told Francis's family that this was not an isolated incident and asked that they speak to her about her behavior at the center. The family hung up, furious, after saying that they intended to report the center to the case manager and that Francis would never be coming back.

- Peer interaction at the center occurs naturally. Older adults in adult day service settings have the right to choose their friends and decide with whom they'd like to associate. There is a point at which socially appropriate behavior is dictated by the responses of the rest of the group. Cliques that hurt other people's feelings are particularly onerous in a small, intense setting like adult day service. Fostering friendships is not synonymous with allowing cliques or rude people to dominate the center. It is also natural for staff to protect people like Virginia from people like Francis but staff also hesitates to correct behavior of this sort for fear of being disrespectful. Staff constantly has to balance their gut reactions with what center policy dictates.
- The Director is in a very difficult position here. His/her first reaction may be, "Thank goodness that's the last time I have to listen to Francis," but he/she must handle the backlash of the family's complaints to the case manager. The way the family and Francis recount the event may reflect badly on the center. Should the Director seek to pacify Francis's family or not? If so, what approaches would continue to show respect yet address the problem? This situation could jeopardize future referrals to the center if the case manager simply accepts the version of events Francis's family tells. The Director needs to evaluate the consequences of any action taken and weigh what is good for the center against what may "feel right," which is also deserving of respect. One responsibility is to work through her feelings and try to ensure that the case manager understands the whole situation.
- There may be repercussions at the center created by Francis's absence. In that case, it would be necessary to explain things to Francis's friends in a way that does not reflect badly on anyone.
- Managing the environment at the center to prevent this type of catastrophic reaction can produce stress for the staff. Staff struggles with the desire to keep things normal and the need to watch over

and protect more frail clients. What about the possibility of being hit? Is it "okay" for staff to be hit once in awhile/ever? What about clients being hit or shouted at by other clients? It is unrealistic for staff to believe that they must control every event that takes place at the center? Constant vigilance does not mean that bad things don't happen. Given these realities, the staff needs to feel confident that they are doing everything possible to create the best atmosphere for everyone and that some things must be dealt with after the fact and prevented from happening repeatedly.

CONCLUSION

These case examples and associated reflections illustrate how adult day service staff face moral dilemmas daily, sometimes without realizing it. In fact, the very act of preparing this chapter generated a new awareness of how much normative ethics pervades our adult day care environment. Very often moral analysis takes the form of "thinking out loud" during a staffing and developing a plan that includes consecutive courses of action based on outcomes of discussions with and actions taken by the family. The thought process includes input from multiple staff members such as the nurse, social worker, personal care worker, and director. It takes into consideration family dynamics, temperament of the client, past interactions, seriousness of the situation, reasonableness of the request, and ways to get a favorable result with the least amount of stress for all concerned. Sometimes, the end result is far from ideal and the staff has to face the frustrations of that experience and find ways to make the best of it or to seek alternatives to resolve the troubling situation. But ultimately our only choice may be to learn to live with ambiguity and uncertainty. The key to providing an ethical day services program is to anchor even the simplest actions—calling a client by name, taking clients' skills and abilities into account when planning the daily schedule, communicating openly and honestly—in a moral framework.

CHAPTER 15

Is Home Care Always the Best Care?

Daniel Kuhn

As a social worker in a clinic at a state- and federally-funded Alzheimer's disease center, I have spoken to thousands of family caregivers over the past 12 years. Troubling ethical problems emerge from the fact that often these older spouses and adult children, mostly women, find themselves alone, responsible for meeting all the needs of their disabled relatives. As Alzheimer's and related dementias progress over a period of 3 to 20 years, the disabled person's needs consume increasing amounts of the caregiver's time and energy. A recent survey reported that caregivers who reside with relatives with Alzheimer's disease spend an average of 100 hours weekly devoted to some type of caregiving responsibility (Alzheimer's Association and National Alliance for Caregiving, 1999). Although the vast majority of persons with dementia are cared for at home, some caregivers clearly pay an enormous price for this arrangement.

Alzheimer's disease inevitably takes its toll on those with the disease and on their family caregivers. The disease may last anywhere from three to twenty years and the rate of progression varies from person to person. Even with help from other relatives, friends, and paid helpers, the burden of responsibility usually rests squarely upon the shoulders of just one or two family members. Some caregivers rise to the occasion in remarkably positive ways and learn to cope successfully with a series of challenges. However, other caregivers become secondary victims of the disease, with dire consequences for themselves and those under their care. Numerous studies indicate the deleterious effects of caring for a relative with dementia at home. The risks to one's physical, mental, social, and financial well-being have been consistently documented (Clipp & George, 1990; Harwood, Barker, Cantillon, Lowenstein, Ownby, & Duara, 1998; Neundorfer, 1991; Schulz, O'Brien, Bookwala, & Fleissner, 1995).

For many reasons, most older adults prefer home care to care rendered in facilities. A study by Mattimore and colleagues (1997) found that a vast majority of seriously ill adults was unwilling to live in a nursing home or would "rather die" than go into one. Moreover, a new study by Gambassi and colleagues (1999) reports that nearly half of nursing home residents with Alzheimer's disease die within two years of admission due to preventable factors such as immobility and malnutrition, nearly double the mortality rate found in residents without the disease. It is no wonder that public distrust of nursing homes persists even though the nursing home industry in the United States is highly regulated and some nursing homes offer outstanding care to both residents and their families. In spite of the growing number of alternatives to nursing homes such as assisted living facilities, home care remains the preferred option in most cases. An important question then is: Should such caregivers continue their demanding roles and responsibilities at home?

Unfortunately, home care can be an unhealthy and dangerous option for both the caregiver and care recipient. Just as numerous studies have documented high levels of distress among caregivers of persons with dementia, the consequences for care recipients can also be detrimental. Abuse and neglect of the person with dementia signals caregiver distress. For example, a caregiver may rely on excessive physical or chemical means to restrain the person with dementia, a practice clearly forbidden in nursing homes (Omnibus Budget Reconciliation Act, 1987). In other cases, a caregiver may be financially dependent upon the person with Alzheimer's disease despite providing poor or inadequate care, and therefore cannot consider alternatives to home care. The first-ever National Elder Abuse Incidence Study (National Center on Elder Abuse, 1998) reports that in 1996 over 60% of the estimated 450,000 elder abuse and neglect victims living in the community evidenced cognitive impairment and two thirds of the perpetrators were their adult children or spouses.

Given these facts, should other options and living arrangements be encouraged and, if so, by whom? Can both the caregiver and care recipient benefit by changing the site of care? How is this decision to be reached, particularly if the caregiver is the surrogate decision-maker for the disabled person? Such questions are laden with competing interests of both parties as well as the interests of other concerned relatives, friends, and professionals. Value conflicts seem inevitable. Three cases involving individuals with Alzheimer's disease and their families illustrate the complexity of making these difficult decisions.[1]

CASE ONE: AN ELDERLY COUPLE

Al, an 83-year-old man with advanced dementia, was cared for at home for three years, primarily under the direction of his 91-year-old wife, Leda. The couple had been married eighteen years, this being the second marriage for both of them following the deaths of their first spouses. Al had a son and daughter and Leda had a son, all of whom lived in the local area. Additional assistance to Al and Leda came from family members and helpers from several private home care agencies. Over time the paid help had proven to be generally unreliable, inconsistent, and in a few cases, prone to theft. Leda appeared emotionally exhausted but she remained adamant in her desire to care for Al at home. They had been devoted to each other throughout their marriage and Leda noted that she wanted "to keep a close eye on him here at home." When he became incontinent and dependent upon a wheelchair, family members strongly encouraged Leda to move Al to a nearby nursing home. Hospice care did not appear to be an option due to his uncertain prognosis. With much apprehension and guilt, Leda eventually agreed to the idea and Al was relocated a nursing home in their neighborhood.

Although in some ways Leda was relieved by Al's absence from home, she was also depressed over his deterioration and anxious about living alone. Overall, family members were satisfied that the nursing home staff offered slightly better care than the paid helpers at home, but they also wondered if the decision to place Al in a facility was the right one for both him and Leda. Within three months of admission to the nursing home, Al developed a urinary tract infection and he was hospitalized. His infection cleared up but his dementia worsened markedly during the hospitalization. Thereafter, he seemed oblivious to everyone and his surroundings. When he developed another urinary tract infection a few weeks later, his family and physician agreed that the medical problem should not be treated aggressively. Al died quietly a few days later at the nursing home. Leda had been expecting his death but was grief stricken. Just six weeks after Al's

---

[1] The couple described in the first case study, Al and Leda Kuhn, are the author's grandparents.

death, she suddenly died at home from what the physician called "natural causes." Everyone else who knew her seemed to think that she died of a broken heart.

When Al was near death, Leda told her family, "He was the best man I have ever known." Her wish to care for him at home expressed that feeling. The family knew that he was a fiercely independent man, a stoic, who would hate being in a depersonalized place such as a nursing home where no one knew him. But they also knew that Al would have wanted to put Leda and her needs first, to do what was good for her. An old-fashioned gentleman, he would have wanted to "take care of his woman." At this point in their lives, however, it was hard to know exactly what taking care of Leda might mean. Taking care of Al's personal needs was taking its toll on Leda, physically and emotionally. As he declined, she declined too, although what she was doing fit her definition of a loyal spouse.

What was good for Leda was to honor the kind of man that Al had been in the past—one who would have hated the nursing home. It was also good for Leda to have Al with her where she could care for him as she had always done and where she knew he would want to be. On the other hand, Leda could hardly carry on because of her frailty. What would have been good for her was to have a consistent and caring individual to provide his day-to-day care so she could assist him and offer the emotional connection that only she and other family members could provide. But that ideal was out of reach because the available assistance was unreliable. The rest of the family had different goals: Al's comfort and relief for Leda. Initially, the nursing home seemed to offer the opportunity to achieve both goals. Often, in trying circumstances such as these, families struggle to meet many competing needs simultaneously. And just as often, there is no singularly correct answer.

Leda felt compelled to advocate for Al by initially resisting the nursing home plan. She downplayed the detrimental effects that caregiving had on her. She saw no dichotomy between serving her needs and Al's needs. Is it indeed possible to separate the needs of both spouses who seem so inextricably linked? Could Leda speak authoritatively for Al when, in fact, she seemed so fragile? If so, why should her fragility matter?

Years later, family members still wonder whether they chose the best course of action. When they made the nursing home decision, they assumed that Al would not survive much longer no matter where he lived. If only Al's children had known he would live for only a few months after he left home, they would have moved in with him and Leda. But, of course, they could not have known. They hoped that by moving him to the nursing home he would be more comfortable. This goal was partially achieved. At the same time, they hoped that Leda would experience some measure of relief, but this goal was not met. For Leda, few benefits were readily available. Leda wanted to continue to care for Al at home. She could not do this without steady and reliable help every day. What Al would have wanted for her, that she take steps to preserve her own well-being, was also no longer possible. At the time the family made the decision to place Al in the nursing home, continuing his care at home no longer seemed viable and yet the alternative also seemed laden with risks.

How does one respect the values shared by people like Leda and Al? Who speaks for those with Alzheimer's disease when they can no longer speak for themselves? Who makes decisions about the best place or best people for rendering care? Can family caregivers fairly represent the interests of those with dementia in light of their special role in the situation? Should caregivers be expected to sacrifice themselves completely, always putting the needs of a loved one with dementia first? Is "good enough" care in a nursing home better than inadequate care at home? Such complex questions require time for discussion and reflection in order for families to live with the consequences of any decision. Perhaps it is not always possible to balance the interests of all parties.

Another set of questions relates to the role of government. How should taxpayers support families in their role as primary caregivers? Does any moral "blame" rest with social policies? For example, should hospice care as a benefit of Medicare be limited to the last six months of life, even in the face of a slow and certain death due to advanced dementia? Is government's lack of support for a comprehensive, community-based long-term-care system responsible for the poorly paid and poorly trained labor force of most home care agencies? The private decisions that families make about home care versus institutional care are seldom addressed within this broader social context. And yet the personal choices family caregivers make on behalf of their disabled relatives are inextricably linked with public policies and programs such as Medicare and Medicaid.

The moral pain that so many people experience as they face illness, dementia, and death can rarely be remedied by signing advanced directives or resorting to other legal or quasi legal methods. In such uncertain circumstances, families can try to understand that there is no "correct" decision. There may be no particularly good decision either. What there will be is a decision that all can try to live with because it makes as much sense as possible at the time. Al, Leda, their children, and grandchildren knew what they valued most, but age, frailty, dementia, other conflicting demands, and inadequate help from paid caregivers meant that they had to settle for the best they could do, all things considered. In this case, no values were trampled and no one was ignored. Family members asked questions of one another. They weighed their options and attempted to understand what the consequences of each of these options might be. Ultimately—but not without pain—they were able to take responsibility for their hard choices. This was the best they could do together under the circumstances.

CASE TWO: A MIDDLE-AGED COUPLE

Another case involving a couple in their fifties presents some related but different issues. When one partner in a marriage has Alzheimer's disease, major changes take place in the marital relationship (Wright, 1993). The well spouse typically must assume a leadership role as the mate with the disease is no longer capable of being a full, active partner in the marriage. Shifts in roles, responsibilities, kinship relations, and friendships are inevitable (Kuhn, 1999). When Alzheimer's disease occurs in midlife, these changes are completely unexpected for all concerned. A radical transformation of a couple's lifestyle slowly takes place while the terms of the marriage are often recast by the well spouse in order to accommodate the demands of the disease.

Betty was diagnosed with Alzheimer's disease at age 52, following a three-year history of progressive memory loss and word finding difficulty. There was no family history of the disease. Both of her elderly parents and two older siblings lived abroad. At the time of her diagnosis, she had been happily married to Clark, age 53, for 29 years and they had two children, ages 28 and 25, who lived in distant cities.

Betty was highly intelligent, fluent in several languages, and still taught language classes on a part-time basis at the time of her diagnosis. In fact, she continued working for another two years as she kept her diagnosis secret from all but family until it became clear to others that she could not continue with her career. She was remarkably aware of her impairments but also self-critical and depressed. An antidementia drug was ineffective in improving or stabilizing the symptoms of her disease and other drugs did not seem to help her mood. There was considerable tension in the marriage as she frequently blamed her husband for her distress. By all accounts, he appeared understanding and remarkably patient with her in the face of difficult circumstances.

When Betty stopped working she became increasingly anxious, talkative, and uninhibited at times with whomever she encountered in public. She often became agitated with Clark, insisting that he be with her at all times. She first attended an activity program at a nearby senior center and then an adult day care center. However, she had to discontinue participation at both places due to her high anxiety, constant interruptions of staff, and desire to go home.

A paid helper, a middle-aged woman, was hired on a private basis, five days weekly, eight hours per day. The helper was increased to six days per week after nearly a year. The helper would drive Betty around in a car every day and they went on errands and long walks together. Betty and the helper became friends. About two years after the helper was introduced into the home, Betty's dementia worsened to the point of bowel and bladder incontinence. This change was both physically and emotionally taxing for Clark. Betty was often unable to recognize him and sometimes referred to the helper as Clark. She continued to be anxious and clinging in his presence at all times. Clark was grief-stricken over her decline. Meanwhile, he continued his career "as a form of therapy." He completed an application at a nearby nursing home in anticipation of relocating Betty in the future and her name was placed on a long waiting list. The rest of his family had urged him to explore this option.

About a year later, Betty's name came up on the waiting list and with a week's notice Clark reluctantly made arrangements for Betty to move. She was now 59 years of age and it had been nearly ten years since the onset of her disease. Clark remarked that, "A lot of little things happened during that year that led to the decision. The incontinence was just a part of the picture." He felt torn by guilt and by the need for relief. He spoke of guilt over being unable to continue caring for her at home where she could have one-to-one care. He also felt guilty over taking away any power she had in decisions affecting her life, including the most important one about her living situation. However, he also realized that he could not continue with her at home unless he became "like a robot"—devoid of feelings for her except as someone he used to know and love. He felt that he was constantly "on call" and there was no way to escape his distress except through work. Furthermore, Betty now had no recollection of him "except as a theoretical person, no longer a reality."

Clark continues working full-time and sees another woman, a long-time friend of theirs who is widowed. His family is supportive of this relationship. At first, Betty was extremely upset about the move to the nursing home but gradually settled in. She found a male resident in the nursing home whom she refers to as Clark on occasion. She no longer recognizes Clark when he visits her daily. He says he visits mainly to ensure that the staff is paying attention to her needs.

Spouses of people with advanced dementia often express the feeling of being in a state of limbo—not quite married but not quite single either. Pauline Boss (1999) has aptly described this as a painful and protracted experience of "ambiguous loss." In the course of a long marriage, spouses cannot help but compare the formerly healthy spouse with the one ravaged by the disease. For the well spouse, images of their past relationship and the formerly healthy partner conflict terribly with the present situation. On the other hand, the partner with dementia may have little or no awareness of the dramatic changes that have slowly taken place. At first, Betty seemed well aware of the changes occurring in her life, as seen in her high anxiety and clinging behavior. Yet gradually the disease appeared to erase major parts of her attachment to her past life. Her anxiety remained high but was no longer specific to a particular place or person. From outward appearances, it seemed to make no difference who cared for her or where care was provided.

Some well spouses still perceive a sense of continuity in the marital relationship, while others feel that the disease has rendered the spouse with the disease "like a stranger" (Chesla, Martinson, & Muwaswes, 1994). However, a spouse's definition of "couplehood" invariably changes to some degree (Kaplan, Ade-Ridder, Hennon, & Brubaker, 1995). Clark appears to have adapted to Betty's disease by drawing a clear distinction between her former and current self. In turn, his commitment to care for her at home changed as she lost familiarity with their home and with him as a meaningful partner. As Clark put it, "I saw little benefit in her remaining at home with me when she no longer recognized either her home or me." At the same time, he worried that she could not possibly have the benefits of constant companionship at the nursing home that she received at home and consequently the quality of her life might diminish.

Given the typically slow yet relentless deterioration of one's partner over an extended period of time, Alzheimer's disease often drives a wedge in a marriage and raises many complex questions about personal commitment. What is the well spouse to do about nurturing his/herself in the physical presence yet psychological absence of the partner? Is complete self-sacrifice expected in order to live out the commitment to love one's partner, "in sickness and in health"? In retrospect, Clark rationalizes that perhaps he could have had the paid helper move into their home but he did not want to completely give up his privacy. He also worried about the ability of the paid helper to continue indefinitely in her caregiving role in spite of "boundless patience." In the end, Clark accepted that his caregiving role could continue just as well while she was living at the nearby nursing home. He had been worn down by caregiving at home and his lifestyle had been scaled down to conform to Betty's growing needs. With no immediate family in the vicinity and most friends having drifted away, he found himself quite isolated except for one female friend.

Is the social isolation so often reported by caregivers to be borne silently and without recourse? Or can the commitment to love mean that the person with dementia will be cared for outside one's home by others who are not emotionally connected in the same way as a long-time spouse? Can a well spouse like Clark be allowed to carve out a new lifestyle while simultaneously ensuring that the spouse with dementia receives good care? Does a well spouse's new relationship with a member of the opposite sex constitute an "extra-marital affair"? Can society as a whole, particularly religious institutions, accept such relationships or view them simply in terms of infidelity? For his part, Clark felt like he did the best he could do for Betty at home and he is now doing the best he can for her while she lives in the nursing home. He respects his own distinct and separate interests and feels that Betty would approve of his decisions if she could understand. His transition to a new way life without her has become a priority for the first time in their marriage.

CASE THREE: A THREE GENERATION HOUSEHOLD

A chronic disease like Alzheimer's tends to have a ripple effect upon an entire family system. Those living nearby, at a distance, or in the same household as someone with the disease may choose to be involved or uninvolved but each person must ultimately decide upon a position. Motivations for involvement or lack of involvement are often rooted in one's personal history as well as one's current situation. If the person with dementia has no spouse but has adult children, then at least one of them typically steps forward to assume the role of primary caregiver. In most cases, a daughter or daughter-in law will take on this role in spite of other competing demands such as a marriage, children, and a career. Elaine Brody (1985) popularized the phrase "the sandwich generation" to describe middle-aged women who accept responsibility for the care of both the older and younger generations. The time and energy required to juggle the needs of so many individuals at the same time often is beyond anyone's capacity. The far-reaching effects of caregiving, for better or worse, are further intensified if the person with Alzheimer's disease resides with his or her extended family.

Carrie was 77 years old when she was diagnosed with Alzheimer's disease. She had been widowed 7 years and was residing in her own home where she had lived for 54 years. Her 47-year-old daughter, Julie, lived nearby with her husband and their two children, ages 16 and 13. Carrie's two sons lived out of state with their own families but they kept in regular phone contact with her. Julie had always enjoyed a close relationship with her mother and at first assisted her with paying bills and shopping for groceries.

Carrie's memory slowly worsened over the next year to the point that she needed help with cooking meals and personal grooming but she adamantly refused these forms of help by declaring, "I can take care of myself!" When Julie discussed the situation with her brothers, one was sympathetic and the other complained that Julie was exaggerating their mother's needs. A short time later, Carrie fell and broke her hip. Following a hospitalization in which Carrie became disoriented and combative, she reluctantly agreed to live with Julie and her family on a "temporary basis." Julie took leave of her job as a budget analyst for a month to help in her mother's recuperation. However, 4 months later she quit work altogether when it became clear that her mother needed full-time supervision. Julie's husband was supportive of the arrangement and their two teenagers did not seem to mind at the time.

About a year later Julie suggested that her mother participate in a local adult day care center but she refused, saying Julie was trying to get rid of her and "put her into a home." Carrie spent most of her time watching television and often criticized Julie and the rest of the family for perceived misdeeds. She occasionally blamed someone in the family for stealing from her. According to Julie, her mother's "once sweet personality was fading into history."

Everyone in the household gradually learned to take Julie's negativity in stride except the younger child in the family, who showed signs of unrest at school and with peers. Family counseling revealed that this child was depressed and deeply resentful about the attention devoted to her grandmother. Julie and her husband quickly adopted a new way of doing things in order to rescue their distressed daughter. They insisted upon some practical help and respite from Julie's brothers who had previously backed away from any responsibility; with this pressure, they provided some help. A home helper was also arranged through a state program to provide Julie with some respite three times weekly; this service proved unreliable and was dropped after 6 months. The family hired private help to allow Julie and her husband to get out of the home and socialize with friends. Although their daughter's mood and behavior improved, Julie and her husband began to argue a lot and felt distant from each other.

By now Carrie had shared Julie's home for nearly 5 years and was becoming increasing impaired by her disease. She required total *assistance with bathing and dressing, and was often hostile toward Julie. When Carrie again fell and broke her other hip, it was an unexpected opportunity to consider another living arrangement. Julie wanted to continue home care, yet everyone else wanted to place Carrie in a nursing home. Julie agonized over the decision but agreed to let Carrie "try out" a nearby facility. Carrie protested the decision but her wish was not honored. Two years later she still resides at the same facility, although she is now severely impaired and must use a wheelchair. Julie or her husband visit Carrie daily. Julie's marriage is back on track and both of her children appear well adjusted and are away at college. Julie has returned to her career but points out, "Taking care of mom was the toughest job I'll ever have."*

In this extended family, the decision made by Julie and her husband to move Carrie into their home had many benefits for her, but the risks to the rest of the family soon became clear. In particular, their daughter acted out the tension in the family and was emotionally distraught for a long time. The strength of the marriage was also tested in extraordinary ways by the caregiving situation. The loss of income by Julie's taking leave of her career also imposed considerable constraints. There were no government tax credits to compensate them, even in a small way. With little outside support, Julie's family managed to provide her mother with good care at home for five years, but the price was a high one at times for everyone involved.

Julie has no regrets, as she felt that she had a unique opportunity to give her mother something valuable in her greatest time of need. Even with the upset caused in her marriage and her younger daughter, Julie believes that it was a worthwhile experience for her family, as it pulled everyone closer together in the long run. At times she doubted that she had the tenacity to continue and worried about the family breaking down. She credits her spouse for his compassion in "dealing well with a bunch of hard-headed women from three different generations."

Carrie's initial wish to remain in her own home and her later wish to remain in Julie's home were vetoed by others under the guise of "temporary" relocations. What say, if any, should Carrie have had in these decisions, in light of her poor memory, impaired judgment, and other diminished skills? Did her need for safety override her right to autonomy? What right or power did she have to impose her wishes upon the rest of the family that ultimately was responsible for her well-being? Are there limits to autonomy under such circumstances?

Balancing the needs of everyone involved in a caregiving situation is a challenge fraught with many ethical considerations. Due to the threats to personal autonomy inherent in Alzheimer's disease and corresponding reliance upon others, people with the disease cannot always expect that their desire to remain at home can be honored indefinitely. Likewise, family caregivers cannot expect that they have the necessary personal, social, and financial resources to carry out their desire to provide home care indefinitely. Some spouses and families have the means or find the means to care for a loved one with Alzheimer's disease at home until the end of the illness, but this effort should be considered nothing less than heroic. Nearly five million Americans now have Alzheimer's disease and the number affected is projected to rise to 14 million by 2050 in the absence of effective preventive measures (Evans et al., 1992). The need for social policies to support families in their role as main providers of care to loved ones with the disease will become even more pressing in the years ahead. Societal values and decisions thus far concerning disabled people in need of care and their families reflect an established American tradition to keep caregiving a private matter for the most part. A radically transformed health care and social service system would enable family caregivers to exercise choice and set ethical limits that cannot be done now without great moral pain.

REFERENCES

Alzheimer's Association and the National Alliance for Caregiving. (1999). *Who cares? Families caring for persons with Alzheimer's disease.* Washington, DC: Author.

Boss, P. (1999). *Ambiguous loss: Learning to live with unresolved grief.* Boston: Harvard University Press.

Brody, E. M. (1985). Parent care as a normative family stress. *The Gerontologist, 25,* 19–29.

Chesla, C., Martinson, I., & Muwaswes, M. (1994). Continuities and discontinuities in family members' relationships with Alzheimer's patients. *Family Relations, 1,* 3–9.

Clipp, E. C., & George, L. K. (1990). Caregiver needs and patterns of social support. *Journal of Gerontology: Social Sciences, 45,* S102–S111.

Evans, D. A., Scherr, P. A., Cook, N. R., Albert, M. S., Funkenstein, H. H., Smith, L. A., Hebert, L. E., Wetle, T. T., Branch, L. G., Chown, M., Hennekens, C. H., & Taylor, J. O. (1992). The impact of Alzheimer's disease in the United States population. In R. M. Suzman, D. P. Willis, & K. G. Martin (Eds.), *The oldest old* (pp. 283–299). Oxford: Oxford University Press.

Gambassi, G., Landi, F., Lapane, K. L., Sgadari, A., Mor, V., & Bernabei, R. (1999). Predictors of mortality in patients with Alzheimer's disease. *Journal of Neurology, Neurosurgery and Psychiatry, 67,* 59–65.

Harwood, D. G., Barker, W. W., Catillon, M., Lowenstein, D. A., Ownby, R., & Duara, R. (1998). Depressive symptomatology in first-degree family caregivers of Alzheimer's disease. *Alzheimer's Disease and Associated Disorders, 12,* 340–346.

Kaplan, L., Ade-Ridder, L., Hennon, C., & Brubaker, T. (1995). Preliminary typology of couplehood: "I" versus "we." *International Journal of Aging and Human Development, 40*(4), 317–337.

Kuhn, D. (1999). *Alzheimer's early stages: First steps in caring and treatment.* Alameda, CA: Hunter House Publishers.

Mattimore, T. J., Wenger, N. S., Desbiens, N. A., Teno, J. M., Hamel, M. B., Liu, H., Califf, R., Connors, A. F., Lynn, J., & Oye, R. K. (1997). Surrogate and physician understanding of patients' preferences for living permanently in a nursing home. *Journal of the American Geriatrics Society, 45,* 818–824.

National Center on Elder Abuse. (1998). *The National Elder Abuse Incidence Study: Final report, September 1998.* Washington, DC: U.S. Department of Health and Human Services, Administration on Aging.

Neundorfer, M. M. (1991). Coping and health outcomes in spouses' caregivers of persons with dementia. *Nursing Research, 40,* 260–265.

Omnibus Budget Reconciliation Act (OBRA). Public Law 100-23. (1987). *Subtitle C, nursing home reform.* Washington, DC: Government Printing Office.

Schulz, R., O'Brien, A. T., Bookwala, J., & Fleissner, K. (1995). Psychiatric and physical morbidity effects of dementia caregiving: Prevalence correlates, and causes. *The Gerontologist, 35,* 771–791.

Wright, L. K. (1993). *Alzheimer's disease and marriage.* Newbury Park, CA: Sage Publications.

CHAPTER **16**

A Good Death? Finding a Balance Between the Interests of Patients and Caregivers

Stephen Ellingson and Jon D. Fuller

Mr. T was a 76-year-old man who lived with his wife in a small, run-down house. She was thirty years younger, and they had met during a difficult time in her life, when she was new to the United States, did not speak the language, and had no money. Marrying Mr. T had solved these problems, and she was grateful. The marriage over the ensuing years was not an easy one. He was a very demanding husband and verbally abusive. Still, a sense of obligation for all he had done for her kept Mrs. T with him to the end. Mr. T suffered a stroke, leaving half of his body paralyzed. He was confined to his bed or wheelchair, and had to be fed through a gastrostomy tube. His wife had to attend to his daily functions as he lost control of both bowel and bladder. He suffered from diabetes and dementia and thus required constant monitoring. To make matters worse, he adamantly refused to participate in his care and continued to be verbally abusive to Mrs. T. He also demanded that he be allowed to die at home under her care, and he refused to consider placement in any kind of care facility.

Mrs. T remained devoted and managed to keep him at home. During the day she worked full time as a nurse's aide in a local nursing home, and at night she cared for her husband, often working around the clock. She hired a part-time caregiver to help while she was away at work. The physical, emotional, and psychological stress of caring for her husband was tremendous and seriously compromised her quality of life. An excerpt from a letter she wrote to her health care providers speaks of the difficulties of caring for a terminally ill patient at home:

> I have been changing the caregiver almost every month. No one can't last longer than a month, they couldn't take care of him, he demanded too much to both caregiver and me. For example: He sat in the wheelchair for a few hours, he then wants to go to bed, we just put him to bed not even ten minutes, he wants to get up again. We explain to him that we will let him up about two more hours. He doesn't like it, he is trying to get up by himself and he gets mad, yelled and demands to get up. . . . It comes to the point that is too much for us to take care of him. Some days I was so down I couldn't open my eyes, then by the time I am home I have to help my husband. . . . I am exhausted.

Mrs. T continued to care for her husband for nearly three years after his stroke. He remained at home under her care until he died in a hospital bed in their living room.

What is a "good" death? The case of Mr. T raises this question in a disturbing way. Was his a good death simply because it occurred on his terms—in his own home, under the care of his family? What about the adverse effects of his terms on his family and caregivers?

As a society, we call a death "good" if it seems to fit neatly into our culturally approved images. These images are of a death that is painless, short, and leaves the dying person with his or her dignity; one that comes without warning, preferably during sleep; one that has been rationally considered by the patient well before the end and follows his or her advance directives. Or perhaps a good death comes not only without pain, but also at home, amidst loving family and friends, after old arguments have been patched up and good-byes have been said.

Yet often death does not occur so peacefully. The process may be long and accompanied by great physical, psychological, and emotional pain. Some patients refuse to participate in their own care. Others, like Mr. T, make nearly impossible demands on their caregivers, fueled by rage and frustration at their loss of control and independence. Many dying people refuse to go quietly into the night, and thus they experience deaths that do not fit our socially accepted ideals of the good death. What lessons can be learned from these "bad" deaths that will help professionals in the field provide better care, improve their research, and design new public policies on terminal care for the dying at home and in institutions?

This essay presents the cases of Mr. T and Mr. A, two men who did not experience "good" deaths. The discussion will do the following: (1)

demonstrate the difficulties created by our culturally approved conceptualizations of death; (2) suggest that we must deromanticize death and develop more realistic assumptions and expectations about death and care for the dying; (3) examine the challenges of balancing the four oft-cited values of care (autonomy, justice, nonmaleficence, and beneficence); and (4) outline an alternative ethic of care for the dying that takes seriously the interests of the community.

Americans' culturally approved understandings of death and care for the dying are flawed, and these flaws worsen the experience of dying for both patients and caregivers. First, our views of how people should die are grounded in the values of individualism—autonomy, independence, self-control, choice. Deeply held and enduring notions of the "rugged individual" and self-reliance, genres of popular culture that celebrate the lone hero, and institutions like the free market that place responsibility for success or failure on the shoulders of the individual— all powerfully shape Americans' understanding of the self (Bellah et al., 1985). These notions influence not only how Americans live but how they die. Death is conceived as a deeply personal event or process that only the individual experiences. So it follows that the person should be allowed, is even entitled, to experience death on his or her own terms. Thus, the demands of some dying patients that "everything be done" and the wishes of others to be left alone so they can die quickly and not be a "burden" on family should be honored. The health care system legitimates this individualistic focus on dying through the legal structures of informed consent and advance directives. Moreover, many scholars of aging and death and many health care workers have reinforced the legitimacy of individualism through their advocacy and actions to protect patients from paternalism, neglect, and abuse and to ensure that patients' rights, interests, and desires receive attention.

The strong emphasis on individual autonomy is important, but it ignores the communal or collective nature of death and dying (Holstein, 1997; Hardwig, 1990, 1993; Jecker, 1993). The emphasis may lead both patients and caregivers to forget that the choices of the individual also have consequences for others (e.g., family members, health care workers, other dying or ill patients). In fact, this approach to death places caregivers, family members, and the dying person in potentially antagonistic relationships where the interests of and responsibility for the good of others must be surrendered to protect the perceived interests and needs of the individual who is dying. The costs of doing so may be very high: the destruction of family relationships and a diminished quality of life for the family (especially if the care creates long-lasting health and financial problems for family members), "burn-out" of caregivers, unavailability of resources for other patients, and, ultimately, poor or insensitive care.

These costs may seem trivial when compared to the gravity of impending death facing a terminally ill person, but only if they are viewed through the individualistic, patient-centered lens. When viewed through a community-oriented lens, the patient-caregiver relationship and the attending costs take on a different valence. Instead of measuring a good death solely by how closely caregivers fulfill the wishes of those who are dying, we also should consider the degree to which doing so threatens the stability and integrity of the whole community. When autonomy automatically takes precedence over other values, when the collective bases for providing care are progressively undermined, then we need to rethink our moral approach to care. Care for dying people will be enhanced only when our society ensures that the health and welfare of families and professional caregivers is maintained. If our collective resources (human capital, finances, the emotional and psychological strength of caregivers) are not protected, then society will not be able to care for dying people effectively, let alone with any degree of compassion and the desire to preserve their dignity.

The case of Mr. T illustrates the danger of acceding to the wishes of the dying person without regard to the consequences for the larger community in which Mr. T is embedded. Mr. T's every demand was met by Mrs. T or the parade of home care workers, without including their needs or interests in the calculus of care. Mrs. T may have acted heroically to care for an abusive, self-centered husband, but her own health was jeopardized, perhaps permanently, by the demands of care. What is more, as Mrs. T's health deteriorated, her ability to hold down two jobs was compromised and thus the financial resources necessary for care were threatened and Mrs. T's own future was jeopardized. Is it moral to seriously harm the lives of the living to care for the dying?

John Hardwig (1990, 1993, 1995) and Nancy Jecker (1993), medical ethicists, argue that the practice of medicine must join the prevalent ethic of patient autonomy with an ethic that includes the interests, needs, and well-being of the family. This new ethic is based on the presumption of equality, which suggests that "the interests of patients and family members are to be weighed equally; medical and non-medical interests of the same magnitude deserve equal consideration" (Hardwig, 1990). The ethic is also based on a presumption of the scarcity of resources—specifically, that there are limits to palliative care and limits to the level of sacrifice we can demand of families (especially many women who are already burdened with other familial demands on their time, energy, and resources). Hardwig (1990) also argues that we must reconceptualize our understanding of patient autonomy: "Autonomy does not mean entitlement without regard for others. Autonomy is the responsible use of freedom and is therefore diminished whenever one ignores, evades or slights responsibilities. . . . If then I am empowered to make decisions about 'my' medical treatment, I am also morally required to shoulder the responsibility of making very difficult moral decisions. The right course of action for me to take will not always be the one that promotes my own interests."

Mr. T should not have been given the kind of absolute power he exercised over his wife and his health care workers. Rather, his strongly felt desires about particular types of care should have been balanced by an equal consideration of the abilities of his caregivers to meet these demands and the ability to meet them without sacrificing the welfare and long-term interests of the larger community. If family members and/or home care workers are unable to set limits on unreasonable, medically suspect, or dangerous patient demands, then an advocate (e.g., case manager, medical social worker, physician, attorney) for both professional and familial caregivers should intervene. Our practices and the very structure of home care for the dying are immoral if they coddle abusive patients and fail to protect the interests and well-being of caregivers, who are often in subordinate positions.

An ethic of responsible care for those who are dying not only requires that we consider both autonomy and justice for the patient, but also that we consider the alignment between autonomy and the values of nonmaleficence and beneficence. Another case of a "bad" death illustrates this concern, and also highlights a related flaw in Americans' understanding of death.

Mr. A was a 76-year-old man with a deadly gastric carcinoma, which had infiltrated his esophagus. He lived alone in a small, one-room subsidized apartment. He led a very simple life, keeping to himself and enjoying his cheeseburgers from McDonalds. Mr. A's only aspirations were to continue his simple life. Unfortunately, his cancer threw him into the world of medicine. Mr. A initially contracted pneumonia, which undoubtedly was contracted from aspirating gastric contents into his lungs. His esophagus was obstructed and would only allow passage of liquids. After his initial pneumonia was successfully treated, Mr. A was sent home with liquid food supplements and warned not to eat solid food again. However, Mr. A continued to eat his cheeseburgers and continued to have recurrent aspiration pneumonia and esophageal obstructions for which he was hospitalized numerous times. He became a major frustration to the health care teams in the hospital. Mr. A suffered from cognitive impairment, and he seemed unable (or unwilling) to make the connection between eating solid foods and his recurring health problems. While he would request that "everything be done" upon each hospitalization, he would not follow the team's recommended treatment regimen on discharge. In addition, once the esophageal obstruction was relieved he would leave the hospital against medical advice, asserting his rights and desires, only to return a few days later with a new obstruction.

Frustration continued to mount as the gap between the goals of the patient and the goals of the treating team became apparent. It was clear that the health care team wished Mr. A would acknowledge his predicament—his impending death—and not only follow the recommended treatment but also agree to be placed in a hospice to die. In fact, Mr. A lacked an understanding of his fatal illness and lacked the capacity to understand the team's recommendations.

Unfortunately, Mr. A had no one at home to help him manage. Even though he desired to stay in his home to the end, he was not able to manage independently. He ultimately returned to the emergency room a final time seeking assistance from the choking sensation in his throat. The gastroenterologists alleviated the obstruction, but then he was admitted to the hospital against his wishes and was placed under a conservatorship. In a short time, he was placed in a hospice against his will, and he died a month later.

The case of Mr. A identifies a second flaw in Americans' understanding of death: the expectation that we can address death rationally. The idea of the autonomous, rational decision-making individual is at the center of how dying persons are treated. Yet death is not rational. Dying often is accompanied by intense emotions—frustration, anger, depression, resentment—for both patient and caregiver. These emotions, and more generally the experience of dying or caring for one who is dying, may lead individuals to act in ways that defy conventional rationality or easy means-end calculation. Attempts to reason with a dying person with dementia or review palliative care procedures with a patient who has no interest in participating may place caregivers in a position in which they must choose the medical values to preserve and the medical values on which to compromise, with little help from the person who is dying.

Professional and family caregivers must recognize that death is not fully rational and alter their expectations about the course that treatment will take. We should expect the dying person to sometimes act as a tyrant (like Mr. T) given his or her level of pain, the loss of control, the depth of anger or depression in the face of death (see Webb, 1997). But the situation does not require that caregivers give in to this tyranny. When the issue of control is central, as in the cases of Mr. T and Mr. A, caregivers must find ways to help the dying patient be a participant in the decision-making process, while also helping the person to understand that what it means to die is to lose complete control over the course of one's life. The lesson is difficult to learn and to teach, but that should not prevent family members and professional caregivers from trying.

The case of Mr. A highlights the challenge of balancing patient autonomy with the moral imperatives of justice and nonmaleficence when the patient is cognitively impaired but not so impaired as to prevent his ability to articulate his wishes for care. Yet because Mr. A was unable to understand the consequences of his choice to continue to eat solid food and reject the recommended treatment plan (repeated bouts of esophageal obstruction and pneumonia and the subsequent costly medical interventions), the medical team was confronted with a difficult ethical decision. Following Mr. A's wishes to have the obstructions cleared and then to return home would preserve his autonomy and allow him to remain in his familiar world. However, continuing to do so made some medical resources unavailable to other patients in the emergency room. It also raised the following question: Would continued treatment of his symptoms without the opportunity to prevent their recurrence be more harmful than taking action to alleviate the pain of his cancer-induced problems?

The medical team acted rationally without demanding that Mr. A act rationally. When continued efforts to explain his treatment options and to reason with him failed, the team decided that Mr. A's interests and the interests of the community (the medical staff, other patients, the hospital) would be best served by placing him in a hospice. Autonomy was tempered with justice, and one hopes with an authentic concern to do no harm to the dying man.

It could be argued that institutionalizing Mr. A actually did more harm than good because it contravened his wish to return to his apartment after treatment and thus led to a death that was not on his terms. However, a collectivist approach to end-of-life-care regards nonmaleficence as entailing more than maintaining a patient's short-term happiness or psychological comfort. This approach pushes us to broaden the meaning of "do no harm" to include actions that protect the welfare of the larger community and provide at least a minimal degree of physical comfort to a patient who insists on harming him- or herself. In other words, concerns to meet the nonmaleficence requirement should be balanced by concerns to meet the demands of justice and beneficence (alleviating suffering or acting to minimize harm). Seen in this light, the medical team's action may be the better moral choice. The resolution of Mr. A's situation can be seen as a necessary compromise of conflicting medical values but one consistent with a community or collectivist orientation toward death.

These two cases illuminate what can happen when patients and caregivers operate with particular understandings of death and dying. When image and reality do not conform and cannot be aligned, patient care becomes extremely difficult, and the demand to engage in moral trade-offs is heightened. Adopting a more collectivist orientation toward care for dying people does not solve the problems or make care easier, but it changes the kinds of moral dilemmas caregivers must face. It also frees us from acting within the constraints of the "good" death and a rational-actor, individualistic orientation. The challenge lies in formulating new strategies to care for those individuals who will not or cannot die peacefully and in finding ways to preserve the autonomy and dignity of the dying person while protecting the interests and needs of the community.

ACKNOWLEDGMENTS

The authors thank Martha Holstein and David McCurdy for their comments on earlier drafts.

REFERENCES

Bellah, R. H., Madsen, R., Sullivan, W. M., Swidler, A., Tipton, S. T. (1985). *Habits of the heart: Individualism and commitment in American life.* Berkeley: University of California Press.

Hardwig, J. (1990). What about the family? *Hastings Center Report, 20*(2), 5–10.

Hardwig, J. (1993). The problem of proxies with interests of their own: Toward a better theory of proxy decisions. *Journal of Clinical Ethics, 4*(1), 20–27.

Hardwig, J. (1995). SUPPORT and the invisible family. *Hastings Center Report, 25*(6), S23–S25.

Holstein, M. (1997). Reflections on death and dying. *Academic Medicine, 72*(10), 848–855.

Jecker, N. S. (1993). Being a burden on others. *Journal of Clinical Ethics, 4*(1), 16–20.

Webb, M. (1997). *The good death: The new American search to reshape the end of life.* New York: Bantam.

CHAPTER 17

Case Managers Meeting to Discuss Ethics

Gail McClelland

Several years ago a few case managers at the Milwaukee County Department on Aging became concerned by the lack of any forum in which they could discuss stories of their day-to-day work in providing services to elders living in the community. Workers particularly wanted to share with each other the narratives of those cases that raised questions about the client's right to self-determination, and about safety, confidentiality, cost of service given limits of financial resources, termination of services, the client's use of drugs or alcohol, or clients' mental health problems.

Several workers believed it was important to come together to critically examine the content and purpose of their work. Supervisory staff agreed that we should meet in order to pursue this goal. At the most rudimentary level, our "ethics discussion group" connoted a level of consciousness or conscientiousness about doing our work reflectively, as well as a commitment to pursue further education in ethics as it relates to our work.

Within a short time the group expanded. It now includes additional case managers, a unit supervisor, the department nurse, and, by invitation, a case manager in private practice with experience in geriatric ethics. This person offers a unique perspective, given that she works outside the department.

The composition of the group provides varied perspectives and is nonhierarchical. Individuals rotate the responsibilities for chairing the meeting, acting as secretary, and providing public relations for each monthly meeting. Meetings occur at an established date and time in our office at the Department on Aging. The meeting is open to any worker having an ethical concern about a case and willing to discuss it with the group.

An abbreviated outline for the case presentation includes a brief description of the elder's medical, psychological, and social levels of functioning. It is available to enable the worker to discuss the case. The format is unstructured. The worker prepares a short summary of the case prior to presentation and states the cause(s) of moral concern or distress that has brought the case up for discussion. Workers are encouraged to invite the elder, the elder's family members and significant others, other agency professionals, and any other providers.

In telling the story of the case and presenting the ethical problem, workers support, affirm, and encourage one another in their efforts to serve the elder and assure that every possible service and case management strategy has been utilized to provide all the services needed by the elder. People at the meeting discuss resources, case management methodology, medical and psychiatric diagnoses, medications, and how best to coordinate with other agencies and service providers. They assist each other in making decisions on complex ethical issues.

In reviewing many individual cases over time, a pattern of ethical concerns in serving elders in the community has emerged. These concerns include gaps in service needs in specific areas of the community, breakdowns and inadequacies in working with other systems serving elders, and need for clarification in matters of departmental policies and procedures specifically related to liability, confidentiality, elders' right to self-determination, and termination of services. The group recognized it needed a mechanism for conveying these concerns to administrative staff. Two people from the group now meet regularly with the agency's administration to keep them informed.

The group's concerns are not just case management practice issues of everyday work with elders. The discussion group has become the place where critical thinking about attentiveness and decision making involved in doing our daily work has merged with narratives recounting the details of that work. The group reached consensus that our name remain "ethics discussion group," not "case consultation group," to best reflect what actually occurs. The group's current challenges are how to expand in size and scope and how to disseminate practice wisdom gained in the group to other workers in the Department.

The ethics discussion group at Milwaukee County Department on Aging encourages critical thinking and facilitates decision making for workers providing long-term-care services to elders living in the community. It allows time and space to be formally set aside to tell each other the stories of our daily work, to support each other in doing this work when it is difficult and perplexing, as well as improve the quality of care given to those we serve.

Perhaps the best possible way to illustrate the effectiveness of the group's process is by case example. This will demonstrate who is involved in providing care in the community setting, in what capacity and how the different providers interact or fail to interact with one another, and how decisions are made in the delivery of care.

> *Ms. C is a 74-year-old woman who came to the attention of the Department as a result of her frequent calls to the police department reporting crime in her neighborhood. When police gained access to her home, they found her house to be cluttered, packed to the walls and to the ceiling with all varieties of stuff, with barely a discernable path through the house for her navigation. An elder abuse and neglect worker conducted the initial assessment of the woman's need for community care.*

In relating to the narrative of this case within the context of the ethics discussion group, it is important to note that the people describing the case are doing so from their own professional worldview. In this case, the officers reported a "nuisance" caller who needed homemaker services—their stated goal being to reduce the number of calls she was making to them regarding her crime-ridden neighborhood. In their investigation, there were no real thefts and officers believed that she was imagining the alleged thieves she reported.

The public health nurse and elder abuse worker responded in turn to calls from the police. Ms. C would not allow the public health nurse to enter her home. The nurse reported no cause for concern about the elder's physical health, but was concerned about the potential health hazards her housekeeping standards posed. The nurse referred the case to elder abuse staff, believing the woman to be self-neglecting in her daily living habits. This professional gained access to the home; when presented with the level of clutter, she threatened the client with removing her from her home, and suggested the need for an immediate wholesale cleanup of her household. When Ms. C responded with a threat of harm to herself, the worker offered a compromise—acceptance on the client's behalf of a deep-cleaning homemaker service. This worker's statements about the case in discussion were definite: Ms. C's housekeeping standards were clearly below community norms, and posed a threat to her own and the community's health and safety. She therefore had the right to use whatever professional force was necessary to mitigate this threat.

The case was subsequently transferred to the next worker, who was responsible for ensuring that the previously agreed-upon services were completed. In addition, this worker was responsible for completing the next level of assessment beyond the initial "crisis" response. She reported that Ms. C's medical level of functioning was satisfactory. Ms. C was in very good physical health with the exception of hypertension, for which she took medication according to schedule and which her physician monitored. Ms. C's psychological level of functioning was impaired. Because Ms. C cried frequently during the interview and expressed hopelessness about her current living situation, the worker was concerned about possible depression and referred Ms. C to outpatient psychiatric care. Ms. C was socially isolated and fearful, living in a neighborhood that had a high incidence of crime. Financially, Ms. C was secure. She continued to live in a dangerous neighborhood because the house had been her home throughout her entire life. She was born and raised in the house, and three generations of her family had lived on that block and nearby streets. Members of her extended family had built the houses in which they resided, attended Mass in the church on the corner, owned the shops, and drank in the taverns speaking their native language. Over the years, persons of a different ethnic background who spoke a different language slowly displaced these neighbors. Ms. C was single and had never married. She attended college and worked as a professional at a nearby hospital until her retirement. She lived her entire life in her childhood home with her parents, caring for them in their elder years through sickness until their deaths. She was resistant to moving from her home, her neighborhood, and her community because they were expressions of her identity, her history, and her life as it was lived. Because of her financial status, Ms. C was ineligible for all but one government-funded program; she was waitlisted for homemaking services. In the meantime, Ms. C spent several thousand dollars for the deep-cleaning homemaking service.

Most participants at the ethics discussion group were satisfied with the outcome of this case. Community response and care was provided to an elder in the community who was difficult to serve and reluctant at first to accept help. The discussion was not lively—for the most part the group was in consensus.

Several months later the group reconvened. Police officers insisted that the Department strongly urge Ms. C to accept psychiatric hospitalization. She had called the police 25 times in the past month regarding imaginary thieves, thus using too much police time in a neighborhood rampant with "real crime." Emergency medical response team members reported similarly that Ms. C had called them 12 times in the past month with vague somatic complaints that, upon investigation, seemed to be symptoms of anxiety and fear. These professionals felt that the individual needs of one member of the community were jeopardizing the overall health and safety of the entire community because time spent responding to her meant a delay in responding to other callers. Participants also expressed concerns about the high cost of such responses.

The group suggested that, with her next call, a team response, including an elder abuse worker, would attempt to invoke the legal provisions for forcible admission to the mental health complex under the state's protective placement or emergency guardianship statutes. The public health nurse reported that several months after the initial deep-cleaning service, housekeeping standards had returned to previous levels, which were clearly a threat to personal and public safety despite Ms. C's continued overall good health. Deep-cleaning service personnel reported that, despite an ongoing need, Ms. C had discontinued service. Ms. C claimed that service staff under-appreciated her despite the fact that she had given so many of her household and personal items to them during their efforts. Clearly, staff reported, Ms. C had overestimated the value of her "junk" which the workers accepted in their efforts to cheer her in her depressive state. Ms. C, taking the advice of the initial worker in this case, obtained psychiatric care. The psychiatrist's prognosis of Ms. C's obsessive-compulsive disorder was that it was "hopeless." Further investigation into Ms. C's financial status revealed that she had more assets than allowed by government standards to enable her to qualify for public assistance programs in long-term care.

Based on the values and professional expertise of most members of the discussion group, the plan for subsequent intervention was as follows: Upon receipt of the next call to paramedics or police, an elder abuse worker would invoke temporary guardianship or protective placement statutes, on the grounds that Ms. C's housekeeping standards were an immediate threat to her physical health. Upon hospitalization, guardianship would be pursued so that Ms. C could be placed in a supervised living environment such as a group home or nursing home. Furthermore, Ms. C had adequate financial resources to pay for the legal services required for the implementation of this plan. Payment for these services would be her responsibility despite the fact that she never requested them.

Much discussion in the group ensued. Not all parties agreed with the plan. Were cost to the community in police and paramedic services, unsuccessful treatment of her late-life onset mental illness, and failure to maintain healthy living standards enough to warrant removal from the community? Was this plan a reaction to the care providers' frustration and failure at not being able to treat this woman's mental health problem successfully or clean her house adequately? Given this woman's financial status, does the public Department on Aging have any obligation to provide long-term ongoing services to her beyond the scope of elder abuse/protective service's crisis-oriented responses? If the case has been previously closed on several occasions because implementing a cleanup was unsuccessful and there was insufficient cause to force this situation to change, is the Department now obliged to reopen the case? If the unclean environment threatens the physical health of the worker, does the worker have a right to refuse this case? If a high incidence of crime in the neighborhood threatens the worker's personal safety, does the worker have a right to refuse the case? What standards determine whether the house is unclean and the neighborhood unsafe? Which community-care providers do not have a right to refuse this case? Why or why not? Does this woman's age factor into our decision to remove her? Would we make the same decision for someone younger? Does a longitudinal view of the person's situation result in a different response? If this household status evolved over 75 years and several generations of accumulations resulting in the same squalor, or if there were abrupt revolutionary change in the person's functional ability, does this change our response? Has the confidentiality of the person been violated by the very fact that this group is discussing her situation without her express consent? Does knowledge of the person's previous functional status and contributions to the community affect our decision? Does higher status "earn" her more entitlement to continued living in the least restricted community setting? Did the cleaning staff have a right to accept any "gifts" from Ms. C? How are they responsible, if at all, for the services being discontinued, if Ms. C claims that their unappreciativeness resulted in her refusal to accept services again, and now that is the very reason for her removal from the home? In the future, Ms. C refuses to accept homemaking services from any individual of a particular race. Should the agency she employs try to accommodate this bias?

Initial responders, police and paramedics, were clear in articulating their role in providing services to Ms. C. She did not need their services, and they referred her to social service professionals with the expectation that these staff would assist Ms. C in cleaning her house and obtaining psychiatric care, thus eliminating her calls to them. Social service professionals in turn referred the problem of cleanup to a home health care agency, whose homemaker staff are the least trained and educated about the complex issues of mental health that affect a change in this person's behavior and household status. How much of the failure of the homemaker staff efforts resulted from cultural and generational differences about possessions and cleaning methods? How did these differences affect the outcome? Ms. C grew up with marginal financial resources; she saved, was extremely thrifty, and found a use for household items beyond their intended time. She would not purchase "garbage bags" at the store, for example, but would wash and recycle other plastic bags from previous purchases for this use. She could demonstrate that bed linens from 40 years ago, when worn thin, were subsequently sewn into pillowcases, then in turn were salvaged and used as rags. These conservation methods were a source of Ms. C's pride. Failure to appreciate or understand these practices was an insult to her. The woman cleaning Ms. C's house would rather purchase something new; she did not see any reason to use cleaning products and procedures that were not the most up-to-date and time and energy efficient. Furthermore, this staff person was being paid to clean, not to validate the history and etiology of Ms. C's rag collection. How did these cultural and generational differences affect the outcome of Ms. C's refusal to continue to employ the cleaning staff?

The discussion group employed bargaining and negotiation techniques. Workers who were insistent on detaining Ms. C in the hospital upon her next call for help agreed to delay their plans, while other team members encouraged her to again accept services. Initially, however, the Department formulated a protocol that enabled workers to provide ongoing services to those in need despite financial ineligibility for funded programs. In part, this was accomplished by recognizing the overall cost to the community at large of not attending to someone's need.

Case discussion led to several interesting points. Participants agreed that different types of case management functions could achieve care plan goals. Some goals are obtained by crisis response and short-term involvement. Success achieved here is often immediate. Other cases require providing sustained and ongoing services, ideally by the same person over time. Success here takes a much longer time to achieve. Attributes and skills of service providers differ, depending on the type of care needed by the individual. Ms. C required sustained long-term care. Qualities such as attentiveness, ability to perceive and acknowledge progress in small increments, a focus on the person's strengths despite her continued losses, and a genuine interest in knowing and appreciating that person's history were essential to implement the care plan successfully. Listening to Ms. C's stories about her life was absolutely critical in effecting a change in her living situation and overall quality of life. By listening, another person validated her life; as a result, Ms. C could begin to accept suggestions about alternatives to her marginal situation.

In contrast, workers who believed that the best course of care was to access involuntary treatment for Ms. C used another approach to accomplish their goal. They needed to obtain information from a number of sources, including the person herself, and document her disabilities and failures in all areas of functioning. They needed sufficient evidence of Ms. C's deficits to demonstrate her need to be enrolled in the long-term-care system and to permit swift access to involuntary care in a treatment facility.

These differences in skills and perceptions are often the manifestation of a larger core value system of beliefs held by workers. The ethics discussion group provides a forum for workers to express their conflicts in a non-threatening space and define their differences in perceptions and values to reach a consensus on how care is to be delivered. Sometimes the group discussion's only function is to illuminate the fact that these differences exist.

This particular case discussion uncovered some sources of moral distress to workers who had experience in providing long-term care to consumers. If a worker strongly believes that advocacy on behalf of the consumer to maintain the least restrictive living environment is good, the worker will inevitably be in conflict with many members of the community—that same community which holds the worker to high ethical standards. Is the identified "client" here the family, neighbors, landlords, other professionals, or the consumer? How does the worker balance the demands made by other persons regarding the care plan? How does the worker handle the stress of maintaining a balanced plan?

How does the individual worker, trained by profession to identify needs and then provide services to satisfy them, work in a delivery system where there is an overall shortage of services and funding for services, but an aggressive recruitment program to identify potential consumers and assess their needs? Is this effort creating a dependency in elderly consumers on a formal service delivery system instead of encouraging consumers to find solutions to problems and resources for their needs in the rest of the community? By encouraging this kind of dependency, what message is being conveyed about the strengths of elders in our community? Are these the initial stages of denormalizing aging?

In this case, the workers attempting to access involuntary care for the person stated that they could not achieve this end due to Ms. C's "failure" to meet the standards for involuntary care. In other words, Ms. C could not be subjected to hospitalization or other treatment unless she consented. The group then agreed that other workers involved in the plan of care would work with Ms. C for a limited time to engage her and encourage her to accept needed services. These workers were successful in that attempt through the use of effective case management strategies grounded in their beliefs. Qualities which assured that success included day-to-day persistence, recognition of Ms. C's strengths and ability to apply them to care plan goals, authentic engagement in life review with Ms. C, continued advocacy on behalf of Ms. C despite complaints and protests about her, and effective communication skills regarding differences in existing cultural and generational attitudes and values. It was not just the employment of highly effective case management strategies that caused the positive change in Ms. C's situation, but fundamental beliefs and attitudes underlying them held by the workers.

Ms. C's social isolation, as well as her anxiety and depression, decreased once workers implemented the care plan. Calls to the police and paramedics decreased dramatically, then ceased completely. Through the successful achievement of long-term-care case management goals, Ms. C purchased additional homemaker services, cleaned her home, then sold it, and is now residing in her own clean apartment in subsidized housing for elders.

This case example demonstrates the use of the ethics discussion group at the Department on Aging. It is an opportunity for workers to engage in open discussion, in a nonthreatening environment, about the differences in values encountered in supporting elders residing in the community. Ideally the discussion should continue until the group reaches consensus. This type of interchange results in improved services and an improved quality of life for the elders we serve.

CHAPTER 18

Who's Safe? Who's Sorry?: The Duty to Protect the Safety of HCBS Consumers

Rosalie A. Kane and Carrie A. Levin

First, do no harm. This is a major tenet in medical ethics. It is also the first statement of the ethical principle of beneficence, that is, doing good, which holds that ethical professionals act so as to benefit their clientele and, at the least, so as to do no harm.

The laudable goal of doing no harm has been extended to the ideal that the care and service plans developed for home- and community-based services (HCBS) for older people be designed to maximize those consumers' physical safety and protection and to minimize the likelihood of preventable negative events, such as falls, injuries, or relapses. The social workers, nurses, and others who hold up safety as a goal may be striving to do no harm. But, such professionals may have lost perspective on the nature of their own agency in helping individuals plan their lives, and they may be assuming too much responsibility for their clients' lives. They may have also lost perspective on the facts, that is, what actually constitutes safety and what actually constitutes risk.

Home- and community-based services (HCBS) have sprung up as alternatives to nursing facilities and are popular for the very reason that they offer clientele the care they need in environments that are more homelike and less restrictive than a nursing facility. Older people choose these options and they remain popular alternatives, in part, because of older persons' desire to manage and direct their own care and lives, and in part because of a desire for privacy, continuity, and familiarity in lifestyle. Protecting HCBS clients ultimately may mean declining to serve them in their own homes because the plan seems unsafe. Protecting HCBS clients ultimately may mean reshaping assisted living settings through regulations until they mirror more restrictive settings like nursing homes, or (in a continuation of the impetus that encouraged placement in assisted living settings) declining to retain a person in assisted living because he or she seems to be unsafe without the greater protection of a nursing home. Paradoxically, therefore, the desire to do no harm and hold safety above all may actually result in harm for consumers, at least in the sense of disrupting their lives.

DEFINING HARM

Harm comes in different forms. One type of harm is physical, affecting one's health and physical safety. The jury is by no means out that all efforts now made on behalf of physical safety are justified in their own right. Harm may also be done to psychological well-being, creating anxiety, depression, a sense of being bereft and without hope. Harm may also be done to social well-being, cutting people off from relationships and activities they value and creating difficulties for those who wish to form new relationships. Those who argue for safety above all tend to emphasize physical safety. The very act of constricting freedom and choice for individuals and preventing them from taking risks may create psychological harm. Less subtly, the environments and programs favored because they appear to be safe rarely nourish the spirit, the psyche, or the intellect.

In this chapter, we consider the full range of harms that may occur to people needing long-term care, namely physical, psychological, and social harms. We also consider that removing the right to take risks from other human beings may in itself be a harm that should not be lightly undertaken. Two justifications for restricting individual's rights to take risks are sometimes made: (1) without that restriction, harm is likely to come to others; and (2) without that restriction people are likely to harm themselves (typically because cognitive impairment or mental illness have rendered them unable to make a judgment). Both justifications can be valid in some instances, but, we argue, are used too readily and with insufficient evidence to restrict people who receive long-term care.

The most exquisitely difficult ethical dilemmas that arise in HCBS concern the proper boundaries between promoting freedom for older people and avoiding interference with their life goals versus acting responsibly to promote the older person's health and safety. These are anguishing dilemmas for professionals. The case files of ethics committees that have sprung up in HCBS are littered with examples wherein professionals wrestle consciously and conscientiously with the problems of striking the right balance between safety and freedom. Often, the professional has the painful sense that he or she is joining the forces pushing unwilling clients towards nursing homes, yet it seems to be for their own good.

These ethical dilemmas are exacerbated by the profound ambivalence that so many people feel about tradeoffs between their freedom and safety. Older people, like people of all ages, want to be *both* free and safe. Older HCBS consumers, who often are aware of their increased risks and diminished capabilities, can have great difficulty making a forced choice between the two values. In one study of more than 800 elderly HCBS clients, about a third chose freedom, a third chose safety, and a third vacillated indecisively between the two (Degenholtz, Kane, & Kivnick, 1997). Professionals express similar ambivalence. One study involving care providers, advocates, and public officials showed respondents overwhelmingly agreeing with the proposition that older HCBS clients should be free to act against professional advice regarding risk-taking without the program withdrawing from the scene. When asked to elaborate the circumstances under which such client risk-taking would be permissible, almost all responded with a variant on "when it does not jeopardize their own safety and those of others" (Kane, 1995). Professionals endorsed informed risk-taking, but apparently only when it was risk-free!

In this chapter, we further dissect the concept of consumer risk-taking and professional responsibly in HCBS. We then turn to possible ways for professionals to negotiate these ethical minefields, including an exploration of the relatively new concept of *managed risk contracting* or *negotiated risk*. We argue that active steps need to be taken to preserve and promote the right of competent older people to make decisions about their care in general, not just narrow decisions about specific procedures. (Currently, it is easier to refuse a recommended amputation than a recommended nursing home placement.) However, some safeguarding procedures and perhaps even some regulation need to be in place to govern any contractual mechanisms for risk-taking of older HCBS clients.

Rights to Risk-Taking

One ethics source book defines risk as "an adverse future event that is not certain but only probable" (Shöne-Seifert, 1995). People who are competent decision-makers ordinarily make autonomous decisions about the risks they wish to take based on the magnitude and the likelihood of expected harms and benefits associated with each course of action. There may, of course, be limits to a person's right to take informed risks. Obviously, one should not implicate third parties in one's risk-taking. For example, the person who wishes to risk smoking around his or her oxygen cannot properly endanger others in a common living setting by choosing to incur risks. The insulin-dependent diabetic who fails to stick to a diet, on the other hand, may injure only herself. Yet, some would argue that this noncompliant individual has no right to repeatedly drive herself into diabetic coma if, in so doing, she harms others by drawing resources away from them. Without getting into the more abstract arguments about finite resources for health care, one could certainly argue that a person who has a weekly health crisis in an assisted living setting takes valuable and often limited staff time away from others.

Let's assume a consumer's desired risk-taking will cause no harm to others. Let's further assume that the consumer has decided, after thoughtful decision-making, that the benefits of following the risky course of action outweigh the potential harms to the self. The consumer may yet not be free to follow her preferences. Care providers might still argue that they cannot allow people under their care to assume certain risks because they, themselves, would then be negligent in their duties. For this reason, home care agencies or HCBS case managers sometimes terminate cases rather than manage them at a lower intensity of service than they think proper (Kane & Caplan, 1993). For certain technical procedures, for example, administration of intravenous fluid or treatment of wounds, the consumer has no privilege to waive technical standards of competence in the performance of the procedures. The provider is not off the hook for negligence because the consumer has consented to, say, reusing a needle. What about the quadriplegic consumer who cannot take his own medicine and prefers to have his housekeeper administer the medications rather than eat up the resources for his HCBS plan with expensive visits from a licensed nurse? Providers struggling to define the boundaries of their responsibilities versus the consumer's right to informed risk-taking may hotly debate this issue. Or, the ethical tension may at least temporarily be resolved at a policy level by rules that require specific training to perform certain tasks.

To take another example, regardless of a resident's informed choice, staff of an assisted living program often obsess over whether they would be negligent to retain someone in their setting whose needs seem to exceed the program's service capability. Such a dilemma typically involves a risk, not a certainty. The resident *might* fall, and *if* she were to fall at night, the staffing level would be inadequate to transfer her back to bed. The resident *might* wander out because of insufficient staff supervision and, if so, *might* sustain an injury, which *might* be serious. However, in jurisdictions where assisted living programs are legally required to eject anyone who reaches a certain level of need, the consumer's prerogative to take certain risks has been preempted. For example, many states permit assisted living residents to receive "help with self-administration of medications," but technically expect the resident to leave if no longer capable of that ambiguous self-administration. In May 2001, *U.S. News and World Report* described how this rule negatively affected an assisted living resident whose stroke left her unable to remember her medication regime, but otherwise was an excellent candidate for assisted living according to her family, the assisted living residents and her physician (Shapiro, 2001).

The great variety of prohibitions and permissions that govern licensed HCBS entities suggests that conventional wisdom is in flux and abounds in confusion about how much protection should be built in programmatically. We need to incorporate safeguards to ensure that autonomy not be legislated or regulated out of long-term care altogether. Because the regulatory arena for both home care and assisted living is changing rapidly, it is important to ensure that these options remain viable. Most individuals with care needs have a strong desire to stay in their own homes. If this is not possible, most will choose to enter the least restrictive long-term-care facility possible. This is why assisted living facilities have become a very popular alternative to nursing homes in the United States today. Home care and assisted living are alternatives that frail elders choose knowing that they will not be completely safe, but they take these risks willingly in order to retain a certain degree of autonomy. There is the potential in developing rules and regulations that these types of popular alternatives will be "regulated away," and all that will be left are nursing facilities—the most regulated types of health care institutions in this country.

Thus, the rights of a consumer to take informed risks are modified by the moral, legal, and regulatory responsibilities of health professionals and care organizations. However, the moral foundation for legal and regulatory constraints on consumer risk-taking needs constant examination. Professional orthodoxy, risk-aversion, and guild motivations may all conspire to reduce the freedom of consumers to make changes in the interests of their own goals.

Deconstructing Consumer Risk-Taking

The slogan "better safe than sorry" covers a wide range of circumstances. A certain amount of deconstruction is needed to parse what the concept of risk encompasses. Also useful would be a common language for discussing risks and risk-taking. We argue that the following should be considered in any appraisal of risks to an HCBS consumer:

Type of Risk to Be Avoided

As stated above, risks may be physical, psychological, or social, including financial. For the most part, care providers bring physical risks to consumers' attention while tending to discount psychological and social risks. Even when considering physical risks, we should surely view differently the risk of having a particular health indicator become elevated (which, in turn, is a risk-factor for a health problem) versus the risk of a specific disease or injury. For example, preoccupation with maintaining cholesterol levels in people over 85 with no history of cardiovascular disease may be short-sighted.

In the psychological or social sphere, risks may be more than trivial. For example, a high risk of painful depression, loss of role, loneliness, and lack of purpose may accompany some care plans. Usually, however, care providers are in the business of presenting risks to physical health and safety and rarely would review social or psychological risks and advise people, for example, to avoid a nursing home because they seem at high risk for substantial human misery.

What about the risk of death, to some the ultimate harm? Viewing death as the result to be avoided at all times belies the fact that most people receiving HCBS of the intensity where these freedom-protection tradeoffs are likely to surface are often very old and have shortened life expectancies. Perhaps a 99-year-old brittle diabetic would rather take her chances with a double chocolate brownie once a week. After all, chocolate brownie or not, her expectancy for further years of life is limited.

Severity of Risk

Some risks are severe, even life-threatening, whereas others are relatively trivial. Surely, the severity of the condition or circumstance being risked must be taken into account. For example, taking some risks—for example, crossing a busy, wide intersection alone despite severe macular degeneration and a slow gait—can result in serious injury or death. Insisting on walking to the bathroom alone despite the same circumstances carries a much lesser risk, though for people with some health conditions a fall can begin a serious decline. Being in a bathroom with an internal locking door carries with it the risk that the individual thus protected may be less quick to receive help should they suffer a fall, a heart attack, or a spell of dizziness. It seems quite unlikely that the bow to normal life and privacy occasioned by the locking bathroom door creates an unacceptably severe risk.

Likelihood of the Risk

Some severe risks are, fortunately, quite unlikely. Perishing in a fire is one such unlikely risk, as is being hit by lightening, though in both cases the consequences of the adverse event are dire. Often, professionals and, for that matter, family members of the older person with the disability concentrate on the severity of consequences, say, if an older person with some dementia is alone in the home and becomes prey to a dangerous criminal rather than on the likelihood of the risk actually happening, which often is slight.

Risks to Others

What if the risks are to others in the housing setting, community, assisted living building, or nursing home? A risk to others is typically taken more seriously than a chosen risk to the self. The archetypal risks to others are fire (caused by unsafe smoking or unsafe use, for example, of cooking equipment) and driving. Thus, there seems to be a good justification for restricting smoking and cooking to times and places where the individual can be observed and assisted, and prohibiting use of an automobile for those whose memories and judgment are impaired. In contrast, using a shower may put the same individual in danger of being scalded or injured but is unlikely to harm others. The important considerations here are the likelihood and severity of the risk, and the possibility of mitigating both the likelihood and severity of the negative event (controlling the water temperature and flow, non-slip surfaces to reduce likelihood, and pull-cords for summoning help to reduce severity). The chocolate brownie for the diabetic apparently carries no risk to others at all, though some might argue that if he or she is truly courting diabetic coma with each slice, he or she will be using resources that could have better been allocated to others. This argument about harming others by using too many resources is often applied in a facile manner, however. Unless this particular person had experienced a few recent crises that demanded the attention of staff, the risk seems altogether too hypothetical to be given much weight.

Quantifying Risk

Risks associated with HCBS plans are notoriously difficult to quantify. In contrast, the difficult matter of advising patients about risks of medical procedures is almost easy. Although science is far from exact, it often is plausible to provide the potential consumer with information about death and complication rates following a surgical procedure or a drug intervention and even to elaborate on the circumstances that exacerbate or minimize the likelihood that the particular person will experience a bad outcome. Similarly, it often is possible to provide information about the likely course of action if the surgery is rejected or the medicine not taken.

In contrast, long-term care typically deals with many small consecutive or repeated decisions rather than one big decision. For example, the likelihood of falling, difficult to predict at best, is related to multiple decisions involving independent ambulation or transfer in all their differing circumstances. The consumer who is advised to curtail activities to prevent falls may adopt a partial strategy, perhaps with less risk avoidance than providers prefer but more caution than she normally would adopt. The likely consequences of highly individualized strategies to entertain or avoid health risks are almost impossible to calculate with any precision.

Negative Effects of Avoiding the Risk

These effects, like the original risk itself, are also not a certainty, but merely a prediction. They, too, can be classified in terms of type of effect, for example, physical, psychological, social, or financial. They, too, can be examined in terms of their likelihood and their severity. Negative effects of avoiding the risk can limit the freedom of the individual and may also cause additional strain or decrease quality of life. If an individual in her own home or an assisted living facility is not allowed to bathe alone because her providers fear that she may slip and fall, this can potentially cause her emotional harm. She may lose dignity by having to ask for assistance. She and her family members may also be strained financially because she will have to pay a provider to assist her with bathing. Especially if this woman has no prior history of falling in the bathtub, the negative effects may be greater than allowing the risk. Another negative effect in this situation may be that the woman will have to burden her family members or friends in order to receive the assistance that the provider believes she needs. This burden can be the physical burden on the family member or the psychological burden of having to ask for assistance. There is risk at every moment in every individual's life. How do we know where to draw the line?

Case managers, hospital discharge planners, and home care providers are often in the role of recommending nursing home placement as the safest bet for an individual who seems to be at risk. Seldom, however, do they evaluate the risks associated with the recommended placement. Rather, they concentrate on the observable risks encountered in the current home situation or if the person were to return home from the hospital. There well may be physical as well as other kinds of risks associated with the more restrictive alternative that have not been considered. For example, there may be dangers of losing functional abilities through disuse, or of the resident being hurt by a combative resident, or of institution-borne infections. Truly assessing the risks involved in a nursing home placement requires particularization regarding the risk factors to which the individual referred to a nursing home is prone, regarding the nature and track record of the nursing home, and even regarding the unit and room where the individual will be housed. Nobody making a placement has time or knowledge to consider such risks, nor does he or she usually learn about the results of the placement. The individual moved to a nursing home because of fear that she might fall in her apartment could have fallen and been severely injured in the nursing home within weeks of admission, but this event would not help inform the discharge planner's decision-making formulae.

Role of Providers

Long-term-care choices differ from choices about many discrete acute health decisions because the providers may still be active in the case after their advice is ignored. In this sense, HCBS resembles primary care, but with much more intensity and intimacy of involvement than is usually the case between patient and physician. If home care providers, care coordinators, or assisted living providers are present on an almost daily basis, they may find themselves impelled to renew the subject of their own concerns regularly. It is always easier to honor autonomy in the abstract than when one must confront a client who is in a dangerous situation. Providers have a genuine sense of responsibility and experience real tension between respecting autonomy and being negligent. Where do we draw the line? How should we draw the line? For example, a client in her early 70s who has difficulty seeing because of complications of diabetes has been in her bed for over a week when a case manager stops by to check on her. The visiting nurse who monitors the situation believes that the woman is in danger of losing her foot because the small sores that she has had for the past month have been left untreated and have turned into large open wounds. The older woman refuses to seek medical treatment from a health care professional because she believes only in herbal remedies. Because the woman is in severe pain caused by what is perhaps an infection in her open wound, she has not been able to get out of bed for over a week. She has been lying in her own feces and urine and the visiting nurse wants her to go to the hospital. The woman refuses, which puts the nurse in a very difficult situation. She does not want to simply abandon her client, but sees that she is in real danger. Health care providers are often placed in these difficult situations and there are no clear-cut ethical rules governing what they should do.

Ingredients of Informed Risk-Taking

Almost as a tautology, informed risk-taking requires a source of trustworthy information. The consumer also may require time to digest that information and consider the implications. At issue is whether and under what circumstances care providers are a good source of information about the riskiness of various courses of action. And, if not the care provider, who should provide such information? Should it be provided in writing? With a witness? Will all those trappings create such an aura of dread and fear that it unduly influences the deliberations of the consumer? Yet, without such a formal process, how is it clear that the consumer has been informed and how do professionals and care organizations protect themselves from legal liability?

Informed risk-taking also requires a competent individual who is capable of understanding the trade-offs and making the choices. Many older adults are capable of making certain decisions, but not others. Just as with any informed consent, a client must be given information and decisions should be made on an individual basis. There is a danger that when older adults disagree with their providers, this can be taken as incompetence when it really is only disagreement. A first step that needs to be taken when considering any type of risk is an assessment of the possible negative effects, as well as the alternatives.

Many long-term-care consumers suffer from some degree of impaired memory or judgment that may render them incapable of making a decision to take chances in the name of autonomy. It still may be feasible to develop a process by which an agent weighs the benefits and harms of various courses of action on behalf of the individual with severe dementia, but the rationale for such a process is based on a different set of assumptions than respect for autonomy, such as a desire to promote happiness. However, just as we examine risk on a continuum, cognitive impairment must also be seen as a progression. There is reason to believe that people with mild cognitive impairment can appreciate some risks and accept them knowingly. Unfortunately, however, probably because of the propensity to protect, little research has been done to examine the nature of the trade-offs people with early Alzheimer's would make and the reliability of their decisions.

Managed or Negotiated Risk Contracting

Managed or negotiated risk contracting is a term that came into vogue in the 1990s as many state HCBS programs started to give explicit recognition to notions such as "dignity of risk" in their supporting legislation or program rules. In the state of Oregon, the concept has had the most widespread application. As developed there, managed risk contracting is an orderly process for examining and resolving issues that arise when providers become concerned about the risks that their clientele are assuming (Kapp & Wilson, 1995). Managed risk contracting as it has evolved in Oregon has several steps:

- defining risks and provider concerns;
- defining probable consequences of the consumer's behavior or condition;
- identifying the preferences of everyone involved, which includes the at-risk consumer, one or more care providers, and possibly one or more family members;
- identifying possible solutions;
- choosing a solution.

Ultimately, the person incurring the risk is perceived as the ultimate decision-maker (assuming competency and no inordinate risks to others), but the search is always for compromise solutions. The plan is documented in writing and signed by the consumer and other relevant parties to the agreement.

Managed risk agreements in Oregon have evolved particularly in the assisted living setting, which by law is a congregate care setting that is expected to maximize values of privacy, dignity, choice, independence, and normal lifestyles. It is structured so as to encourage people with nursing-home levels of disability to live in their own self-contained small apartments with features and amenities that encourage independence but also court danger, for example, because of roll-in showers, refrigerators and cooking appliances, and locking doors. Assisted living programs in Oregon charge less than nursing homes, receive less in public payment, and are not staffed for constant attention even if the environments were conducive to such surveillance. As individual residents are perceived to be at some risk because of their own behavior—e.g., not waiting for bathroom assistance, violating special diets, going out on their own recognizance, imperfectly managing self-medication regimens—formal managed risk contracting is sometimes considered. At times, the managed risk contract is put into effect because the consumer's preference counters the providers'. For example, the provider might prefer to administer all medications, whereas the consumer prefers to self-medicate either to keep independent or to avoid extra costs associated with accepting more help. At other times, the managed risk contract clarifies what kind of assistance can be expected in the setting. For instance, the consumer might be content to be accompanied on all walks, but the provider may not have the staff to do so.

In an ongoing study, we asked about 60 assisted living providers to comment on their views of managed risk contracting as a mechanism for clarifying and perhaps resolving some of the ethical conflicts arising over safety/freedom tradeoffs. We found vastly differing enthusiasm for the concept, ranging from high to unwillingness to touch it with a 10-foot pole. Regardless of the respondent's stance, few providers believed that a managed risk agreement is a legally binding document. Indeed, we have not identified any case law that is directly on point to clarify the topic and suspect that a managed risk agreement would provide little protection in the case of a legal challenge.

Proponents of managed risk contracting believe that the very act of identifying the issues is salutary and may, in fact, lead to creative compromise solutions. Managed risk contracts are a tool that encourages and structures discussion among all parties involved. Often family members, residents, and providers have not all sat down together to discuss the issues. This is one way of getting the discussion started that allows each party to voice his or her preferences. Opponents believe these contracts are not worth the paper on which they are written. Some opponents indicated that they saw formal managed risk contracts as a failure in care planning. They asserted that managed risk contracts are unnecessary because discussions of risks and preferences should be a regular and ongoing part of care planning. We also identified a small subset of providers who were using the mechanism to clarify the risks *providers* were willing to take. For example, the managed risk agreement might read that the consumer would be permitted to smoke in a defined area of the building but, if he dropped the cigarette, he would need to smoke outside. Certainly, the establishment of progressive steps in a provider's willingness to tolerate the risky behavior and the ultimatum approach (three strikes and you're out!) distorts the original consumer-empowering intent of managed risk contracting.

Examples of Managed Risk Contracts

At present, no official "legal" format exists for managed risk contracts, and there are few models circulating in the community. Individual providers and public payment programs have created approaches to managed risk contracts that suit their specific needs. Some assisted living facilities have managed risk policies or declarations in their resident handbooks or as part of the orientation material that prospective residents receive (Figure 18.1). Most create individualized managed risk agreements as situations come up, and some use both devices. That is, they include general language to alert residents and families that risks

> Assisted Living Facilities in Oregon operate on the principle of MANAGED RISK. Managed risk allows elderly or disabled persons the choice of living more independently than allowed in some institutional settings such as nursing facilities. With the increase in independence comes some risk to the resident. Listed below are some of the features at _____ and the risk each may present.
>
> 1. locked and keyed private apartments where staff members do not interrupt residents unless a resident calls for assistance or a planned intervention has been arranged; hallways and doorways are not monitored
> 2. non-restraint policy increases the risk of falling for those residents who are unsteady on their feet
> 3. unsupervised snack area which allows residents who are on restricted diets the chance to stray from their diets
> 4. concludes with a statement that the resident is the final decision-maker unless there is a guardian

FIGURE 18.1 Language from admissions material at an Oregon assisted living setting.

may be taken in this facility, but if the risks go beyond normal, they execute a managed risk agreement.

Figure 18.2 shows a hypothetical managed risk agreement based on some that we collected from Oregon Assisted Living Facilities. This particular firm has developed a pattern for managed risk agreements that identify the problem or issue, the resident's concerns, the provider's concerns, the list of possible solutions generated, and the chosen solution.

Figure 18.3 shows an example of a managed risk contract developed by a free-standing case management organization in Illinois. The agency has developed a format that includes a standard statement on the top that explains the nature of a managed risk agreement, followed by a specific managed risk agreement for a particular client. The specific document makes it clear that the doctor would prefer a different plan and also specifies risks to the individual. In this particular agency, the risks are often articulated generally as the risks of staying at home rather than accepting residence in a nursing home.

Resident's Name: Henrietta _____ Date:

Parties involved in discussion:
Henrietta _____, Henrietta's son, the AL nurse, and Henrietta's case manager.

Managed risk issue/problem:
Henrietta is an insulin-dependent diabetic with physician's orders to follow the American Diabetic Association's recommended diet. Henrietta however, loves to eat candies such as gum drops and peppermints in her room as well as cake with white frosting in the dining room. Henrietta asks staff members to purchase sweets for her outside the facility. She frequently requests dessert after meals. Henrietta refuses to eat diabetic desserts stating that they are not made for human consumption.

Resident's concerns:
Henrietta wishes to be allowed to eat candy in her room and desserts in the dining hall.

Consequences of the risk/providers' concerns:
Refusing to follow the diabetic diet can place Henrietta at severe health risks including possible diabetic exacerbations, coma, and even death.

Possible alternatives to minimize the risk:
1) Henrietta could refrain from asking for non-diabetic desserts in the dining hall; 2) Henrietta could refrain from eating sugar candy in her apartment; 3) the facility could increase the variety of diabetic desserts offered in order to find one that Henrietta likes; 4) Henrietta can get special diabetic candies from the local market; 5) Henrietta could be permitted to do as she desires after being informed of the health risks involved with being non-compliant with the ADA diet.

Agreement:
The AL will offer more varieties of diabetic desserts including diabetic candies. Henrietta will try diabetic desserts and will help the cook find new recipes for diabetic desserts that look more appealing. If Henrietta insists on eating a particular dessert that is not on her diet at a meal, the dining staff will remind her that it is not recommended, but will not prevent Henrietta from eating the dessert. This agreement will be reviewed by _____.

Signatures:

_____   _____
Resident   Date

_____   _____
Representative of facility   Date

_____   _____
Family (if applicable)   Date

_____   _____   _____
Other (as applicable)   Role   Date

Source: Adapted from a variety of corporate tools with an emphasis on approaches used by Assisted Living Concepts, Portland, Oregon.

FIGURE 18.2 Example of a managed risk agreement in assisted living.

RISK STATEMENT FORM

I, _____, understand that I have the right to self-determination. I have chosen to remain at home and refuse to go into a nursing home. I understand that Dr. _____ has recommended a nursing home that provides 24-hour care and supervision but that s/he has agreed to home care at my preference.

My care manager has discussed the following risks, which I understand and am willing to accept:

1. My dizziness may result in a fall.
2. Not being able to see clearly to take my medications by myself may aggravate my congestive heart failure and result in hospitalization. I understand that my daughter is no longer able to continue medication set-up as she has previously done.
3. Not being able to easily prepare food may result in a loss of nutritional status.
4. Not being able to use my oxygen when I need it may result in hospitalization.

_____   _____
Client signature   Case manager signature

_____   _____
Date   Date

Client's functional and cognitive assessment status attached.

Source: Based on a form developed by Alternatives for the Older Adult, Rock Island, Illinois. Client described is also fictional but based on real situations.

FIGURE 18.3 Example of managed risk statement used in home care. Some clients choose to make decisions that are contrary to the recommendations of the physician, the family, the care providers, or the case manager. Such decisions may put the client at risk of injury or harm. This "Risk Statement" has been developed to highlight the client's impairments and the particular risks that may occur if the client chooses to remain at home against the doctor's, family's, or case manager's recommendations. The client's signature indicates informed consent; that he/she understands the risks and consequences that his/her decisions may have, and that he/she is willing to accept the risks.

WHEN THINGS GO WRONG

Everybody can congratulate themselves on being sensitive to consumer preferences as long as no untoward events occur. When things go wrong, especially in publicly-funded programs, there is a natural tendency to seek someone to blame (Kapp, 1997). The true test of an approach in which consumers can make decisions to take chances comes after the negative event. When the fall occurs, does the consumer get a chance to rise and fall again? In the worst possible scenario, when the consumer dies as a result of the course of action pursued, will providers be held culpable? Even if they are not blamed, will they feel responsible in a way that detracts from their effectiveness?

The more long-term care mirrors normal life, the more things can go wrong. Depressed people will have more access to weapons that could potentially harm them. Die-hard smokers on oxygen will have the opportunity to become human torches (an event that is more likely to kill them than injure others nearby). People may leave their homes or assisted living setting, suffer a health event (e.g., a fall or stroke), and die unattended. Should care providers be held responsible for each such negative event regardless of its rarity and the fact that they had discussed the possibility with the consumer?

COGNITIVE IMPAIRMENT AND SURROGATE RISK-TAKING

The most difficult scenario concerns cognitive impairment, the very scenario in which most risks occur. Some family members express confidence that they know what kind of risks their relative would prefer to take, and some lay claim to greater freedom for their relatives with Alzheimer's disease. Do family members have the right to assert that mother would rather be at home, even if at times alone and unsafe, than in an unfamiliar institution? Do they have the right to assert that they would rather have that independent experience for mother? Do they have the right to say dad should remain in an assisted living setting where he might at times wander out and accept the consequences? Should a family member be allowed to negotiate an agreement that the assisted living setting will check the whereabouts of a wandering parent at intervals and call 911 if the parent is missing? Does such an agreement get the facility off the hook if the worst happens? What if family members appear to have a conflict of interest? For example, the more protective plan may erode an expected legacy from the older person.

TOWARDS CLARITY

Resolving the problems that arise when perceived safety and freedom conflict will require new organizational and perhaps legal vehicles. It will be necessary to determine who has a stake in the outcome and who deserves to be part of the deliberations. It will be necessary to develop better ways of engaging consumers in genuine and ongoing consideration of the risks they want to take and the way they want to live. We will need to learn how to distinguish between negligent care and care that respects autonomous risk-taking, between protecting consumers and coercing them into conforming lifestyles. Most ethical problems in home- and community-based care revolve around the safety-protection trade-offs and consumers and providers alike are anguished about what to do. We have already tried making safety (in the eye of the provider) the default position without guaranteeing either safety or other sorts of well-being. A cautious effort to develop a new approach seems worth the risk.

ACKNOWLEDGMENT

The work that led to this manuscript was supported by The Retirement Research Foundation.

REFERENCES

Degenholtz, H. B., Kane, R. A., & Kivnick, H. Q. (1997). Care related preferences and values of elderly community-based LTC consumers: Can case managers learn what's important to clients? *The Gerontologist, 37*(6), 767–776.

Kane, R. A. (1995). *Quality, autonomy, and safety in home and community-based long-term care: Toward regulatory and quality assurance policy.* (Report of a Mini-Conference for the White House Conference on Aging, February 11 and 12, 1995.) Minneapolis: National LTC Resource Center, University of Minnesota School of Public Health.

Kane, R. A., & Caplan, A. L. (1993). *Ethical conflict in the management of home care: The case manager's dilemma.* New York: Springer Publishing.

Kapp, M. B. (1997). Who is responsible for this? Assigning rights and consequences in elder care. *Journal of Aging and Social Policy, 9*(2), 51–65.

Kapp, M. B., & Wilson, K. B. (1995). Assisted living and negotiated risk: Reconciling protection and autonomy. *Journal of Ethics, Law, and Aging, 1*(1), 5–13.

Shapiro, J. (May 2, 2001). A better way to grow old: Alternatives to nursing home care. *U.S. News & World Report,* 64–66.

Shöne-Seifert, B. (1995). Risk. In W. T. Reich (Ed.), *Encyclopedia of bioethics* (Vol. 4). New York: McMillan, pp. 2316–2321.

CHAPTER 19

Addressing Prejudice: A Layered Analysis

David E. Guinn

Mrs. Mann is an 84-year-old woman who has recently suffered a mild stroke that is limiting her mobility. In order for her to go home from the hospital, she needs a daily home care attendant. Chase, the case worker, worked out the details of the home care plan with Denn, Mrs. Mann's daughter. On Mrs. Mann's first day home, Chase learned that Mrs. Mann has ordered the home care worker out of her home, asserting that she didn't want a person of that race (using a racial epithet) in her home. What should Chase do?

Given the unfortunate pervasiveness of racism and ethnic prejudice in the United States, this case scenario is hardly unusual. It is a topic that has arisen frequently in a research project on the ethics of home health care being conducted by the Park Ridge Center in association with the Illinois Department on Aging and community and home care providers. Nonetheless, while recognizing racism as morally wrong, some might ask in what sense—if at all—racism is an *ethical* issue or, at least, an ethical issue with any possibility of resolution. In many cases, the ability to accommodate discriminatory preference (even if this were somehow deemed morally unobjectionable) is precluded by the demographics of the available workforce. Moreover, laws against discrimination preclude hiring workers on a racial basis to satisfy the demands of a client.

Does not the law override ethical considerations—even render them superfluous—in such cases?

These considerations do not exhaust the possibilities for ethical reflection about Mrs. Mann and her caseworker. However, the fact that some would not see an ethical problem in this case is significant because it reveals how profoundly important the way we view a case is in terms of our ability to identify the ethical problems at stake. More significantly, it demonstrates that the perspective we adopt in viewing a moral problem will help determine and shape the actions we take in addressing that problem. The more comprehensive we can make our ethical perspective, the more opportunities for action we may perceive.

In this essay, I will be describing a process of ethical reflection which explores several perspectives which, when taken together, can generate a comprehensive outlook on the problems of Mrs. Mann and her caseworker. It is a process that may be likened to the blossoming of a rose where the complex beauty of the whole is slowly revealed petal by petal.[1] Without exhausting all possible viewpoints, I will identify several different ethical perspectives that have salience for this case and the possibilities for action offered by each. Each perspective originates in one or more popular theoretical orientations in ethics; they will range from those which perceive no ethical difficulty to views that suggest the existence of many ethical concerns.

More importantly, this process of ever deepening reflection will simultaneously demonstrate the inadequacy of some of the more limited, though very popular, ways of considering ethical problems. Ethical discussion and reflection frequently end when people find a perspective which offers them an answer they can live with. A more expansive perspective reveals that there is no single answer. It suggests instead a range of opportunities and possibilities.

NO ETHICAL PROBLEM: THE FORMALIST APPROACH

As noted above, some people might question whether the case of Mrs. Mann presents a serious ethical problem. These people see cases in a very simple way: a conflict involving moral values arises which demands an answer to the question, "What should I do in response to this conflict?" In this case, the question would be, "Should I comply with Mrs. Mann's demand for a caregiver of a particular race?" For someone taking the "no problem" perspective, what I will refer to as a "formalist

---

[1] My thanks to my colleague Martha Holstein for this metaphor.

approach," ethics is a way to resolve this conflict. Where a clear answer to the particular question is provided by law or by circumstances within the case, then there is no longer an ethical problem. You simply adopt the answer given by law or circumstance.

In this case, Mrs. Mann's objection to the race of her caregiver clearly touches a moral value. Discrimination is a moral wrong. The objection, in turn, creates a conflict which must be addressed. Chase must resolve the moral question of whether or not to honor Mrs. Mann's demand. Yet, in this case, it is unlikely that Chase would be able to comply with this demand. First, it is probable that compliance would violate state and/or federal anti-discrimination laws. For example, meeting Mrs. Mann's demands would, ultimately, affect hiring decisions, and hiring on the basis of race is prohibited. Second, in many areas, the available labor pool determines the complexion of the caregiver workforce. In many cases, the caregivers are almost exclusively people of color. In such an area, if Mrs. Mann's objection is that the caregiver is a person of color, Chase could not respond to the objection simply because there may not be any employees of Mrs. Mann's preferred race. Where social conditions preclude choice, such as where there are no home care workers of a particular race available or where the law dictates a practice (i.e., 'decides the question'), there is no viable choice available and, therefore, no ethical problem according to this formalist understanding of ethics.

This formalist approach may arise, in part, because discussions in applied ethics are frequently constructed around dramatic cases in which a person must choose among actions embodying conflicting moral values. This mistakes the method of studying ethics (i.e., its "form") for its content. That is to say, individuals adopting this approach mistakenly assume that the case which is used to illustrate ethical values and conflicts actually defines the whole scope of ethics. If a situation does not fit the mold of a typical ethics case, then ethics has no role in its resolution.

A second reason that the formalist approach may have gained currency is that it reflects the nature of modern professional life. Health care professionals are generally goal-directed individuals constrained by limits of time and resources. They identify the task to be accomplished and seek to accomplish that task as efficiently and effectively as possible. When problems arise that threaten achieving the goals they have set for themselves, professionals seek the most expedient way to overcome those problems. In this case, a formalist approach to ethics views ethics as a means by which to resolve the conflict which gets in the way of accomplishing the task at hand. It is simply one more tool in their professional arsenal.

While a person adopting the formalist approach is correct in believing that ethics can facilitate finding ways to resolve moral conflicts, the approach itself is flawed because it limits our view of the moral concerns that are explicitly raised in the case by the people involved. It looks only at the question expressed by the active conflict in the case and fails to see the other unarticulated moral concerns which may exist. Even on a pragmatic level—the level at which this approach may be justified—the formalist approach is inadequate. It can, for example, fail to identify problems which could result in even greater ethical conflicts at a later date.

For example, the formalist approach to the case of Mrs. Mann follows a simplistic line of decision making. Mrs. Mann objects to her home caregiver on racial grounds. This raises the conflict which Chase must resolve. Since meeting Mrs. Mann's objection may not be possible (i.e., there may not be any workers of Mrs. Mann's preferred race available) and because the effort may violate the laws against discrimination, Chase has no choice but to refuse Mrs. Mann's demand. This answers the presenting conflict of the case under a formalist approach.

But this refusal doesn't end the case. Mrs. Mann is then placed in the position of deciding to accept or refuse the help that is offered. Clearly, in the United States, she has the *right* to accept or refuse home care help. If a patient in the hospital can refuse lifesaving treatment if he or she so desires (true), then Mrs. Mann can certainly refuse care for a non-life-threatening condition. As such, the formalist approach would again view this as settling the case: by law or social context, the client decides the answer to this second question. But does the right to refuse treatment end all of our moral concerns? If we assume that society provides home health care services out of a moral concern for its recipients, does that moral concern end with its refusal? Moreover, what happens to Mrs. Mann when she refuses? If she can't take care of herself, who will? Home care is generally less expensive then hospital care. If she refuses home care and is forced to return to the hospital, who will bear the cost?

For those who perceive ethical problems in this case, the formalist perspective is inadequate. It fails to highlight many of the fundamental concerns that lay outside a simple decisional path of what can or cannot be done in response to voiced conflicts. Moreover, this perspective commands no action on the part of either actor with respect to even the most obvious moral concern—that of prejudice—other than a response limited to acting in compliance with the law. Yet, reliance upon social conditions and legal requirements is common practice in our everyday working lives. Events that call this reliance into question are important reminders of the fallibility of the formalist perspective (Tong, 1997).

AUTONOMY OF THE CLIENT

One of the major revolutions in professional health care ethics arose in the late 1960s and early 1970s with the ascendence of the principle of patient or client autonomy. In place of the then-prevailing ethic of paternalism, in which the health care provider assumed authority over the patient/client to act in that person's best interest, the principle of autonomy asserted that the patient/client should be respected and allowed to exercise authority over all important health care decisions. Many argue that autonomy has become *the* dominant principle in health care ethics, often overwhelming other well-recognized concerns (Campbell, 1994.)

What autonomy means and its ethical consequences are very controversial. As many critics note, the dominant understanding of autonomy views the individual in isolation. This understanding fails to recognize that we all live in the midst of a complex web of relationships which impose a variety of obligations upon each of us and may powerfully influence how we behave (Addelson, 1994; Sandel, 1996; Young, 1990). Yet, the principle of autonomy has an intuitive appeal. It conforms with our experience of ourselves as having an individual identity and our desire to exercise authority over our lives.

Despite the problems inherent in applying the principle of autonomy, in a positive sense it at least moves the discussion about Mrs. Mann's decision beyond a factual account of legal rights to the realm of morals and values. The moral basis for the concept of autonomy transcends a simple view of human agency and control. It's not just that she has the right to make decisions about her life. It is that we recognize that right because we are morally called to respect Mrs. Mann as an autonomous moral agent. Our sense of who we are is, in part, dependent upon our being recognized by others as deserving of attention and respect (Taylor, 1991). To be unseen by others is to have our humanity diminished, to join the class of the invisible man described by Ralph Ellison (1963).

To respect Mrs. Mann means, minimally, to grasp her perspective and the nature of the decisions the agency is asking her to make. We need to try and look at the world through her eyes. In doing so, our understanding begins to get more complex. Home care aides enter the privacy of one's home. Cleaning the home and assisting with the laundry takes them into areas not open to most visitors. They may even be called upon to help the client dress, bath, defecate, or urinate. These are clearly very personal and intimate matters. Insofar as we respect the autonomy of the client, we are compelled to recognize that Mrs. Mann's right to decide who is allowed to enter into these intimate spaces is a very important moral value. These aspects of life touch upon her human dignity.

Unfortunately, while deepening our understanding of the situation, this popular understanding of autonomy by itself doesn't advance us beyond this point. Unless the home care agency gives Mrs. Mann the right to choose a specific home care aide (which they legally cannot do), then her choice devolves into simply choosing whether or not to accept the aide offered to her. The only action required of the caseworker is to accept Mrs. Mann's decision. Indeed, an extreme understanding of autonomy would preclude Chase from even attempting to influence Mrs. Mann's decision.

The concept of autonomy in bioethics emerged, in part, as a response to a recognition of the power differential between patients and physicians. A similar power differential exists in this situation. Chase has enormous power in managing Mrs. Mann's case and developing care plans. Respecting Mrs. Mann's autonomy would include avoiding the use of that power as a means of overcoming Mrs. Mann's self-determined decision. Obviously, Chase should not use coercive tactics to affect Mrs. Mann's decision, such as threatening to commit her to a mental asylum because of her prejudice without evidence of mental incapacity needing treatment. However, given the differences in their positions and the imputed "power" of Chase as a professional, one might argue that *any* intervention creates risks of unduly influencing the client's decisions and intruding upon her autonomy.

This is, however, an extreme position that most people, I think fairly, would reject. It is possible to respect someone else and argue with their decisions. Indeed, arguing with someone, recognizing that they can disagree, can be very respectful. However, the concept of autonomy moves us no further than that. Mrs. Mann's decision is still final.

DUTIES OF PATIENT SUPPORT AND CARETAKING

When the principle of autonomy entered health care ethics, it was not intended to stand alone. Other principles relating to the moral obligations or duties of the health care provider towards the patient and others accompanied it (Beauchamp & Childress, 1979; Veatch, 1981). Among those obligations directed toward patients are two different perspectives which I will refer to as a duty of support and the duty of caretaking. The former seeks to support clients in their individuality. The later looks to the clients' best interest.

A duty of support obligates the care provider not only to acknowledge the client's autonomy, but to actively support the client in the exercise of that autonomy. This duty can be found not only in a principled approach to ethics (e.g., Quill & Brody, 1996), but also in feminist (e.g., Tong, 1997), and communitarian (e.g., Taylor, 1985, 1989) theories that reject the notion that an individual acts totally independent of others. Insofar as we recognize the importance of others in our understanding of the self, then respect for an individual demands relational support. In determining how to act, persons will seek the advice and support of people important to them. If they do not have these types of supportive relationships with living people, they may retreat to the support offered by their pasts: memories of their parents, colleagues and other important figures or influences (Taylor, 1989). The duty of support urges caregivers to serve as this support. It means moving beyond a skeptical distance from the client assuming that the client is capable and qualified to make all relevant decisions, to a relationship which seeks to make sure that the client is autonomously competent to make the decision.

At a basic level, a client cannot exercise autonomy without adequate information. It makes no sense to say that a decision made out of ignorance is meaningful to the client. To understand whether or not Mrs. Mann has adequate information, the caseworker may need to interview Mrs. Mann to understand why she is resistant to having an aide of a particular race and whether or not she realizes that rejecting an aide on racial grounds may preclude her from receiving any assistance. To support Mrs. Mann's autonomy does not mean that Chase cannot try to persuade her to accept assistance or educate her to overcome her apparent racism. Indeed, by offering her advice Chase may be enhancing Mrs. Mann's autonomy by assuring that her decisions are made with a fuller understanding of the situation (Quill & Brody, 1996).

The duty of caretaking, derived from principles such as the duty of beneficence (Beauchamp & Childress, 1979), or from concepts related to feminist ethics and ethics of care (Larrabee, 1993), provides a slightly different approach. Instead of understanding the client as simply an independent rational agent, it points to the caregiver's responsibility to take care of clients who may not be able to take care of themselves. Under a principlist approach, this duty arises out of the position we hold. Caregivers owe this duty to their clients as an element of their professional life. With an ethics of care, an ethical theory of which the duty of care is only one small part, the obligation arises out of the specific relationship between the individual caregiver and a particular client. The particularities of that relationship define and guide the duty. In either case, once we have taken on the commitment to care for another, we have an obligation to do so to the best of our ability according to the best interests of that person.

On this basis, Chase should explore whether or not Mrs. Mann is mentally competent to make the decision to accept or reject care. While the question of competence relates to the question of autonomy, it is the duty of care that pushes us beyond the isolating boundaries of autonomy. Rather than assuming that each individual can and should make his/her own decision, the duty of care asks that we make sure that the individual is in fact capable of exercising this right in a meaningful way. If Mrs. Mann is not competent, then Chase must develop an alternate health care plan with someone who is capable of making decisions on Mrs. Mann's behalf under the law of the state where she lives.

It may also be necessary to explore what Mrs. Mann's rejection of assistance means to her (Kitwood, 1998). For example, her ostensible racism may reflect a denial of the need for home care. It may be that Mrs. Mann is not resigned to the idea of home care. Her rejection of the home care aide (while poorly expressed) may reflect a subconscious rejection of *anyone* intruding into her life at home—or her feeling that a stranger is invading her kitchen, which she has subconsciously connected with her feelings about herself. While these psychological inhibitions, if they exist, might raise questions about Mrs. Mann's decision-making competence, they generally will not rise to that level; in most cases, they are important to identify because they provide the caregiver with the means of reasoning with the client. With this information, Chase could counsel Mrs. Mann about her concerns and help her make the psychological adjustment necessary to accept home care. If these psychological reservations can be overcome, Mrs. Mann is in a better position to make decisions in her own best interest.

This duty of caretaking does not obviate the need to respect Mrs. Mann's autonomy. In the final analysis, in any conflict we give precedence to the wishes of a competent adult client. The duty of care merely gives impetus to a deeper engagement with the care for Mrs. Mann and moral grounding for challenging a superficial claim for autonomy. On the basis of Chase's duty of caretaking, it may be necessary for Chase to reject Mrs. Mann's claim to autonomy if it is evident that Mrs. Mann is not competent to express that autonomy. At a minimum, it supports Chase's efforts to persuade Mrs. Mann to cooperate in her care plans.

A RELATIONAL POINT OF VIEW

Feminists and phenomonologists, among others, have been very critical of "principlist" ethics that stress the importance of principles such as autonomy (Gudorf, 1994; Zaner, 1994). One of the major problems with the whole focus on autonomy and related principles is that it locates the discussion singularly within an isolated individual client. However, humans are social and relational. We do not naturally live alone. We live in the midst of a complex web of relationships. In this case, Mrs. Mann's rejection of assistance would affect not only her, but also her daughter and possibly other family members who have obligations to care for Mrs. Mann. It would also be troubling to Chase, who knows of Mrs. Mann's need for services.

A strictly client centered approach precludes consideration of the interests of others. Moreover, since the principle of autonomy frequently incorporates a valuation of privacy, the involvement of the daughter without Mrs. Mann's explicit consent would ostensibly violate Mrs. Mann's autonomy. A relational perspective compels us to realize that a relationship exists between Mrs. Mann and her daughter and that the decision that Mrs. Mann makes will strongly affect both people. This consideration may justify Chase in involving Denn, Mrs. Mann's daughter, in developing and implementing the care plan. It may also justify calling upon the mother-daughter relationship to influence Mrs. Mann's decision.

This involvement of a family member cannot be done in a rote or mechanical way, nor should it be based on stereotypical assumptions. If the relationship between Mrs. Mann and Denn is troubled or manipulative, Mrs. Mann's rejection of home care may reflect that. It could, for example, be a veiled effort to force Denn into caring for her. Alternately, if Denn has historically been abusive towards Mrs. Mann, it would be inappropriate to invite her to participate in developing a health care plan. Not only would it violate Mrs. Mann's interests, it could destroy her relationship with Chase. Chase might no longer be viewed as a professional offering help, but as an ally of Denn bearing all of the problems of that relationship.

A relational perspective also highlights the relationships that can and do exist between the client and the home care provider. Home care, like other forms of health care, is not an impersonal service. It ideally involves people caring for other people (McCormick, 1994). It involves a personal engagement between the care provider and the care receiver. To provide good care, Chase and Mrs. Mann can (or at least should) have a positive relationship. If Chase can earn the trust of Mrs. Mann, that relationship may help facilitate Mrs. Mann's acceptance of the home aide (Williams, 1993). Similarly, Chase can try to facilitate the development of a personal relationship between Mrs. Mann and the home care aide that may itself overcome Mrs. Mann's possible prejudice.

By moving outside the client focused analysis, relational perspectives also highlight the need to consider the home care aide as a subject of moral concern. Specifically, placing a home care worker in a hostile environment created by prejudice must concern the case manager. Clearly, there are times when this is unavoidable—but it should be addressed. For example, where a patient suffering from severe dementia is racially abusive, it may nonetheless be necessary to ask an aide of that race to attend to the client. This is not unlike the obligation imposed on nurses and doctors to care for an abusive patient. However, the case manager should make all possible efforts to provide adequate training for aides to help them understand that such abuse is related to the medical condition of the client and is not a reflection upon them (Williams, 1993). The aide should also be provided with emotional support to help her deal with this abusive situation.

Moving beyond a strict, traditional client centered focus does not necessarily result in a diminution in client care or attention as is commonly feared. Given the fact that we all exist in relationships with others, incorporating concerns about those relationships within the decision-making process means that problems in the relationships can be addressed rather then ignored. The plan of care can be integrated with the client's life and the lives of others who are significant for her well-being.

THE SOCIAL VIEW

Virtually every major theory of health care ethics recognizes the inadequacy of a purely personal ethics. We live in a complex social/political world which profoundly influences our lives. The concern is to understand the interactive relationship between individual choice and action and larger social concerns. It is in the realm of social analysis that we can begin to grapple directly with questions about Mrs. Mann's apparent prejudice.

It is very easy to recognize prejudice as a moral wrong. We ought to respect each other as fellow human beings irrespective of race, creed, gender, or any other characteristic that is superfluous to our genuine humanity (Koggel, 1998). The law gives this moral wrong tangible meaning. The duty not to discriminate in our hiring practices, as embodied in law, recognizes that such discrimination results in measurable harm to those who are discriminated against by denying them the opportunity for gainful employment in their chosen profession.

However, let us assume that Chase has some flexibility in her assignment of home care workers and that she could assign an aide to Mrs. Mann (or others) in compliance with the client's wishes without adversely affecting job opportunities for others. Say, for example, that there are more jobs available than there are qualified applicants for those positions (which is the current reality). How might this affect our judgment?

To understand the harm in this context, it is necessary to move beyond the individuals involved. For good or ill, our moral obligation to confront individual prejudice is relatively weak. Prejudice is considered a private vice. It is only when prejudice becomes a public act, carried out by the state or an employer whose economic stature makes them part of the public economy, that we have a duty to intervene. We object to prejudice in these cases because it represents a public endorsement and furtherance of the prejudice. Historic prejudice is reenacted in the present and will influence the future. When we act according to the dictates of prejudice, we not only accept its legitimacy, our acts give testimony to all who will see that we deem it valid as a basis for others to act upon as well.

In this regard, we clearly do not want to teach prejudice in our schools and workplaces. We expect our public officials to act against such teaching, educating those practicing prejudice about their behavior and preventing such acts from influencing public attitudes and actions. However, Mrs. Mann is 84 years old. Our ability to intervene and alter her attitudes is limited. Her expression of prejudice is isolated within her home. Therefore, unless she is part of a larger aggregate of prejudiced individuals whose prejudice may ultimately affect the employment opportunities of others, the social benefit of resisting her prejudice may be relatively limited. To what extent can we say that allowing her to choose her home care aide will tend to propagate prejudice in our society? Does even this isolated tolerance of bigotry legitimate prejudice, for example, in the eyes of other clients or employees? Or might they view it as simply the tolerance of an illness of aging, like other ills?

At the same time, failure to provide home care assistance could result in Mrs. Mann being forced into an institutional care setting where the financial costs of care might be far higher. In an age of ever increasing scarcity, this, too, is an issue of ethical concern. Do the benefits of resisting prejudice *in this case* outweigh the costs?

More problematic, prejudice is a socially constructed or imposed condition. Mrs. Mann acquired her prejudice as a member of this society. This education may have occurred in a hundred trivial ways: in the books she read, in the movies she saw, in the lives of the people around her. It may have been the result of a personal trauma when, for example, she was the victim of a violent crime perpetrated by a member of that race toward which she has unfairly generalized her anger. In this latter case, imposing an aide might make her feel traumatized again. In either event, to what extent should Mrs. Mann be held culpable—or penalized—at this stage of her life?

Looking at prejudice in a different way, this problem arose because Mrs. Mann objected to her home care aide because of her race. But what if her prejudice resulted in favoring an aide of that race? For example, what if she preferred a person of color because she thought they were best suited to act as 'menials' and 'servants' around the house (Williams, 1993)? Are there systems in place to identify this type of prejudice? Is this type of prejudice "better" than the other? If not, is it fair to sanction one and not the other?

Finally, we need to reflect upon the ways in which our approach to Mrs. Mann may differ from the way we approach what may be identified as a cultural or religious conflict. If Mrs. Mann were Jewish and she maintained a kosher household, would we consider a request by her that she be assisted by a Jewish home care worker a display of prejudice or would we seek to accommodate her interests under the guise of religious tolerance? Does Mrs. Mann's race or ethnicity make a difference? For example, what if she was an ethnic minority seeking a home care worker of the same ethnicity? Would we accommodate this interest in recognition of multiculturalism?

In attempting to answer these questions, a distinction can be drawn between the prejudice of members of a privileged class directed against a minority or oppressed class and discrimination by the client who is a member of a religious or cultural minority. The latter is generally far less socially harmful than the former simply because, by definition, the latter groups lack significant power over others in the community. Their actions do not carry the social endorsement of being deemed a norm for society that is present in the acts of a member of the majority (Minow, 1990). That is not to say that this discrimination may not cause harm, but rather that it causes far less than that practiced by the majority. Moreover, because minorities are themselves frequently the subject of discrimination, allowing limited discrimination in favor of their own ethnic or religious group may be considered remedial to the harm they have suffered at the hands of the dominant society (Young, 1990).

The crucial point is that if such a distinction is to be made, it should be done explicitly so as to avoid confusing the two situations. Every act has an expressive element. For Chase to act upon the request of any client communicates some type of acceptance. The content of the act needs to be clarified by making it explicitly clear what her specific act means. Is she supporting religious pluralism or multiculturalism—or tolerating prejudice?

Social analysis views are extremely hard to evaluate and often end in frustrating compromises. It is generally easier to identify with and have sympathy for the individual we are working with than it is to adopt the interest of society as a whole. Moreover, it will often be the case that social concerns raise not just one issue, but many that are ill-defined and conflicting. For example, recognizing that prejudice is socially constructed results in understanding Mrs. Mann as both victim and victimizer—she is the victim of her indoctrination in prejudice and victimizer in her treatment of the proposed aide and in her public acts in support of continued prejudice. We cannot address one side of this balance without affecting the other. Nonetheless, we must take social interests seriously.

A PROCESS OF REFLECTION

There are many ways of looking at an ethical conflict. Each, in isolation, provides its own analytic tools and suggests a particular course of action to address the problems it identifies. However, as I hope I have demonstrated, each in isolation is inadequate to deal with the rich complexity of human life.

In working through this case, I have demonstrated a process of ethical reflection which can be used to develop a richer and more complex understanding of the ethical problems of the case from which a plan of action can be developed. Starting with the client as the initial focal point of analysis (with the idea of rights and moving into the idea of client self-determination), I have progressively added layers of concern about the role of the caregiver, the family, and society. This structuring of the process or the use of the analogy of layers does not reflect or advocate a hierarchy of values, with any one having greater or lesser authority. It is simply a way of relating a variety of viewpoints as interrelated fields of inquiry, like concentric circles on a flat field.

This process, in many ways, resembles the efforts of narrative ethics to understand that our actions only make sense within the context of the life story we are living out. The layers of analysis are simply tools to tease apart the rich complexity of a person's life. The layers ultimately remain intimately linked and intertwined. Their meaning(s) can only be understood in the context of a specific life and those touched by that life within the broader context of our shared society.

A final recommended course of action (and there may be more than one that may be morally appropriate) will depend upon the detailed specifics of the case. It will often require a careful balancing of many conflicting values drawn from each of these "layers" of concern. Any solution may be flawed—the lesser among necessary evils. However, understanding a situation in its full complexity may provide opportunities not only to answer the question asked, but also to address the consequences of answering the question in that way. It may allow Chase not only to decide whether or not to respect Mrs. Mann's wishes, but also to address the problems this may create for the prospective home care worker or Mrs. Mann's daughter—concerns which might have been missed in a more narrowly focused analysis of the ethical problem.

Even cases in which the answer appears to be defined and answered by certain basic criteria like law and/or practice can benefit by a layered analysis. While the law or the nature of the labor market may preclude Chase from meeting Mrs. Mann's demands for another home care worker, looking at the other moral concerns present may provide opportunities to address those values in ways not identified by the legal/practical mandate. Understanding why she is rejecting the home care aide may help in negotiating with her over her refusal. Involving her daughter in discussions and/or trading upon the development of a relationship between Chase and Mrs. Mann may similarly achieve acquiescence. These tactics can be identified as morally appropriate only through a careful layered analysis of the case. In other situations, these actions could be morally inappropriate as being manipulative and not respectful of Mrs. Mann's moral standing.

Morally troubling cases are rarely simple. A deeper understanding of a problem like prejudice will not provide an easy answer, but it may provide a greater range of options for those compelled to deal with such problems.

REFERENCES

Addelson, K. P. (1994). *Moral passages: Toward a collectivist moral theory*. New York/London: Routledge.
Beauchamp, T. L., & Childress, J. F. (1979). *Principles of biomedical ethics*. New York: Oxford University Press.
Campbell, C. (1994). Principlism and religion: The law and the prophets. In E. R. DuBose, R. Hamel, & L. J. O'Connell (Eds.), *A matter of principles?: Ferment in U.S. bioethics*. Valley Forge, PA: Trinity Press.
Ellison, R. (1963). *Invisible man*. New York: Random.
Gudorf, C. E. (1994). A feminist critique of biomedical principlism. In E. R. DuBose, R. Hamel, & L. J. O'Connell (Eds.), *A matter of principles: Ferment in U.S. bioethics*. Valley Forge, PA: Trinity Press.
Kitwood, T. (1998). Toward a theory of dementia care: Ethics and interaction. *Journal of Clinical Ethics, 9*(1), 23–34.
Koggel, C. M. (1998). *Perspectives on equality: Constructing a relational theory*. Latham, NY: Rowman and Littlefield.

Larrabee, M. J. (1993). *An ethic of care: Feminist and interdisciplinary perspectives.* New York and London: Routledge.
McCormick, R. A. (1994). Beyond principlism is not enough: A theologian reflects on the real challenge for U.S. biomedical ethics. In E. R. DuBose, R. Hamel, & L. J. O'Connell (Eds.), *A matter of principles: Ferment in U.S. bioethics.* Valley Forge, PA: Trinity Press.
Minow, M. (1990). *Making all the difference: Inclusion, exclusion, and American law.* Ithaca, NY: Cornell University Press.
Quill, T. E., & Brody, H. (1996). Physician recommendations and patient autonomy: Finding a balance between physician power and patient choice. *Annals of Internal Medicine, 125,* 763–769.
Sandel, M. (1996). *Democracy's discontent: America in search of a public philosophy.* Cambridge, MA/London: Harvard University Press.
Taylor, C. (1985). Atomism. In *Philosophy and the human sciences: Philosophical papers 2.* Cambridge: Cambridge University Press.
Taylor, C. (1989). *Sources of the self.* Cambridge, MA: Harvard University Press.
Taylor, C. (1991). *The ethics of authenticity.* Cambridge, MA: Harvard University Press.
Tong, R. (1997). *Feminist approaches to bioethics: Theoretical reflections and practical applications.* Boulder, CO: Westview Press.
Veatch, R. (1981). *A theory of medical ethics.* New York: Basic Books.
Williams, O. J. (1993). When is being equal unfair? In R. A. Kane & A. L. Caplan (Eds.), *Ethical conflicts in the management of home care: The case manager's dilemma.* New York: Springer Publishing.
Young, I. M. (1990). *Justice and the politics of difference.* Princeton, NJ: Princeton University Press.
Zaner, R. M. (1994). Experience and moral life: A phenomenological approach to bioethics. In E. R. DuBose, R. Hamel, & L. J. O'Connell (Eds.), *A matter of principles: Ferment in U.S. bioethics.* Valley Forge, PA: Trinity Press.

CHAPTER 20

Cross-Cultural Geriatric Ethics: Negotiating Our Differences

Harry R. Moody

Mrs. Chu is an 85-year-old citizen of the People's Republic of China who has recently come to live in the United States with her adult children, both immigrants. She has some limited ability to understand English. Mrs. Chu has experienced some health problems and is being cared for at home by her family. She has now been brought to a hospital for tests. The children understand that doctors have definitively diagnosed Mrs. Chu's medical condition as cancer, but the family are adamantly opposed to telling Mrs. Chu right away. It would be disrespectful to talk about death to her this way, they say. Instead, they tell hospital authorities they have their own approach to dealing with these matters, an approach that includes traditional Chinese herbal remedies.

Members of the health care team involved in Mrs. Chu's case are debating what should be done next. A doctor says that he is horrified at the idea of treating cancer with herbal remedies but that he believes he has fulfilled his responsibility by informing the family. What happens next is not his responsibility. A nurse strongly insists that Mrs. Chu has a right to informed consent and that she must be told the truth directly, whatever the family says. Finally, a social worker on the health care team argues that we need to balance the risks and benefits of telling the truth by taking account of traditional Chinese ideas about the family and ideas of health and illness. One member of the team says they should tell Mrs. Chu she has "neoplastic disease," while still another argues that Mrs. Chu is a citizen of China, not the United States, and just as laws differ across countries, so do values differ across cultures, with the conclusion that we should respect other cultures as much as possible.

What should the health care team do now?

The case of Mrs. Chu illustrates a range of ethical dilemmas in geriatric care raised by cultural and ethnic differences. Some believe that rights and values are entirely relative: for example, that the Confucian idea of filial piety and family solidarity is simply different from the Western idea of individual autonomy. In this view, respect for other cultures means accepting the Chu family's version of ethics, whatever that may be.

Others believe that claims about human rights—for example, the right to informed consent—are absolute and universal. For that reason, it is said, we can condemn torture and other acts that dehumanize people, even if those acts are approved by majorities or by custom in another society. The same logic leads believers in universal rights to condemn, for example, female circumcision, a practice that remains common in African societies.

Finally, there are still others who believe that finding "the right thing to do" necessarily involves questions about social context: in this case, questions about the role of an elderly person in the family system. Without dialogue and deeper appreciation of context, this argument goes, broad ideologies such as cultural relativism or a belief in the existence of universal human rights can lead to irresponsible abdications or irresponsible interventions. According to this perspective, communication among all involved in an ethical dilemma becomes the paramount responsibility and is the only basis for finding a resolution acceptable to all parties.

Cultural relativity, human rights, and imperatives of cross-cultural communication are all important considerations in trying to make a decision in a case like the one involving Mrs. Chu. But ethics is above all a matter of practice and decisions. In the last analysis, what do we *do* in the case of Mrs. Chu? Do we come up with different answers for people depending on their ethnic or cultural backgrounds? Does age make any difference at all in a case like this one?

ETHNICITY, ETHICS, AND AGING

In an effort to explore some of these questions, the Brookdale Center on Aging of Hunter College embarked on the project Ethnicity, Ethics, and Aging (1998–2000) which was supported by the Fan Fox and Samuels Foundation. As part of the research effort in that project, the Brookdale Center convened a series of focus groups in New York City, deliberately engaging participants from diverse ethnic backgrounds. What was striking about the results was not so much the predictable differences across ethnic groups but rather the commonalities and similarities that emerged. One of the most important of these commonalities was the prevalence of mistrust of health care professionals on the part of elderly patients and their families.

In the first instance, many statements from focus group participants expressed fatalism and also reluctance to communicate with health care professionals. Some examples of comments follow.

- "In my family we don't talk about bad things—you can jinx fate."
- "Birth and death just happen—we don't discuss those things—they are God's will."
- "I believe in modern medicine, but my grandparents believe in herbal medicine."

Other statements express the need to be heard and also doubt about the willingness of professionals to hear from patients:

- "Families should be consulted, or at least they should be told why certain decisions are made for their sick relatives."
- "Sometimes doctors give the proxy a hard time—when they want to do something else."
- "You don't know what the doctor's attitude is toward black people."
- "Doctors don't make an in-depth assessment of the concerns of the patient. They don't give you first class treatment; they make assumptions about your age, or because you are black, or because you are a woman."
- "They say: 'black women are strong, they can take it.'"

Other statements reflected deep distrust of the motives of the health care system as such:

- "Why would they want to keep anyone alive? The answer: money."
- "The longer a person lives, the more they can use the information for statistics. Treatment is not given for the benefit of the patient but for the benefit of the doctor."
- "Could hospitals be afraid of malpractice suits?"
- "In my family we were poor—we had bad experiences: Medicine is about what is available, not what is good for the patient."

- "My doctor said, 'At a certain age, there is no point in resuscitation.'"

Interestingly enough, these expressions of mistrust came from group participants from all varieties of backgrounds, with other group members often nodding in agreement. Although the members of the groups were from many different backgrounds, religions, or cultures, a common theme that emerged in the focus groups was the human experience of suffering, uncertainty, dependency, and capacity for caring. It is this common human experience—rather than the formulation of ideas about universal rights and obligations—that reaches the level of true universality. Neither empty universality ("principlism") nor stereotyping ethnic groups (referring to, for example, "Asian values") is helpful in achieving the difficult dialogue across cultures that will be necessary for ethics in the twenty-first century.

AGING AND CULTURAL DIFFERENCES

In the closing years of the twentieth century, the United States experienced its second great wave of immigration in that century. Headlines remind us of ethnic fragmentation in places like Rwanda or the former Yugoslavia. Here at home demographic forces are making us aware of enduring differences among ethnic groups. At the same time, a sea change has taken place in culture and philosophy—a development loosely called "postmodernism"—and this change has sharpened sensitivity to differences of all kinds so that questions of multicultural identity become fundamental. The United States has not yet gone the way of the Balkans, but coming to grips with potentially fragmenting ethnic differences is an unavoidable challenge when we consider matters of values and ethics. Deciding how ethnic and cultural differences should affect health care ethics is not an easy task.

Earlier in this decade the political scientist Samuel Huntington (1996) wrote an influential, if controversial, book on cross-cultural difference, titled *The Clash of Civilizations*. Huntington's image is of a world of separate and distinct cultures confronting each other, something like Thomas Kuhn's portrayal of scientific explanation where alternative views of the world are wholly incommensurate with each other. In this spirit, proponents for multicultural "identity politics" sometimes speak as if contrasting values held by different ethnic groups simply confront each other as stark alternatives. Vive la différence, one might say, especially when a politically correct response is to come down in favor of "tolerance." But "tolerance" is too easy a slogan to invoke when difficult decisions are at stake. As the case of Mrs. Chu reminds us, deciding what tolerance ultimately calls for—in practice—is not easy to say.

RECENT HISTORY

In recent years cultural diversity has become a recognized issue in the geriatric health professions (Wieland, Benton, & Kramer, 1995). Baker and Lightfoot (1993) argue that psychiatric care of ethnic elders demands appropriate recognition of ethnic factors in a patient's life history. It can be a grave mistake to assume uncritically that other cultures around the world must share the same high valuation of autonomy and individual choice that predominates in American culture (Blackhall, Murphy, Frank, Michel, & Azen, 1995). Some critics have even gone so far as to argue for a complete version of "ethnic ethics," involving the wholesale reconstruction of moral theory on lines different from the mainstream of Western ethical concepts (Cortese, 1990).

Critics working within the main lines of contemporary bioethics (DuBose, Hamel, & O'Connell, 1994) have urged an alternative basis for ethical reasoning beyond the methodology that has come to be called "principlism": that is, beyond appeal to the "big three" ethical principles (beneficence, autonomy, and justice). On a methodological level, the search for alternatives has led recently to a deeper appreciation of other approaches very different from analytic philosophy. Some of the more influential alternative lines of development for ethical thinking have been feminism (Gilligan, 1982) and African-American perspectives (Flack & Pellegrino, 1992; Secundy, 1992).

Still another point of importance here is that different cultures have different explanatory alternatives for health and disease themselves. Chinese medicine, for example, places stress on the importance of "Chi" as a vital force comparable to Western ideas of immune system equilibrium (Kaptchuk, 1983), while "curanderismo" plays an important role in Latino views of disease and curing (Maduro & Applewhite, 1995). As the postmodern critique of science gains more favor, it is tempting to adopt a more relativistic outlook not only on matters of ethics but on matters of medical explanation as well. The difficulty this presents for public policy is illustrated by the trouble American courts have had in taking proper account of sincere beliefs of Christian Science practitioners who hold a view of health and illness at variance with the dominant medical model. Competent adults have a right to refuse treatment on any ground, but courts have intervened when Christian Science would stop children from receiving conventional medical care.

In the United States there is a long and tragic history of discrimination in health care based on skin color. On the one hand, this history should make us sensitive to the voices of minority ethnic groups (Jones, 1981). On the other hand, that very same history should make us skeptical about the idea of wholly different and incommensurable ethical concepts for people of different race or ancestry. To cite only one example of this point, authoritarian regimes in Asia, ranging from Singapore to Myanmar and China, have sometimes appealed to "Asian values" in their argument that universal principles of human rights provide no legitimate basis for criticizing their societies. Here, as has happened before, ethical relativism easily becomes a slippery slope leading toward acceptance of injustice. If we abandon standards of universal human rights, then what basis do we have, say in the case of Mrs. Chu, for insisting that a patient be truly and fully informed about the truth of a diagnosis? Do we have any basis for criticizing Mrs. Chu's adult children if they maintain a conspiracy of lies? What if they try to implicate health care providers in the conspiracy?

The conventional "liberal" approach to dealing with patients of different cultural background is to insist on the primacy of "equal opportunity": that is, recognition of ethnic diversity among elders (Gelfand, 1994), emphasis on accessibility and appropriateness of service delivery (Damron-Rodriguez, Wallace, & Kington, 1994), or the importance of translation (Haffner, 1992). But the "soft" liberal approach just described does not tell us what to do when confronting a situation like the case of Mrs. Chu. The dominant liberal view favors openness and truth-telling, but does it also require intrusion into family communication patterns if the family, and perhaps even the elderly Mrs. Chu, resist the Western style of cultural openness?

Perhaps a "hard" liberal version (i.e., a commitment to absolute universal human rights) would insist that liberal values prevail whatever the cost. But opponents of this kind of liberalism could point out that other values are at play here, not least of them filial piety and family solidarity. Filial piety in East Asian families is not simply a casual or customary practice but has deep historical roots in Confucianism (Okada, 1988). As a result of this rich and powerful tradition, understanding the elderly Asian patient requires appreciation of the Confucian background that has influenced cultural development in China, Korea, and Japan.

The case becomes even more complicated when we consider that not only ethics but systems of medical explanation may be involved in the case of Mrs. Chu. The family, after all, prefers to rely on traditional Chinese herbal remedies, and, here too, as in the Confucian tradition, we confront a major alternative tradition quite different from modern Western medicine.

What we see in both East and West is the rise of what is increasingly called "complementary," rather than "alternative," medicine. The semantic shift suggests not incommensurable systems but complementary approaches that can be used, pragmatically, in different ways as a specific case demands. Perhaps this pragmatic, complementary approach can also be applied to the resolution of ethical dilemmas when we face opposing imperatives, as in the case of Mrs. Chu. Western health care practitioners have become accustomed to seeing methods like acupuncture or herbal medicine as appealing to young adults or middle-aged baby boomers. But the elderly, especially immigrants from Asia, are likely to have grown up familiar with so-called alternative medicine. Among immigrants, the age profile of those who find alternative medical approaches appealing may be exactly the reverse of what we would see in the Anglo population.

DIGNITY, ETHICS, AND AGING

A major goal of health care ethics is to treat patients with respect and dignity, and this ideal is reflected in policies favoring patient autonomy and privacy. Thus, hospitals try to provide privacy for patients by limiting visiting hours or prohibiting visitors from sleeping overnight. In contemporary bioethics we tend to believe that autonomy is best served when individuals make decisions for themselves without undue influence from others, even on the part of their own families. But curtailing visiting hours or separating a patient from family decision-making can actually be a profound assault on patient dignity. Many non-Anglo families would much prefer more "family friendly" sleeping accommodations. Privacy and autonomy, however admirable as ideals, may clash with what families, especially elders, deem to be ethically appropriate treatment.

Over the past generation, a revolution in health care ethics in the United States has occurred. Because of its influence, we tend to take for granted the idea that telling patients the truth about terminal illness is always the right thing to do. Yet most cultures around the world make the exactly opposite assumption. Talking openly about death could be a profoundly disrupting, even disrespectful thing to do. In the case of Mrs. Chu, her adult children make just such a claim.

The ideal of dignity and respect for age is a powerful, if often neglected, dimension in the field of aging, as a recent volume (Disch, Dobrof, & Moody, 1998) reminds us. Yet, a concern about dignity can itself become a major problem inhibiting doctor-patient communication and therefore damaging care of elderly patients. Galanti (1991) cites the case of a 64-year-old Chinese woman in the hospital after an acute heart attack. The physician at discharge urged her to return after two weeks for follow-up, and the patient agreed but never did so. What probably happened is that the patient did not want to offend the doctor by refusing to his face and causing dishonor. By agreeing, then not following through, she spared everyone embarrassment, though perhaps put her life at risk.

Some blunders in cross-cultural communication are so absurd as to be laughable. For instance, in traditional Chinese culture it is common to think of numbers as "lucky" or "unlucky." Failing to understand the meaning of numbers can cause big problems. In New York, an ethics advocacy group developed a new outreach program on advance directives for Chinese elders and publicized it with a call-in telephone number. Time went on but no one ever called the number. Finally, someone informed that outreach group that the telephone number used in Chinese signified "sudden death."

Another point where courtesy and dignity become an issue is when saying "no" really means saying "yes" and vice-versa. Here cultural norms governing politeness may cause serious misunderstanding. For example, it is not unusual for Middle Eastern or Asian patients to say "yes" in order to avoid the embarrassment of contradicting a health professional and thereby showing disrespect. When cultural norms in favor of politeness or compliance are overlooked, the result can be disastrous. Imagine the case of asking a recent Asian immigrant patient whether a specific painkiller seems to be working. The elderly patient says yes, and the nurse or doctor goes away blithely assuming the dosage is correct.

Galanti (1991) cites the case of Mr. Ling, a 68-year-old Chinese man with second degree burns over his body who persistently refused any pain medication, despite evidence of severe pain. His refusal made worse an associated cardiovascular problem resulting in seriously high blood pressure. In this case the attending physician tried to get the patient to accept pain medication to lower the blood pressure. But Mr. Ling, along with his family, refused, and the nursing staff felt they had to uphold his right to refuse treatment. The difficulty here goes back to a stoic attitude to pain widely shared in Chinese culture. With Asian patients, it may be best for health professionals to anticipate needs for pain medication and not simply wait for a formal request. If there is good reason to be concerned about pain, then patients can be told that the doctor has ordered the medication, and patients may be less likely to refuse because of courtesy. Even if patients do refuse, as in the case of Mr. Ling, there may be ways to negotiate with them and persuade them to accept more aggressive palliative care.

The case and intervention strategy just cited may strike some readers as an example of outright paternalism. But it is not. Negotiation with a patient is not the same thing as overriding that patient's decision. On the contrary, as I have argued elsewhere (Moody, 1992), at the initial level, "negotiated consent" involves advocacy and definition of choices that patients themselves may have given up because of "surplus compliance." An aggressive advocacy stance, therefore, may well involve challenging a patient's "spoken choice" if that choice is compromised by factors that inhibit it, such as fear or pervasive cultural habits like reluctance to communicate.

Above all, negotiated consent means calling a patient's reasons into the light of day through dialogue. What happens through that dialogue is not known in advance. If Mr. Ling's (cultural) stoicism proves more powerful than his (cultural) deference to authority, then he still exercises his right to refuse pain medication, and the medical staff must oblige. But we should not opt for silence and blind acceptance of spoken choice as the sole preferred mode of showing respect for patients unless we have compelling reasons to do so (sometimes we do, of course).

The real point is that any dialogue with Mr. Ling, or Mrs. Chu, or members of their families, will be a dialogue not only between individual agents (professionals and patients) but also a dialogue across cultures. We need not reify culture or stereotype "Asian patients," but we can recognize cultural tendencies and recurrent barriers to communication. From the standpoint of negotiation and communicative ethics, cultural differences become an occasion for communication and clarification, not a trump card that cuts off debate about right and wrong, as would be the case for simplistic versions of cultural relativism and, ironically, also with an abstract and impoverished notion of patient autonomy.

The most important point to be made in the case of Mr. Ling is the most obvious point of all: It is a case of pain management, for good or ill. In fact, the American health care system does a very poor job of pain management, as project SUPPORT and other empirical studies have recently shown. In a system that does a poor job of managing pain, does it really make sense to encourage patients to "freely" disregard options for palliative care? A hollow concept of patient autonomy that is independent of culture and history is likely to lead to perpetuation of injustice and mindless preservation of the status quo. Oppressed people will sometimes "freely" make choices that reflect the limited alternatives available to them in concrete circumstances. The alternative is not arrogant paternalism, but a serious dialogue that recognizes, and crosses, the cultural differences that are part of our global society today.

With these considerations in mind, we can return to the case of Mrs. Chu and make certain concluding observations about the case.

First, respect for Mrs. Chu's dignity and position in the family is a prima facie ethical imperative. Such a prima facie imperative can be rebutted and overcome, but we are wise to proceed cautiously in communicating with Mrs. Chu, and we should certainly not disregard family members. The medical profession's admonition "First, do no harm" means to think carefully before intervening in a family's customary or culturally sanctioned form of life. The nurse's suggestion that the health care team should inform Mrs. Chu directly, no matter what the family may say, is wrong.

Second, we should reject the doctor's "hands off" claim that, once having informed the Chu family, he has fulfilled his duty in the matter. Contrary to what he says, what happens next is very much his responsibility. There is actually a Chinese saying that maintains that should we save the life of another person, we then become responsible for that person ever after. Whatever that saying may ultimately mean, it reminds us that life-and-death interventions invoke ongoing responsibilities that cannot be lightly disregarded.

Third, we should be skeptical of the social worker's proposal to "balance risks and benefits," in the utilitarian manner. It may prove very difficult to reach such a conclusion in cases where cultural expectations lead to different experiences of what a "benefit" may actually be. The power of an ethics of rules and principles is to give us guidelines for action instead of trying to predict outcomes or calculate risks and benefits in obscure ways.

As for the health care team member who advocates "telling the truth" by obfuscation ("You have neoplastic disease"), we can only dismiss this as a self-serving rationalization. From a legal point of view, if Mrs. Chu is receiving health care within the United States, then she is subject to the laws of this jurisdiction, not her country of origin or citizenship. When the health care team grasps at straws in this way, it is surely a sign of failure to come to grips with the underlying ethical conflict.

The preferred solution in the case of Mrs. Chu is to adopt a posture of "negotiating our differences," an approach endorsed by those who favor mediation in medical ethics. But "mediation" doesn't mean simply "splitting the difference." On the contrary, the process of mediation, like communicative ethics more broadly, is an ethical enterprise. Negotiation means holding out for certain ethical ideals—such as patient autonomy—while at the same time recognizing competing values, such as family solidarity in the Confucian tradition. To negotiate does not mean to abandon one's own values, but it means acknowledging that one is not in a position to enforce those values at the cost of competing claims. In Mrs. Chu's case, a culturally sensitive approach to her condition might mean acknowledging a complementary role for herbal medicine in her treatment plan. Even in the matter of truth-telling, compromise is possible. There are forms of communication that can gradually convey to Mrs. Chu the truth of her diagnosis without disrupting communication patterns within the family.

Having recommended negotiation and mediation in the case of Mrs. Chu, it is now time to utter a final word of caution. The practice of negotiation does not stand alone. Among some immigrant groups the idea of "negotiation" may be more associated with the marketplace than with medical settings, where traditional paternalism ("Doctor knows best") tends to prevail. If we are to avoid the perils of the new American medical marketplace (with the rise of managed care and other changes) while also escaping the dangers of traditional paternalism, then we will need recourse to powerful ethical ideals. Here, I fear, even "negotiated consent" is not enough. Negotiation needs to be balanced by greater priority to ideals of dignity and demands of social justice rather than individualized autonomy or truth-telling, particularly when autonomy or truth-telling proves incompatible with dignity and self-respect.

The emphasis on social justice reminds us that, even within the framework of "principlism," conflicts between beneficence and autonomy do not stand alone. Just as individual liberty and equality need to be balanced by fraternity, so conflicts between individual beneficence and autonomy need to be balanced by consideration of the wider historical and cultural context. Concern about ethnicity is precisely such a consideration. But the danger of "ethnic ethics" lies in the prospect of cultural fragmentation and relativism in which universal rights and principles simply vanish from sight—truly, a "night in which all cows are black," where no protest or intervention on behalf of justice is even possible.

To avoid moral darkness, we need to keep in mind what diverse ethnic groups share in common—a concern for the dignity of elders—and also what all groups face under America's increasingly chaotic and ethically opaque health care system. This is a key point and one that helps us avoid the danger of "diversity" becoming a slippery slope leading toward fragmentation and interethnic conflict.

Today, more than ever, groups divided by color or language or cultural ancestry need to make common cause around ideals of justice and the common good: a reminder of the unity that transcends our differences. This reminder is in the spirit of the ancient Chinese saying that when the Tao (Spiritual Truth) disappears, morality remains. When morality disappears, law remains. When law disappears, force remains. When force disappears, then chaos rules all. In a world where chaos and force are all too evident, the appeal of law and morality must be embraced by a unity in which our differences do not disappear but are reconciled by all that we hold in common.

REFERENCES

Baker, F. M., & Lightfoot, O. B. (1993). Psychiatric care of ethnic elders. In A. C. Gaw (Ed.), *Culture, ethnicity, and mental illness*. Washington, DC: American Psychiatric Press.

Blackhall, L. J., Murphy, S. T., Frank, G., Michel, V, & Azen, S. (1995). Ethnicity and attitudes toward patient autonomy. *Journal of the American Medical Association, 274*, 820–825.

Cortese, A. (1990). *Ethnic ethics: The reconstruction of moral theory*. Albany: State University of New York Press.

Damron-Rodriguez, J., Wallace, S., & Kington, R. (1994). Service utilization and minority elderly: Appropriateness, accessibility and acceptability. *Gerontology and Geriatrics Education, 15*(1), 45–63.

Disch, R., Dobroff, R., & Moody, H. R. (Eds.). (1998). *Dignity and old age*. New York: Haworth Press.

DuBose, E. R., Hamel, R. P., & O'Connell, L. J. (1994). *A matter of principles?: Ferment in U.S. bioethics*. Valley Forge, PA: Trinity Press.

Flack, H. E., & Pellegrino, E. D. (1992). *African-American perspectives on biomedical ethics*. Washington, DC: Georgetown University Press.

Galanti, G. (1991). *Caring for patients from different cultures*. Philadelphia: University of Pennsylvania Press.

Gelfand, D. E. (1994). *Aging and ethnicity: Knowledge and services*. New York: Springer Publishing.

Gilligan, C. (1982). *In a different voice: Psychological theory and women's development*. Cambridge, MA: Harvard University Press.

Haffner, I. (1992). Translation is not enough: Interpretation in a medical setting. *Western Journal of Medicine, 157*(3), 255–259.

Huntington, S. (1996). *The clash of civilizations and the remaking of the world order*. New York: Simon & Schuster.

Jones, J. H. (1981). *Bad blood: The Tuskegee syphilis experiment: A tragedy of race and medicine*. New York: Free Press.

Kaptchuk, T. J. (1983). *The web that has no weaver: Understanding Chinese medicine*. New York: Congdon and Weed.

Maduro, R., & Applewhite, S. L. (1995). Curanderismo and Latino views of disease and curing. *Western Journal of Medicine, 139*, 868–874.

Moody, H. R. (1992). *Ethics in an aging society*. Baltimore, MD: Johns Hopkins University Press.

Okada, T. (1988). Teachings of Confucianism on health and old age. *Journal of Religion and Aging, 4*(3–4), 101–107.

Secundy, M. G. (1992). *Trials, tribulations, and celebrations: African-American perspectives on health, illness, aging, and loss*. Yarmouth, ME: Intercultural Press.

Wieland, D., Benton, D., & Kramer, B. J. (1995). *Cultural diversity and geriatric care: Challenges to the health professions*. New York: Haworth Press.

V
Policy

CHAPTER 21

The Science and Ethics of Long-Term Care

Larry Polivka

As a researcher and policy analyst in aging, I have been puzzled by the wide and arguably growing gap between, on the one hand, what we know about the long-term-care preferences of the elderly for community-based alternatives to institutional care and about our capacity to provide these alternatives cost effectively and, on the other hand, the kind of care, mostly institutional, we have in fact made available. Even though over the last several years we have learned how to make community-based programs affordable and effective, long-term care remains dominated by nursing homes in the vast majority of states. This failure to use what we know to change long-term care in ways vastly preferred by those at greatest risk of needing care (the frail elderly) reflects less a gap in knowledge than a lapse of moral imagination.

We have not paid sufficient attention to the ethical dimension of the debate over health care policy for the elderly, especially the frail elderly with chronic conditions and impairments requiring long-term care. We have been absorbed with cost-containment, efficiency, and cost-effectiveness issues and have tended to pay little attention to the many ethical and moral assumptions inherently related to these issues, which are most commonly treated as technical matters. I am referring to such assumptions as the notion that autonomy is not important to the impaired elderly and should not be used as a criterion in the development of long-term-care policy. I think this situation is a manifestation of what Taylor (1991) has described as the domination of "instrumental reason"—pure, self-verifying rationality in the conduct of contemporary policy studies and in policy making.

Instrumental reason, as described by Taylor, has dominated our thinking about long-term-care policy and practice. Many of us, I think, have long believed that we were just one or two extensive studies short of having the evidence needed to make a conclusive case for the cost-effectiveness of home- and community-based alternatives to nursing homes and the creation of a consumer-oriented long-term-care system, as if justification of such a model rested singularly on its cost-effectiveness. I am now convinced, however, that we cannot rely on either cumulative learning from multiple research projects or a "big bang" breakthrough (the big study) to achieve a basic change in long-term-care policy. The science of long-term care will not do the work of the moral imagination in the development of a long-term-care system that is fundamentally responsive to what the frail elderly and their caregivers want and deserve.

In fact, we already have a body of research that demonstrates the capacity of community-based programs to serve the seriously impaired in a cost-effective fashion. These studies have found that, by making available certain services to high-risk recipients in increased quantities (e.g., number of nurse visits or hours of homemaker services), community programs may reduce nursing home use. Findings reported in recent articles by Jette, Tennstedt, and Crawford (1995), Greene and colleagues (1995), Weissert (1995), and Weissert and associates (1997) indicate that certain mixes of clients and services have the potential to reduce nursing home use substantially.

While we need to continue to conduct research studies on long-term-care options, we should not expect that the results of research alone will create sufficient conditions for a profound change in the direction of long-term-care policy. Such change will require a collective change of heart that is fundamentally dependent on the creation of a clear moral vision for long-term care. Research can help us identify the most efficient and consumer-responsive methods of achieving policy priorities inherent in a moral vision. Research is not, however, a substitute for the kind of moral reasoning we need to undertake as a community and as an aging society.

As I will discuss later, adult communities of people who are, respectively, developmentally disabled and physically disabled have substantially changed their systems of care over the last 25 years. They have done this through advocacy initiatives to change the way society views the disabled. They have used research to make pragmatic program decisions and to evaluate outcomes. They have not, however, relied on research to shape fundamental policies. For this, they have articulated and acted on a moral vision that maximizes the rights of people with disabilities to define and control their own destinies. The examples from these two communities about the role of moral reasoning in achieving change can serve as a model for revolutionizing long-term care for the elderly.

THE CURRENT SYSTEM

Many states began to develop in-home and community-residential programs in the 1970s in the hope that they would eventually lead to a substantially reduced dependency on nursing homes and a far more balanced system of long-term-care services. However, the percentage of public long-term-care expenditures going to nursing homes (80–90%) is essentially the same now as it was when the first community-based programs were implemented (Kane, Kane, & Ladd, 1998). The very large increase in the Medicare home health care program, which has grown from 1.6 million beneficiaries in 1986 to 3.6 million in 1995, does not seem to have done much to change the economic dominance of nursing homes in long-term care (Ladd, Kane, & Kane, 1999). On the other hand, without the increase in the Medicare home health care program, nursing home dominance might have been even greater in many states, reflecting the stagnation in public funding for nonmedical home- and community-based care.

Some policy analysts and advocates who work on aging issues, including myself, assumed that, with the decline of general-revenue funding for community-based programs, states would shift to Medicaid waiver funding sources. Waivers would replace state general revenue and maintain the momentum in the development of community-based programs that had been generated in the early and mid-1980s. This assumption, however, was largely unwarranted.

Data do not support the notion that Medicaid waiver funds have been used in place of state general revenue funds to continue the expansion of community-based programs for the elderly (Polivka, 1999). Waivers have instead been used in most states to maintain existing community-based programs, while general revenue funds were increasingly shifted to the politically popular areas of education and criminal justice.

Bruce Vladeck, former administrator of the federal Health Care Financing Administration, recently noted that very little has been accomplished over the past fifteen years in the implementation of home- and community-based programs for the elderly, even as the demographic pressures and demand for services have continued to build inexorably.

He acknowledges the trends described above, by pointing out that "almost all the growth in Medicaid and home- and community-based services has been among the non-elderly populations eligible for such care" (Vladeck, 1998).

The absence of substantial progress in the development of community-based long-term care for the elderly over the last several years is made even more egregious by what we know about the nature of life in most nursing homes for many residents. Nursing homes have improved over the last ten to fifteen years and they are the only feasible option for some small percentage of the most impaired elderly, but they were not designed to nurture autonomy or provide a high quality of day-to-day life. Most of us dread the specter of nursing home placement for ourselves and our loved ones, and would prefer to remain at home with supportive nursing and homemaker services, or live in as homelike and noninstitutional an environment as possible.

PUBLIC POLICY AND DIFFERENT PERCEPTIONS OF DEPENDENT POPULATIONS

What then accounts for the discrepancy in the kinds of publicly-funded long-term care available to the impaired elderly and that available to persons with physical or developmental disabilities? We usually hear that this discrepancy is largely a function of differences in the kinds of physical or cognitive impairments experienced by these populations, differences in the extent of involvement in their own care, and differences in commitment and the amount of advocacy in which the respective populations are engaged. These are important differences, but the real reason is that the aging research and advocacy community does not have a coherent, compelling moral vision and ethical theory that can compare to the development/normalization model that has guided policy and practice in the disability community since the early 1970s.

The community of persons with developmental disabilities has long benefitted from well-organized, intensive advocacy initiatives at the federal and state levels. These initiatives have historically been guided by a moral vision and ethical framework (a theory of rights and obligations) grounded in the normalization principle, which holds that while individuals with developmental disabilities may be different from others, these differences should not be viewed negatively and should be accommodated by a society prepared to support and nurture them as autonomous individuals.

Advocates in the independent living movement have largely recast disability as an oppressed-minority-group status, which has allowed the disabled to advocate for a more responsive and supportive environment and to generate sources of self-empowerment. By comparing the independent living orientation of nonelderly disabled with the perception of dependency imposed upon and acquiesced to by many disabled elderly, Kennedy and Minkler (1999, p. 94) show how disability is, in substantial part, socially constructed: "We speak of the disabling environment. This concept places the locus of disability not solely within individuals who have impairments but also in the social, economic, and political environment. By this argument, people are impaired but the environment is disabling."

Kennedy and Minkler contrast this perspective with the currently dominant view of the disabled elderly: "Whereas 'access' and 'full participation' have become key concepts for the younger disabled population, for disabled elders, the rights of families and professionals, and of the disabled elders themselves, tend to be far more circumscribed." In this way, "aging professionals, elders, and society in general appear to have traded earlier, limited views of aging for an even more limited view of what it means to be old and disabled" (p. 101).

TOWARD AN ETHICS OF LONG-TERM CARE

During the past few years I have often thought about what kind of ethical framework would begin to do the kind of work for the impaired elderly that the developmental model and normalization principle have done for the developmentally disabled for almost 30 years. I have found helpful a complex, interpersonally oriented notion of autonomy and also the efforts of feminist ethicists to develop a theoretical framework for an ethics of care.

The concept of autonomy integral to the conventional ethics of acute care emphasizes the role of informed consent by a competent, unimpaired patient confronting relatively precise decision-making events involving specific medical procedures and short-term treatment strategies.

This conventional notion of autonomy, which is based on the fundamental liberal values of freedom and the integrity and dignity of the self (the bases of identity in Western culture), has played a critical role over the last two centuries in defining what it means to be a person in Western societies. Individual autonomy provides the framework for the legal concepts of competency, consent, and confidentiality. After years of legislation and litigation, these concepts have emerged as hard-won tools for ensuring that individuals have the right to be presumed competent (rigorous criteria must be met to prove incompetence) and to control what is done to and for them (consent and confidentiality). These rights, if effectively enforced, protect autonomy and help preserve the individual's sense of self—of who she or he is.

This approach to informed consent and confidentiality, however, is not an effective means of preserving autonomy in long-term care, where the lives of patients are shaped less by discrete decision-making events than by daily routines and styles of caregiving. The effective application of informed consent in long-term care is dependent on continuous, undistorted communication between the impaired person and his/her care providers. This approach has been referred to as a process model of informed consent, as contrasted with the event model of informed consent in acute care (Agich, 1993).

In the absence of continuous, undistorted communication in long-term-care settings, Moody has noted that we have the "colonization of the life-world in old age, where the last stage of life is emptied of any meaning beyond sheer biological survival. . . . This whole development is part of a social and historical process, not all a matter of individual choice. Therefore it is not surprising that the traditional ethics of individual autonomy has been helpless to halt this erosion of freedom. The ethics of patient autonomy may insist on informed consent or encourage advanced directives. But those very instruments are compromised by the institutional structures and the systematically distorted communications in which the elderly receive care" (Moody, 1992, p. 115).

In *Autonomy and Long-Term Care,* Agich (1993) makes a sophisticated argument for autonomy as the core value governing long-term-care policy and practice. His argument is based on a critique of the concept of autonomy that includes many of the same concerns raised by Moody. The concept of autonomy derived from liberal theory with its heavy emphasis on individual independence, nonintervention, and rational decision-making does not provide a practical framework for an ethics of long-term care. It is too abstract and removed from the complex realities of long-term care. Agich's view of autonomy is grounded in a situated perspective that focuses on interpersonal relations, institutions, culture, and other contextual factors that shape the development of the self.

Agich's emphasis on communication and negotiation reflects his intention to identify ways of protecting and expanding opportunities for autonomy in the complex "real world" of long-term care. A person's evolving sense of self and the need to choose activities and projects consistent with his/her sense of self does not end with frailty and long-term care. Autonomy in long-term care is preserved by listening to and taking seriously the unique life stories of the impaired person and providing the kind of support that helps that person maintain his/her identity despite impairment and illness. This positive interpretation of autonomy is based on the recognition of human interdependence and the limitations inherent in the liberal theory model of complete independence, especially in the context of long-term care.

Long-term care, therefore, must include a broad range of options and alternatives in order to maximize the opportunities for choices and actions that are consistent with the impaired person's sense of self and the need to create opportunities for the person's continued development. Even nursing homes, the most limited long-term-care environment, should be designed to maximize opportunities for autonomy, offering supportive substitutes for the activities the impaired person values but may no longer be competent to perform without assistance.

I don't think the more complex notion of autonomy, as described here and as distinct from notions of autonomy found in biomedical ethics, has ever been adequately recognized as a value to be achieved in the development of long-term-care policy and practice. In my experience, respect for the need and desire of frail elderly people to remain as autonomous as their impairments allow by providing supportive, nurturing environments and services has been, more often than not, compromised by the needs of policy makers and providers to achieve short-term bureaucratic or fiscal goals and the implicit notion that autonomy may well not be an appropriate or achievable goal for the dependent elderly.

Autonomy among the dependent elderly cannot be recognized and supported in the absence of the kinds of nurturing relationships mandated by an ethics of care, which prepares us to protect the vulnerable, including dependent older people. Tronto has noted, "Throughout our lives, all of us go through varying degrees of dependence and independence, of autonomy and vulnerability. A political order that presumes only independence and autonomy as the nature of human life thereby misses a great deal of human experience, and must somehow hide this point elsewhere" (1994, p. 135).

Marilyn Friedman has noted that an ethics of care which incorporates mutual recognition of autonomy and vulnerability, fosters a respect for persons which is " . . . not the abstract respect owed to all persons in virtue of their common humanity, but a respect for individual worth, merit, need, or, even, idiosyncrasy. It is a form of respect which involves admiration and cherishing, when the distinctive qualities are valued intrinsically, and which, at the least, involves toleration when the distinctive qualities are not valued intrinsically" (1993, p. 270).

Friedman admits that we cannot respond to everyone in their particularity, including each person's unique needs and preferences and capacities to act autonomously, and that a comprehensive ethics of care (autonomy and vulnerability) may operate somewhat differently at the levels of society (of public policy formulation) and the individual relationship.

According to this framework, rule-based equal respect for the frail elderly needing long-term-care services would require the equitable allocation of public resources to long-term-care programs. At the level, however, where decisions are made about how to spend and administer the allocated resources, the focus shifts from the general to the particular; from the frail elderly as a group to the frail person who is dependent on day-to-day care and intimate, responsive relationships with others, which are essential to an acceptable quality of life in any long-term-care setting.

The kind of ethical framework for the care of the frail elderly outlined here can be linked to the emergence of the human rights movement over the last half century. I think that efforts to improve care of the elderly can be strengthened by making them part of the evolving human rights agenda which increasingly constitutes the moral criteria we use to judge the behavior of governments toward their own citizens and those of other nations. Respect for the autonomy and dignity of each individual, which are the guiding values of the human rights movement and the ethical framework for the care of the frail elderly that I am recommending, is based on what the social theorist Paul Heelas (1996) calls the ethics of humanity which has emerged in Western culture over the last 200 years. According to the great sociologist Emile Durkheim in his late 19th century work, *Suicide* (as cited in Heelas, Lash, & Morris, 1996):

> As societies become greater in volume and density, they increase in complexity, work is divided, individual differences multiply, and the moment approaches when the only remaining bond among members of a single human group will be that they are all men (*sic*). Under such conditions the body of collective sentiments inevitably attaches itself with all its strength to its single remaining object, communicating to this object an incomparable value by so doing. Since human personality is the only thing that appeals unanimously to all hearts, since its enhancement is the only aim that can be collectively pursued, it inevitably acquires exceptional value in the eyes of all. It thus rises far above all human aims, assuming a religious nature. (p. 211)

It was only after the savagery of World War II, however, and in response to the growing awareness of the evils of racism and murderous nationalism, that the need to recognize and protect individual rights, including autonomy and equal opportunity within a community of humankind, began to emerge as the framework for a universal ethics of humanity. This is expressed in "The Preamble of the Universal Declaration of Human Rights (1948) . . . 'Whereas recognition of the inherent dignity and of the equal and inalienable rights of all members of the human family is the foundation of freedom, justice and peace in the world . . . ;' and Article 1 states, 'all human beings are born free and equal in dignity and rights. They are endowed with reason and conscience and should act towards one another in a spirit of brotherhood' " (Heelas, 1996, p. 208).

Many religious traditions offer spiritual foundations for an ethical framework for the care of the frail elderly. Regardless of one's religious orientation, however, the application of a human rights perspective, based on an ethics of humanity in long-term-care policy and practice, could help generate the moral passion that I think will be necessary to create a just and compassionate long-term-care system.

APPLYING AN ETHICS OF CARE TO LONG-TERM-CARE POLICY AND PRACTICE

Our current policies and programs for the frail elderly are not designed to protect their autonomy and the provision of basic care is far from adequate. Most publicly supported long-term care is provided in nursing homes, where patient autonomy is a low priority and the quality of care is shaped by the impersonal bureaucratic routines described by Agich. In short, our treatment of the frail elderly falls far short of our stated respect for autonomy, as defined more narrowly by an ethics of justice or more broadly by an ethics of care. Given the current and growing emphasis on reducing public expenditures and replacing publicly administered programs with privatized alternatives, which are presumably responsive to the efficiency maximizing operations of the market, this gap threatens to widen as members of the huge baby boom generation reach their 70s in the next two-to-three decades.

An ethics of long-term care, based on the work discussed in this chapter, would recognize the need to balance the protection of autonomy with the realities of dependency and interdependency in the provision of long-term care for the frail elderly. A critique of our current long-term-care system from the perspective of an ethics of care, which incorporates Agich's concept of complex autonomy and a commitment to what Hofland calls the "right to flourish," would discover, at a minimum, that the current system does not accommodate a wide range of dependency nor does it maximize autonomy. Such a critique should be designed to draw on the findings of the Retirement Research Foundation's project on personal autonomy in long-term care (Hofland, 1995, and chapter 2, this volume).

The first of the four major findings from the project was, "Personal autonomy is seriously and unduly restricted in many long-term-care facilities. Most nursing home residents report that they value autonomy highly and want more control over everyday aspects of their lives and care including their personal space, room, and day-to-day lifestyle. Both professional and paraprofessional staff members agree that it is important for residents to exercise control over everyday matters, but staff members sometimes doubt that it is possible in the present regulatory and reimbursement environment" (Hofland, 1995, p. 22).

Rosalie Kane (1995) has described a number of steps that could be taken through the regulatory process to enhance rather than restrict the autonomy of persons in long-term-care facilities. She notes, "Expectations embodied in regulations that require residents or their agents to have the opportunity to participate in their care plans have the potential to enhance autonomy. Such provisions offer residents a chance to provide input into and question the care plan. On a systemic level, regulations requiring resident councils, requiring mechanisms for appeal of care decisions, requiring the residents be consulted on room or roommate changes all have the potential effect of increasing residents' voices and power within the facility" (p. 79).

Other autonomy enhancing regulations include requiring that residents be permitted to make telephone calls to whomever they choose and talk to them privately, call their primary care physicians and specialists and speak to them alone, wear their own clothing, be offered choices of food, and choose bedtimes and rising times.

Kane notes that:

> Perhaps the most controversial way that regulation can enhance autonomy is by mandating minimal requirements for privacy and dignity of the environment. Arguably, such standards are needed for anyone to exercise autonomy when unrelated adults live together in a group situation. (1995, p. 80)

The second project finding was that there is often a substantial mismatch between resident and staff perceptions. Long-term-care facility staff members often make paternalistic assumptions that they know what residents like and want, but actually they often do not know. Kane and her colleagues (1990) found that nurses' aides and residents differed considerably in how each group ranked the aspects of day-to-day life which were most important for residents to control. The two items rated highly by most residents were trips out of the facility and use of the telephone, whereas nursing assistants most frequently rated organized facility activities, such as bingo and arts and crafts, as important, and least frequently rated using the telephone as important (Hofland, 1995, p. 22).

The third project finding was that procedures to assess decisional capacity are seriously flawed and often biased against the elderly. Decisional capacity is frequently treated as a global, all-or-nothing phenomenon rather than as specific to a particular decision. Capacity can fluctuate as a function of anxiety, depression, grief, or a short-term confusional state. Too often, assumptions of incapacity and actual legal determinations of incompetence result from the mere presence of advanced age, frailty, poor health, eccentricities, or a medical diagnosis, such as Alzheimer's disease or a related dementia. Moreover, once an older person is labeled as incapacitated and a guardianship has been instated, staff often wrongly assume that the person is incapable of making any choices or decisions (Hofland, 1995).

The fourth project finding was that, although nursing assistants provide the bulk of direct care in facilities and are critical for support of resident autonomy, their task-oriented work approach greatly limits opportunities for the exercise of autonomy. Aides usually see their work as implementing routines for such tasks as lifting, turning, dressing, feeding, waking, and communication between aides and residents (Hofland, 1995).

Kane (1995, p. 24) suggests several solutions to this dehumanizing situation including:

> Initial and continuing education and training for aides that include discussions of enhancement of resident autonomy in their everyday work would be a good starting point. Also important are the involvement of aides in the development of care plans, modeling of appropriate behavior by senior and professional staff, and assignment of aides to specific residents so that the aides come to know, care about, and feel responsible for these residents. Most important, autonomy must become a central goal of care, and autonomy-enhancing efforts must be rewarded through regulatory and reimbursement mechanisms.

We have only begun to tap the potential of programs designed to accommodate dependency by providing resources for the exercise of autonomy. We have learned enough from our limited initiatives, however, to know how such resources can be effectively employed. Adequately funded in-home and congregate-care (assisted living and adult foster homes) alternatives to institutional care, including forms of consumer-directed care, can provide opportunities for autonomy and interpersonal connection far beyond those currently available. This is true even for those who are seriously disabled, including people with Alzheimer's disease, who should not be limited to locked units in congregate settings.

The kind of ethical framework that I'm recommending here, an ethics of care with a focus on autonomy, would support the development of a long-term-care program for the frail elderly patterned after the current system of care for persons with developmental disabilities. That is, long-term care for the frail elderly would include a wide range of in-home and congregate-care alternatives to nursing homes and consumer-directed care, including cash-based programs; they would be available to all who preferred this form of care and were minimally eligible. No one would be forced to enter a nursing home because no appropriate alternative program was available. According to this policy scenario, the percent of funding for nursing homes would be reduced from 80% of all public funds to under 50% over the course of a decade.

The development of such programs should not be governed by cost-effectiveness criteria only; the effectiveness criteria should incorporate an ethics of care framework based on the value of autonomy in the lives of dependent people, including the frail elderly. Just such a framework was implicit in the original vision for the development of in-home programs and the assisted living program for seriously impaired and publicly supported residents in most states. This vision featured a commitment to quality-of-life values, including autonomy, privacy, and dignity, that are more achievable in a person's own home or in a homelike, rather than institutional, environment. It is now time to develop what was implicit in the original vision of community-based care as an explicit ethics of care with a focus on autonomy and extend it across the spectrum of long-term-care programs.

REFERENCES

Agich, G. (1993). *Autonomy and long-term care.* New York: Oxford University Press.

Dillon, R. (1992). Care and respect. In E. B. Cole & S. Coultrap-McQuin (Eds.), *Explorations in feminist ethics.* Bloomington and Indianapolis: Indiana University Press.

Friedman, M. (1993). Beyond caring: The de-moralization of gender. In M. Larrabee (Ed.), *An ethic of care: Feminist and interdisciplinary perspectives.* New York and London: Routledge.

Greene, V. L., Lovely, M. E., Miller, M. D., & Ondrich, J. I. (1995). Reducing nursing home use through community long-term care: An optimization analysis. *Journal of Gerontology, 50B*(4), S259–S268.

Heelas, P. (1996). On things not being worse, and the ethic of humanity. In P. Heelas, S. Lash, & P. Morris (Eds.), *Detraditionalization* (pp. 200–222). Cambridge: Blackwell Publishers.

Heelas, P., Lash, S., & Morris, P. (Eds.). (1996). *Detraditionalization.* Cambridge: Blackwell Publishers.

Hofland, B. F. (1995). Resident autonomy in long-term care: Paradoxes and challenges. In L. Gamroth, J. Semradek, & E. Tornquist (Eds.), *Enhancing autonomy in long-term care: Concept and strategies* (pp. 20–31). New York: Springer Publishing.

Jette, A., Tennstedt, S., & Crawford, S. (1995). How does formal and informal community care affect nursing home use? *Journal of Gerontology, 50B*(1), S4–S12.

Kane, R. A. (1995). Autonomy and regulation in long-term care: An odd couple, an ambiguous relationship. In L. Gamroth, J. Semradek, & E. Tornquist (Eds.), *Enhancing autonomy in long-term care: Concept and strategies* (pp. 69–84). New York: Springer Publishing.

Kane, R. A., Freeman, I. C., Caplan, A., Aroskar, M. A., & Urv-Wong, E. K. (1990). Everyday autonomy in nursing homes. *Generations, 14*(Suppl.).

Kane, R. A., Kane, R. L., & Ladd, R. C. (1998). *The heart of long-term care.* New York: Oxford University Press.

Kennedy, J., & Minkler, M. (1999). Disability, theory and public policy: Implications for critical gerontology. In M. Minkler & C. Estes (Eds.), *Critical gerontology: Perspectives from political and moral economy.* Amityville: Baywood Publishing Company, Inc.

Ladd, R. C., Kane, R. L., & Kane, R. A. (1999). *State LTC profiles report, 1996.* Minneapolis: University of Minnesota School of Public Health.

Moody, H. R. (1992). *Ethics in an aging society.* Baltimore: Johns Hopkins University Press.

Polivka, L. (1999). Long-term care at the turn of the century [Review of the book *The heart of long-term care*]. *The Gerontologist, 39*(3), 368–373.

Taylor, C. (1991). *The ethics of authenticity.* Cambridge: Harvard University Press.

Tronto, J. C. (1994). *Moral boundaries: A political argument for an ethic of care.* New York: Routledge.

Vladeck, B. (1998). The future of home- and community-based care. Paper presented at the American Society on Aging 44th Annual Meeting, *Charting a Course for the Age Boom,* San Francisco, CA.

Walker, M. U. (1992). Moral understandings: Alternative "epistemology" for a feminist ethics. In E. B. Cole & C. Coultrap-McQuin (Eds.), *Explorations in feminist ethics* (pp. 165–175). Bloomington and Indianapolis: Indiana University Press.

Weissert, W. (1995). Unpublished report prepared for the Commission on Long-Term Care, Tallahassee, Florida.

Weissert, W., Lesnick, T., Musliner, M., & Foley, K. (1997). Cost savings from home and community-based services: Arizona's capitated Medicaid long-term care program. *Journal of Health Politics, Policy and Law, 22*(6), 1329–1357.

CHAPTER 22

Paid Family Caregiving: A Practical and Ethical Conundrum

Martha B. Holstein and Phyllis Mitzen

Families, in particular women, have ushered babies into the world, soothed feverish adults, and tended to the dying. For most of our history, family caregiving was a central fact of life. Today, long-term-care policy in the United States is built around the informal care provided by wives, daughters, daughters-in-law, and sometimes sons. Public policy, which tries to balance the responsibility of individuals, families, and the state in meeting human needs, has treated home care as a residual public responsibility available primarily through Medicaid.

For the past decade or so, social and economic changes have challenged the long-held assumption that women would be available to care for the sick and the dying. Women are in the labor force in ever-growing numbers; they often have children later and so are caught in the middle between obligations to their own immediate family and to the generation now old. It may be that younger women—the "baby boomers"—will be less likely to have a strong sense of obligation as a result of the cultural values that dominated as they grew into adulthood. In spite of these changes, women now provide 72 percent of the "informal" care; to do so they often must reduce the hours they work for pay, rearrange their work schedules, take time off without pay (the option available to them under the Family and Maternal Leave Act), or quit their jobs to resolve conflicts between work and caregiving.

We offer this set of articles on paid family caregiving for several reasons. As a start, the topic is laden with ethical questions that point to the limits of autonomy understood as free and unfettered choice and the power of external forces like the gender-biased labor market or public policy to occasion a morally problematic environment. We also offer this discussion because paid family caregiving will continue to surface as a matter of practice and policy as the need for home care workers accelerates and the availability of such workers declines. Further, there are clear "camps" on this issue, providing an example of how thoughtful people can interpret evidence and weigh values differently, but there is also considerable uncertainty as people struggle with conflicting values. Is it exploitative to ask women to spend thirty to forty hours a week providing care to an elderly relative? Is such caregiving morally similar to the care we provide to our children in nuclear families? How are we to decide which family members to pay? Is it unjust to pay some family members and not others? Do some situations, like dangerous neighborhoods or language requirements, make it necessary to pay family members rather than bring in outside workers?

These essays with their opposing points of view also suggest another feature of note. Where one sits can shape what one notices and finds compellingly important. An administrator, accountable to the legislature or the director of an agency and likely to be skewered by the media, will see things in a different light than a researcher who is accountable to his or her colleagues for careful design and execution of a study examining issues related to paid family caregiving.

As you read these two perspectives, we ask you to think about the following questions:

- How would you try to assure that caregiver and care recipient share a common understanding of their responsibilities to one another and the day-to-day moral world they want to occupy?
- Is there anything morally troubling about paying family members to do "what they would do anyway"? Does eldercare differ, in morally important ways, from caring for our children?
- What remedies can you think of that would address the problems of gender justice that caregiving raises?
- Whose moral evaluation of the situation counts? How do we uncover this evaluation?
- Using your moral imagination, can you envision a third way of caring for people who need help that addresses the difficulties with and benefits of paid family caregiving?

The Case Against Paid Family Caregivers: Ethical and Practical Issues

C. Jean Blaser

Paid family caregiving can be the best of care and, unfortunately, the worst of care. In their essay, Simon-Rusinowitz, Mahoney, and Benjamin will detail how paying family for the care of elderly family members can be the best of care and a benefit to client, the family, and society. This essay will detail how paying family can produce the worst of care, and why taxpayers should not support such payments.

This position is based on experience derived from managing the Community Care Program in Illinois, which provides home- and community-based care to over 35,000 older people a month. Eligibility is based on a need for care, as measured by a standardized instrument termed the Determination of Need. The instrument assesses functioning with fifteen activities of daily living and instrumental activities of daily living, and for each activity with which the older person has difficulty, the availability of family and informal supports is addressed. Need for care is determined by a look at those activities with which the applicant has difficulty and lacks necessary assistance. In this way, the program is designed to complement and supplement family support, but not replace it.

In the first years of the program, as a result of a policy decision by another state agency, a significant portion of the caseload was served by family members who were paid as personal care attendants. When the program was transferred to the Illinois Department on Aging, detected abuses led the department to close that subprogram, allowing no more clients to have personal care attendants, and to allow payments only to contracted agencies. Since that time, however, a number of agency providers have elected to hire family members as "preferred" workers, assigning them to care for an elderly family member. As a result, the department has a considerable history to draw upon regarding the problems that can occur when a family member is a paid caregiver.

EXPLOITATION

Advocates may argue that a policy of paying the family caregiver supports and strengthens basic family values. On the other hand, it can be argued that such a policy exploits family values by paying the family member less than the going "market" rate for provided services.

Under the banner of "consumer-directed care," states can reduce the costs of home- and community-based care by providing vouchers or direct payments to clients who, in turn, hire their own workers, termed personal care attendants. By avoiding the administrative costs of recruiting, hiring, training, and supervising workers, the cost per unit of service is substantially reduced. The cost is further reduced by not having to pay mandated fringe benefits such as unemployment and workman's compensation, although most states may pay Social Security taxes on behalf of the client. And, of course, no health insurance, retirement benefits, sick leave, or vacation are offered. Indeed, the states are careful not to pay for these benefits lest they be open to a charge that these workers are state employees and subject to all the benefits state workers enjoy.

It is a well-established fact that reimbursements to home care workers are inadequate in most areas of the country. In these times of full or nearly full employment, workers can demand and receive higher wages. Because fewer are willing to accept the low salary and lack of benefits paid to personal care attendants, there is a severe shortage of home care workers.

However, family workers, who can be considered to be a subset of the larger class of personal care attendants, can be an exception to this general finding. Family members are more likely to be trapped into accepting such employment because they are unable to recruit and hire a nonfamily worker. Faced with the prospect of placing their family member in a nursing home, these family workers will sacrifice higher wages to care for their family member at home.

One such family member detailed this problem in a public hearing on providing a "living wage" for home care workers. She reported a long and fruitless search for a competent and reliable worker. After many experiences of workers not showing up, not performing the requested tasks, or even stealing from the client, she reluctantly decided to quit her higher paying job with benefits to stay with the client as a paid family worker. She was paid minimum wage and received no benefits for this sacrifice. In addition, she again faced the difficult task of finding a replacement whenever she was ill and unable to work, her car broke down, or she needed respite. She felt trapped by a system that did not value caregiving and did not provide sufficient reimbursement to attract a qualified and quality workforce.

In a society that already exploits the in-home worker, the policy of paying family to provide the care simply continues the exploitation and, in fact, may remove any incentive to change. If family members agree to provide the care at a less-than-adequate wage, and if the policy that allows them to do so can be cloaked in the "feel good" language of consumer choice, the pressure to increase wages and benefits for all in-home workers is reduced. And, with other potential workers able to obtain jobs with higher wages and benefits, the client and family are likely to have very little choice but a family caregiver.

POTENTIAL FOR FRAUD AND ABUSE

The above discussion focused on the better side of paid family caregiving, where the family member is more reliable, competent, and caring than a nonfamily worker. On the other side of the picture are instances in which the family member defrauds or abuses the client and program.

While the potential for fraud and abuse exists in any social service program, a program in which family members are paid to provide care creates an environment that is particularly ripe for fraud. The most common type of abuse is financial fraud, where the client and the family member collude to report services that were not delivered, in order to collect payments. In some instances, the benefits of the fraudulent payments are shared. Other times, the older client allows the family member to receive the payment, perhaps through a distorted sense of intergenerational transfer.

A recent example of collusion was detected when a case manager conducted an annual redetermination of eligibility for an elderly woman who had been served by the Community Care Program for five years. The assessment was conducted in the home of the granddaughter, who had been hired by a contracted service agency to care for her grandmother. The client was lying on the sofa and reported she was in great pain and able to do very little for herself. The case manager, who did not speak the language of the client, used the granddaughter as an interpreter and, when the assessment was completed, the client was found to have scored 79 points, which on a scale of 0 to 100 is very impaired and represents less than 4 percent of the service population. As a consequence, the case manager authorized fifty hours of service a week, to be provided by the granddaughter.

An alert home care supervisor, unable to contact the worker or the client at times when the worker was supposed to be serving the bed-bound client, made an unannounced in-home visit and learned from a building manager that the client did not reside in the apartment but, rather, lived in a senior highrise. The supervisor alerted the case manager, who visited the senior housing site and observed the same client participating vigorously in an activity. Upon inquiry, the case manager was advised that the client had lived in the highrise for five years, and was able to function independently. In fact, the supposedly very confused bed-bound client who did not speak English had taken English classes.

In this example, the client and the granddaughter colluded to defraud the state of more than $48,000 in service payments. In other cases, however, the department has found the family caregiver defrauding the state without client involvement. Through a match of service records with state death records, the department has found cases in which the client has died but the family member continues to report services, forging the client's name to the service verification records. In another case, the client moved to another state, but the family caregiver continued to bill the state as if services were still being provided. Unfortunately, these examples are not all that uncommon.

A more troubling problem arises when the older person is coerced through intimidation into signing the service receipt. Most often, the older person is fearful of losing support and is threatened with nursing home placement and so signs for receipt of services. But, in some instances, the older person has been subjected to physical abuse or neglect or financial exploitation. Neglect is the most common type of abuse. Department staff have seen numerous examples of care provided in early morning or late evenings because the family member is holding down another full-time job, or the grandchild is the supposed worker and is using the funds in order to pay for college.

In other instances, the abuse takes the form of financial exploitation. The family member may be dependent on the pension or Social Security check of the client as well as the payment for services to the client. Case managers have reported instances in which the older person is very impaired and in need of more intensive or skilled care than can be provided by the family member, but is denied this needed care because the family member would then lose control of the client's financial resources. Staff who had talked with one such client reported that she begged for someone to get her into a nursing home and away from her daughter, who was the paid caregiver.

INCREASED ADMINISTRATIVE COSTS

With such potential for fraud and abuse, home care providers report having to take extra measures to assure quality service from "preferred" or family workers. First, the agencies report more difficulty in assuring that the workers are trained before they start service and that they participate in required quarterly in-service training sessions. Second, the agencies have had to increase their monitoring efforts, making more calls to the home or making unannounced visits to the home when the worker is supposed to be on duty. Indeed, it is this sort of monitoring that brings to light many of the cases of fraud, as was seen in the case described earlier.

There are limits, however, to how successful such training and monitoring measures can be. In cases in which the family worker fails to attend the required training session or is not providing the care as directed, the agency will often follow its personnel policies for employee discipline and may terminate the worker. When this happens, the worker will simply go to another home care agency and secure employment. The client will then request to transfer to the second agency and request services from the family member. This "employer hopping" can continue until the worker finds an agency that is willing to hire family members as workers and that is less than diligent in monitoring the delivery of services.

Advocates of consumer choice will argue that such behavior is an example of the client exercising the right to choose a family member as worker rather than a stranger. A less sanguine interpretation is that the family member is exploiting the client and the service system. Otherwise, why is the family worker not content to make the same salary serving a different client, while an unrelated worker serves the family member?

Thus, agencies not only incur increased administrative costs in monitoring workers but may lose clients as a result of either refusing to assign workers to care for family members or detecting and acting upon fraud. And, the agencies that do not diligently monitor the delivery of services may be subject to loss of contracts or even payments for damages as a result of poor or nonexistent care.

INCREASED PROGRAM COSTS

In addition to the potential for fraud and abuse of the system and the client, there is the potential program cost of a policy to pay family caregivers. The financial impact of such a policy could be significant. If we are to believe the literature, about 80 percent of the care provided to older people is informal and is provided most often by family members. A systematic program to pay these family and informal caregivers, then, could increase program costs as much as five times, with no increase in actual care provided. In Illinois, where the Community Care Program spends about $100 million a year for homemaker services, program costs could escalate to $500 million to pay for the family care currently being provided.

The above estimates assume the present level of care for the present number of clients and do not account for any likely increase as families who are currently providing total support to an elderly family member learn of the policy and apply for payments. If the standard formula of three equally impaired persons in the community for every one in the nursing home applies, we can estimate that, in Illinois, there are as many as 150,000 older people who would qualify for home- and community-based services (there are about 50,000 older people supported by Medicaid payments residing in nursing homes in Illinois). The above estimated $500 million, which would support about 35,000 people, could escalate to over $2 billion dollars for services.

In states where the home- and community-based services are entitlements, which is the case in Illinois, a new entitlement, for families with older family members in the area, would be created if a formal policy of paying family workers were to be instituted. It is not too difficult to imagine not only a significant number of families applying for the benefit once they learn of it but also family intrigues about who gets to "claim" Granny.

On the other hand, the more usual case is that the state caps the amount of funds available for home- and community-based services. In such states, the limited resources could no longer be targeted only to those who had needs beyond those that the family could meet or who had no family nearby to provide assistance. Instead, the $100 million in the above example, which currently serves 35,000 people, could be reduced to serving fewer than 2,000 people. It is likely that there would be a public outcry when it was learned that as many as 33,000 very needy individuals were going without care, while the families of 2,000 older people were receiving payments for care that had formerly been provided at no charge to the state.

AN ALTERNATIVE APPROACH

The issue of family responsibility has plagued policy makers for decades. Several years ago, as a response to an advocacy effort to establish payments for family caregivers, the Illinois Department on Aging commissioned an opinion survey of the provider network. The results were interesting, with an almost equal number of respondents agreeing with each of the following statements: "strongly support," "somewhat support," "somewhat oppose," and "strongly oppose" paying families to care for their older members. With such a clear lack of consensus, the department sought the middle ground.

Current department policy does not allow direct payment to family members for care but offers services to complement and support the family members in their efforts. Eligibility for services is based upon both impairment and informal support, so that individuals with moderate impairment but no informal supports are eligible, as are those with strong family support but high impairment. In this way, the program acknowledges the need for support and respite for the family. And, if the family is absent or not able or willing to provide assistance, the state will provide for the needed services. With these policies, the family is supported but the negative consequences of direct payments to the family are avoided.

Further, the department recognizes that some provider agencies may elect to assign family members to provide the needed care. For agencies with these sorts of personnel policies, the department requires that they develop and implement specific policies identifying the conditions and limitations on the assignment of family caregivers and engage in more intensive monitoring than is generally required in the program rules. Usually, the agencies' policies allow family caregivers in situations in which an appropriate worker cannot be secured, as when the client has special medical, cultural, or language needs. In addition, the policies often preclude hiring family caregivers who live with the client or who have full-time employment elsewhere.

In an effort to assure culturally appropriate services to older people with limited English-speaking ability, the department has developed the Service PLESE (Program for the Limited English Speaking Elderly) program, which funds twenty small service providers with roots deep in the various ethnic communities. These agencies recruit and train in-home workers from the ethnic communities to serve the elderly members of the community. This project assures that the more than 1,600 non-English-speaking clients in the Community Care Program are served in culturally appropriate ways by workers who speak the same language, removing the need to recruit and pay family workers to achieve these goals.

In summary, then, the Community Care Program is an example of how home- and community-based services can be provided for older people in ways that prevent or delay inappropriate nursing home placement—without the many pitfalls and problems associated with payment to family caregivers. Such options, which build on the strengths of both the formal and informal systems of care, should be pursued.

Payments to Families Who Provide Care: An Option That Should Be Available

Lori Simon-Rusinowitz, Kevin J. Mahoney, and A. E. Benjamin

The critical role of families, especially women, in providing care to elderly relatives (as well as younger relatives with disabilities) is well established. According to the 1990 Survey of Program Participants, 83 percent of community-dwelling people with chronic disabilities under age 65, and 73 percent of these individuals over age 65 rely only on informal (unpaid) care. Assistance with activities of daily living—including eating, bathing, dressing, using the toilet, and transferring from bed to chair, for example, as well as varied household tasks—provided by informal caregivers is often a key factor in determining whether a person with disabilities can live in a community setting or needs to be in an institutional setting (Stone, 1995). Despite this important role, the practice of *paying* relatives who provide this critical care is considered controversial in this country—raising issues of appropriate public-private responsibility, oversight, and fears of exploding public costs for services primarily provided for free. This article will explore why an option should be available to pay family members who provide care to their disabled relatives. While this option may not be appropriate for or desired by everyone, it should be available for those who choose it. The discussion begins with a definition of payments to family caregivers and identifies key benefits of this policy. It continues with a review of research on this topic, and concludes with an overview of ethical and practical issues in designing such an option.

DEFINITION AND BENEFITS

Public-sector payments to family caregivers have recently been envisioned in numerous ways—ranging from coverage of a limited amount of respite care under Medicare to tax credits to individuals who provide dependent care for household members with disabilities. But the way the debate over public payments to family caregivers typically unfolds, and the way we will treat it here, is limited to whether family members should be eligible providers in state (Medicaid) programs delivering personal assistance services. Such programs generally identify unmet needs for these services and then authorize a given number of hours of care to be provided by a home care agency, or in some states, an independent provider. Currently, federal Medicaid policy bars legally liable relatives from serving as authorized providers but permits all other relatives to do so. This discussion highlights the following key benefits to offering payment to families caring for their relatives: improving gender and class justice by placing a monetary value on the labor of a primarily female, low-income workforce; increasing consumer choice and the quality of care; and increasing the worker supply.

Although men participate in caring for relatives with disabilities (Harris, 1998), the bulk of caregiving is provided by female relatives. According to Osterbusch and colleagues (1987), the "feminized structure of family caregiving raises issues of equity because, in order to fulfill what can be viewed as both a private and public responsibility, women must often forgo other opportunities and the freedom to make choices that may be critical for their well-being." The financial aspects of caregiving are likely to affect caregivers' present and future well-being if caregivers discontinue or limit their workforce participation (Pavalko & Artis, 1997). Time away from the workforce limits one's ability to support one's self especially if one is not compensated, however minimally, for work one is doing. In addition, caregivers who leave the workforce will be unable to accumulate retirement savings, contribute to Social Security, and earn Social Security work credits.

This issue is especially important to consider for people who are most vulnerable to becoming impoverished in their later years—low-wage, minority women (Ozawa, 1993). Low-wage workers are most likely to limit or forgo employment for caregiving demands as their "opportunity costs" (i.e., lost or lowered salary) will be less than the costs for higher-wage workers. Thus, an opportunity to be paid for some of their caregiving labor (the same wage level as unrelated workers) could allow these women to provide needed care for a relative with disabilities while addressing their current and future financial needs. For those low-income people with minimal education, work skills, and experience, employment options may be limited. Paying family caregivers will attract some relatives who are outside the workforce, not currently assisting their needy family, and draw them into regular paid employment. For those family members who are employed, paying them for their personal assistance work will make it easier for them to make a commitment to that work, decrease the financial penalty associated with it, and legitimize their work at a modest public cost.

The ability to hire whomever one wants—including a relative—to provide services can empower consumers by maximizing choice and contributing to their satisfaction with services. Initial findings from a federally funded study of personal assistance services in California suggest that for outcomes like client safety and client satisfaction, those self-directed clients who hired family providers had more positive outcomes than self-directed clients with nonfamily providers and clients with agency providers. Some clients with family providers had concerns about being too reliant on family members for help, but overall the study indicated that family caregiving and client well-being were strongly related (Benjamin et al., 1998). Two other studies of home care clients spanning four states found that consumers were happier with their care when they had more control over their services, including items such as choosing their own workers (Doty, Kasper, & Litvak, 1996; Barnes & Sutherland, 1995). A relative may understand a consumer's ethnic and cultural preferences, may speak the consumer's native language and cook ethnic foods that the consumer enjoys. In addition, consumers may feel safer having a relative in their home, rather than a stranger.

Finally, the option to pay family members to provide care for their relatives with disabilities may expand the frequently limited personal care worker supply. While some family members would not consider providing caregiving services to a stranger, they would become a caregiver for a relative for whom they feel affection or filial obligation. In a study of paid family caregivers in Michigan, caregivers explained that the low wages were not enough to encourage them to provide services, and they wouldn't do so unless they truly cared (Keigher & Murphy, 1992). One respondent explained: "If the state told me they would pay me to care for somebody else for the money I am getting, I would say forget it—for that amount of money for what I'm doing? ... There has to be love involved because the money certainly wouldn't make somebody go in and do something like (I do)." Preliminary findings from the California study suggest that perhaps one-fifth of family members paid to assist clients had not done so before entering the program as a paid provider. Thus, they were drawn into service provision at least in part by the remunerative nature of the work. There is other evidence, less easily quantified, that regular payment assures reliable service provision over time. In the California study, family caregivers seem to have longer tenure in the job than unrelated providers (Benjamin et al., 1998).

RESEARCH ON PAYING FAMILY CAREGIVERS

Research on payments to family caregivers has primarily addressed policy and program issues, including the extent of such payment programs and their features (Linsk et al., 1986; England et al., 1989; Burwell, 1986), attitudes of administrators and policy makers about family payments (Linsk et al., 1986), consumer-directed home care approaches, including family providers (Sabatino, 1990), family payments as an incentive to caregivers (Biegel, 1986), and evaluation of specific programs (Whitfield & Krompholz, 1981). Until recently, only one small study (Keigher & Murphy, 1992) addressed the views of consumers and their families. The previously mentioned report on California's In-Home Supportive Services Program, which includes many paid family caregivers, describes views of consumers and providers about this arrangement (Benjamin et al., 1998). Recent research assessing consumers' preferences for a consumer-directed cash benefit, which permits hiring relatives as workers, offers further information from this perspective (Simon-Rusinowitz et al., in press). This discussion briefly reviews findings from key research.

While payment to family members who care for relatives with disabilities is still considered controversial in this country, this practice is widespread here and abroad. Linsk and colleagues (Linsk, Keigher, & Osterbusch, 1988; England et al., 1989) surveyed state programs in all U.S. states and territories in 1985 and 1990 to assess the extent to which jurisdictions permit public payments for family caregiving. In 1985, thirty-five jurisdictions (thirty-three states plus the District of Columbia and Puerto Rico), or 70 percent of those responding, reported permitting some type of payment to relatives who provide home care services. In 1990, thirty-seven jurisdictions (thirty-five states plus the District of Columbia and Puerto Rico), or 69 percent of those responding, indicated permitting some form of such payments.

On a federal level, the Veterans Administration's HouseBound Aide and Attendance Allowance Program provides a cash benefit to veterans with disabilities so they may pay whomever they choose to provide personal assistance, including a relative. A 1987 evaluation of this program reported 220,000 veterans in this program (Grana & Yamishiro, 1987). Finally, many advanced industrial societies have publicly funded programs that provide cash benefits to people with disabilities to allow them to purchase personal assistance and other disability-related services. Some of these programs (in Germany and the Netherlands, for example) provide cash benefits directly to consumers while others offer payments directly to caregiving families (Linsk et al., 1992; Cameron & Firman, 1995).

In 1985, Linsk and colleagues studied payments to family caregivers in the Illinois Community Care Program to guide Illinois policy makers and leaders in determining whether this caregiving arrangement should be expanded, modified, or discontinued. The study consisted of a mail questionnaire completed by seventy-six (of the program's 177) home care agency administrators (who were responsible for hiring and supervising paid family caregivers) and in-depth interviews with nineteen policy experts (Linsk et al., 1992; Simon-Rusinowitz, 1987). This research assessed respondents' views about the policy's impact on home care agencies, consumers, and government agencies and found varying levels of policy support with respondents speaking to both advantages and disadvantages of paying family caregivers. In regard to the impact on home care agencies, respondents focused on agency problems such as difficulties in monitoring and training family workers; however, they acknowledged advantages such as easing worker shortages in difficult-to-serve areas and finding workers for "hard to serve" clients.

The majority of respondents saw advantages of the policy for consumers and their families, including better quality care, improved consumer satisfaction, and economic benefits for consumers and families. Respondents expressed concern, however, about possible negative impacts from mixing business and family relationships and family conflicts affecting caregiving. When asked about the policy's impact on government agencies, the majority spoke about potential negative effects including increased government costs due to what were termed policy abuses (those mentioned were consumers "coming out of the woodwork" to claim the benefit and paid care substituting for care previously provided without pay) and relatives accepting pay without providing services. Conversely, some respondents who had experience with paid family caregivers were unconcerned about these problems and described consumers as typically wanting to maintain their independence, asking for as little help as possible, and sometimes refusing services offered.

In summary, while respondents were generally reluctant to support such a policy, their comments reflected contradiction and confusion about the outcomes of paying family caregivers. At times the same individuals spoke enthusiastically about both policy benefits and disadvantages. In addition, respondents generally focused upon the problem case that created a lasting fear. One agency administrator's explanation typified many respondents: "When the situation works well, it works well, but the few times problems occur they are 'horrible.' " When asked about the frequency of major problems, this respondent estimated two cases out of five thousand. The authors concluded that the option to pay family caregivers should be expanded and encouraged further research to test various models in which this arrangement could be offered.

As background research for the Cash and Counseling Demonstration and Evaluation (CCDE), the University of Maryland Center on Aging has conducted telephone surveys and focus groups with Medicaid personal care consumers in Arkansas, Florida, New Jersey, and New York to assess their preferences for a cash benefit that allows them to hire their own worker versus traditional agency-delivered services (Simon-Rusinowitz et al., 1997; Simon-Rusinowitz, 1987). Each survey asked whether specific program features would make consumers interested in the cash option, including the ability to "hire whomever you wanted to provide services, even a friend or relative." A range of 86 percent to 93 percent of respondents (in all four states) who were interested in the cash option indicated that this feature contributed to their interest in this option.

While the survey asked about hiring a "friend or relative," the focus group discussions explored preferences of consumers and surrogates for either option. Contrary to the primarily positive views of elderly consumer–family dyads reported by Keigher and Murphy (1992), the idea of hiring a relative to be one's worker drew mixed responses from focus group participants in New York and Florida. Older and younger consumers saw both benefits, such as being able to reward a young relative for providing assistance, and possible problems, explaining "It's like buying a car from a relative. When it goes wrong, you're kind of caught." Parents of children with developmental disabilities overwhelmingly supported the idea of hiring a relative, explaining that they would trust a relative more than a stranger and would feel better being able to pay relatives rather than impose on them for care. As the CCDE unfolds, we will learn more about which consumers are interested in hiring relatives as their providers, as well as those who are unlikely to choose this option.

EXAMPLES OF ETHICAL AND PRACTICAL ISSUES

One way to see how a public program that allows payments to family caregivers would work is to examine a real-life example, highlighting how ethical and practical decisions actually play out. Such an example is provided by the CCDE, set to get under way in the fall of 1998. In the four demonstration states, recipients of Medicaid personal assistance services (personal care clients in Arkansas, New Jersey, and New York and home- and community-based services waiver clients in Florida) enter the system much as they did prior to the demonstration. They receive an assessment (or reassessment) that takes account of existing formal and informal supports (including care regularly provided by family members), and thus identifies *unmet needs* for personal assistance services. Unmet needs serve as the basis for a care plan, which spells out the number of approved hours of service that the consumer is entitled to under the Medicaid program. For the demonstration, consumers who have passed through a screening process are then given the option of receiving agency-delivered services (the traditional approach) or their cash equivalent. (Consumers who are not totally capable of self-direction are given the opportunity to select a representative decision-maker to act on their behalf.) Interested clients will then be randomly assigned to the cash treatment group or the traditional system, the control group. The evaluation will measure effects of the cash option on the number and type of personal assistance services received, quality of care, consumer satisfaction, and costs, along with impacts on formal and informal caregivers.

Consumers in the cash treatment group begin by developing a plan for use of the cash. This plan must be approved by their counselor. In general, this Medicaid money can be used for (and only for) personal assistance services including personal care assistants, home renovations, and assistive devices. This is where the possibility of payment to family caregivers comes in. If consumers choose to use some or all of their funds to hire personal care assistants, they are responsible for hiring, scheduling, training, managing, and potentially firing such assistants. Traditional Medicaid rules forbidding the hiring of (legally responsible) relatives are removed, so the clients can hire whomever they wish.

Three aspects of the CCDE support consumers and mitigate against potential problems with hiring family members as personal care workers. These include (1) the availability and in some cases requirement of services of fiscal intermediaries, who can play a vital role in assuring that workers are not open to exploitation, mitigating against the possibility of fraud and abuse; (2) a range of supportive counseling services—including assistance in locating workers and providing back-up—available to consumers as needed and wanted; and (3) regular monitoring.

ADDRESSING THE CONCERNS

Despite such safeguards, those who, like Jean Blaser in the preceding article, oppose paying family caregivers worry about several key issues: exploding demand for benefits, poor quality service, fraud and abuse, and worker exploitation. We conclude with an examination of these concerns.

Exploding Demand

Often the most basic fears regarding public payments to family caregivers center around a perceived "out-of-the-woodwork effect" (wherein people not currently receiving paid personal care would come forward to request it because of the appeal of a cash option). Policy makers are particularly concerned as they realize that the majority of community-dwelling elderly who need assistance to perform basic activities of daily living receive all their help from informal (unpaid) sources (Stone, 1995). Policy makers and program administrators reason that payments to family caregivers could lead some, even many, of these individuals to substitute paid for unpaid care. Policy makers worry that such possibilities would have massive effects on government budgets. But, looking carefully at this case example, we see that care plans are constructed to meet *unmet need*. Existing support from family, neighbors, and friends is taken into account when the number of hours the public program will pay for is determined. It is only after the publicly funded care plan is set that family members enter into the picture as one option for providing this needed care.

Quality Issues

Another set of worries revolves around the quality of care family members might provide. Many people would describe typical family caregivers as being especially knowledgeable about the needs of their relatives and motivated largely by a concern for their well-being. But some fear the exception to this rule, while others question the amount or types of training and supervision family caregivers receive. Much of this concern dissipates after hearing the results of the evaluations of California's In-Home Supportive Services program. According to a report to the state, "the dominant and practically only variable influencing consumer evaluations of provider reliability is the provider/client relationship. Family members and friends are simply more reliable than strangers independent of client functional level and all context of care variables and provider characteristics" (Barnes & Sutherland, 1995, p. 5).

(And we must also keep in mind that paying family caregivers is but one option under the CCDE.)

Fraud and Abuse

Another variant of the above theme is concern over fraud or abuse. Admittedly, fraud and abuse go on to some (one would hope minor) extent under the status quo, and such problems are hardly peculiar to family caregivers; but this concern does deserve attention. The ways the CCDE states have chosen to mitigate against possible abuses are to put effort into initial training, provide numerous avenues for consumer feedback and refine plans for monitoring outcomes. Financial exploitation will certainly be lessened by the availability of fiscal intermediaries to handle (or monitor) the check writing and recordkeeping.

Attempts to prohibit paying family providers seems based primarily on concerns about potential for fraud and abuse, which are largely based on anecdotal evidence. While family fraud is probably exaggerated, the extent of family dedication and sacrifice is often minimized, and that applies equally to family members who are paid. The "family fraud" view also tends to overlook existing fraud and abuse among agency workers.

Worker Exploitation

Finally, public payments to family caregivers could lead to worker exploitation if there were no safeguards (but this would be true in the case of any individual caregiver for that matter). Under the CCDE programs, consumers are required to pay at least the minimum wage and to honor all other labor laws. Fiscal intermediaries will make sure that all taxes are properly withheld and paid. New York State is even pioneering efforts to assure that workers hired under the CCDE program will receive such benefits as health care and vacation time comparable to what they would have received working for local agencies delivering personal care.

On the more positive and proactive side, CCDE programs offer some potential for improving the worker's lot. In the surveys conducted prior to the start of the demonstration, a majority of the Medicaid personal care clients who were interested in the cash option said they thought it was important to be able to pay their workers a more competitive salary (Simon-Rusinowitz et al., 1997). Furthermore, recent exploratory research (Keigher & Luz, 1997) provides preliminary evidence that independent providers can gain great(er) satisfaction from working directly for the consumer rather than having to respond to the priorities of an agency supervisor.

CONCLUSION

Despite the careful planning the CCDE states have done to operationalize one of the ultimate forms of consumer direction and to mitigate against potential problems, some negative incidents are inevitable. This is a cost of freedom. (Although we all know that most of these problems also occur under the status quo.)

The cash option (and payment to family caregivers) is not for everyone. The rigorous evaluation connected with this demonstration will shed a great deal more light on all these issues—helping policy makers determine if these program options are valued and viable. And as many of the concerns about family caregiver payments really apply to any independent (non-agency-based) providers, this information will help clarify when, where, and why public policy should differ for independent providers who are family members and those who are unrelated.

REFERENCES

Barnes, C., & Sutherland, S. (1995). *Context of care, provider characteristics, and quality of care in the IHSS program: Implications for provider standards.* Interim Report to the California Department of Social Services. Institute for Social Research, California State University, Sacramento.

Benjamin, A. E., Matthias, R. E., Franke, T. M., J. Parke E. (1998). *Client- and agency-directed models for providing supportive services at home.* Draft report prepared for the Assistant Secretary for Planning and Evaluation, Department of Health and Human Services. Center for Child and Policy Studies, University of California, Los Angeles.

Biegel, E. (1986). *Family elder care incentive policies: Final report of the Pennsylvania Department of Aging.* Pittsburgh, PA: University of Pittsburgh, Center for Social and Urban Research.

Burwell, B. (1986). *Shared obligations: Public policy influences on family care for the elderly.* Cambridge, MA: SysteMetrics.

Cameron, K., & Firman, J. (1995). *International and domestic programs using "cash and counseling" strategies to pay for long-term care.* Unpublished report. Washington, DC: National Council on the Aging.

Doty, P., Kasper, J., & Litvak, S. (1996). Consumer-directed models of personal care: Lesson from Medicaid. *Milbank Memorial Fund Quarterly, 74*(3), 377–409.

England, S. E., Linsk, N. L., Simon-Rusinowitz, L., & Keigher, S. M. (1989). Paid family caregiving and the market view of home care: Agency perspectives. *Journal of Health and Social Policy, 1,* 31–53.

Grana, J. M., & Yamishiro, S. M. (1987). *An evaluation of the VA housebound aide and attendance allowance program.* Millwood, VA: Center for Health Affairs, Project Hope.

Harris, P. B. (1998). Listening to caregiving sons: Misunderstood realities. *Gerontologist, 38,* 342–352.

Keigher, S. M., & Murphy, C. (1992). A consumer view of a family care compensation program for the elderly. *Social Service Review, 66*(2), 256–277.

Keigher, S., & Luz, C. (1997). *A pilot study of Milwaukee's gray market in independent care: Common stakes in home care of the elderly.* Final project report. School of Social Work, University of Wisconsin-Milwaukee.

Linsk, N. L., Osterbusch, S. E., Keigher, S. M., & Simon-Rusinowitz, L. (1986). *Paid family caregiving: A policy option for community long term care.* Final report submitted to Illinois Association of Family Service Agencies. Chicago: University of Illinois.

Linsk, N. L., Keigher, S. M., & Osterbusch, S. E. (1988). States' policies regarding paid family caregiving. *Gerontologist, 28,* 202–204.

Linsk, N. L., Keigher, S. M., Simon-Rusinowitz, L., & England, S. E. (1992). *Wages for caring: Compensating family care of the elderly.* New York: Praeger.

Osterbusch, S. E., Keigher, S. M., Miller, B., & Linsk, N. L. (1987). Community care policies and gender justice. *International Journal of Health Services, 17,* 217–232.

Ozawa, M. (1993). *Status of older women.* Washington, DC: National Eldercare Institute on Older Women and U.S. Administration on Aging National Information Dissemination Center.

Pavalko, E. K., & Artis, J. E. (1997). Women's caregiving and paid work: Causal relationships in late midlife. *Journal of Gerontology: Social Sciences, 52B,* S170–S179.

Sabatino, C. P. (1990). *Lessons for enhancing consumer-directed approaches in home care.* Washington, DC: American Bar Association Commission on Legal Problems of the Elderly.

Simon-Rusinowitz, L. (1987). *Government participation in long-term care of the elderly.* Unpublished doctoral dissertation. University of Illinois at Chicago.

Simon-Rusinowitz, L., Mahoney, K. J., Desmond, S. M., Shoop, D. M., Squillace, M. A., & Fay, R. A. (1997). Determining consumer preferences for a cash option: Arkansas survey results. *Health Care Financing Review.*

Stone, R. (1995). Forward. In R. A. Kane & J. D. Penrod (Eds.), *Family caregiving in an aging society: Policy perspectives.* Thousand Oaks, CA: Sage.

Whitfield, S., & Krompholz, B. (1981). *The family support demonstration project.* Baltimore, MD: State of Maryland, Office on Aging.

CHAPTER 23

Ethics, the State, and Public Policy: From the Inside, From the Outside

June L. Noel

There is nothing ordinary or usual about creating and building an initiative on "ethics, public policy, and aging" within a state agency. "Ethics and public policy" simply does not fit the traditional ways bureaucracies act and react. Bureaucracies see their missions as concrete—solving tangible problems and developing visible solutions. To do so, they use familiar tools and methods: interpreting law, regulations, and rules, establishing guidelines, monitoring, auditing, and occasionally undertaking evaluations. Precedent guides a great deal of policy justification. Much government time is spent in budgeting and deciding how to use resources to address complex societal problems. At the end of the millennium, it seems that governments spend much time worrying about competing demands, ways to control costs, and how to reduce budgets.

Questions about ethics in the lives of seniors, and certainly ethical questions in public policy, have had little visible place in the official world of state government. Ethics just does not seem to be a topic for auditing and monitoring. Yet, it is apparent that traditional methods of law, rule, scientific administration and management, money, and politics simply cannot sufficiently respond to today's questions.

We live in a new time. There is a new social order—a paradigm shift—emerging from a combination of remarkable longevity, new technologies, new information, the experience of multiple generation families, parental role reversal and an ever-growing "sandwich" generation, various choices for how to live and even how to die, and new quests for the meaning of old age. This is happening as we cope with supposedly dwindling resources. While states recognize these changes, for the most part they and their agencies have not acknowledged the concomitant ethical questions that accompany this paradigm shift to an aging society.

One government department recognized the need to address the ethical dimensions of aging and public policy. The first half of this chapter, "Working from the Inside: The Florida Ethics and Aging Initiative and What It Accomplished," describes the initiative developed by the Florida Department of Elder Affairs. It is ironic that the Department succeeded in moving the fledgling initiative forward by producing "guidelines" in "the Field Guide for Community Initiatives on the Ethics and Responsibility of Aging."

The Department is a multipurpose agency, heavily focused on developing and funding alternative long-term-care programs for local communities. The first half of this chapter concentrates on how the Department sought a community and local focus for this initiative. Most human service providers make ethical decisions each day without recognizing why so many decisions are so difficult. Traditionally our social workers had assumed that adequate resources would answer almost every problem they faced, but extremely high demand, moderate funds, and competing interests inevitably complicated their work. The failure of resources to remedy some problems thus became even more baffling. To understand what was happening, the Department needed to listen to providers and seniors and move beyond traditional sources of information.

The second half of this chapter reflects the period after I left Florida state government in early 1999. In this part, I reflect on accomplishments and weaknesses of the initial project from a different perspective. I explore questions about what more a state initiative on ethics "ought" to do and become. In *Rationing Health Care in America*, Larry R. Churchill (1987) noted that even in philosophical medical ethics, there is a tendency to neglect the macro issues of justice in favor of micro issues, which he describes as individual dilemmas encountered in daily life. To date, the Florida initiative has focused mostly on the micro level. Macro issues surrounding resource allocation and distributive justice, strict safety regulations and higher costs versus more living affordable options, and policies with many unintended consequences still are not framed as ethical questions—but rather as administrative contrivances or as political battles. The exception to this generalization was the yearlong effort to improve Chapter 765 Florida statutes dealing with advance directives.

WORKING FROM THE INSIDE: THE FLORIDA ETHICS AND AGING INITIATIVE— WHAT IT ACCOMPLISHED

History

Having been in state government for 2 decades, I can offer many reasons why an initiative related to ethics, aging, and public policy is unique. It is no secret that state agency agendas are already overcrowded with impossibly complex issues and mandates. Often states adopt mandates without the necessary resources to support them. Just the words "ethics" and "moral reasoning" in a state (or should I say, secular?) setting call forth skeptics and unnerve agency advisors. Some of the images that cause fear go to the roots of American history—our struggle for separation of church and state, prohibitions against intrusion on privacy, and our resistance to government going beyond the boundaries set for it by the people. These worrisome thoughts need to be addressed by exercising good judgment and respecting boundaries.

That is "almost" where we started. First, we announced that we would pursue an initiative. The Department staff then discussed the need for the initiative with the Department's Advisory Council and sought ideas from focus groups. At first, several Department advisers resisted launching this project. Staff had to go to some length to describe the types of questions that required special attention. Yet, there was still disagreement in the Department about launching this initiative. The advisers who argued for the initiative recognized the ethical implications of Florida's demographic characteristics. Our large, complex, and multicultural population begged for exploration of the pluralistic moral values that exist in our communities. Several of the advisers argued for the need for a fresh look at our charge and mission.

From this debate with advisers, the Department established useful boundaries. The Department would not take positions on ethical questions. Positions and opinions were to be left to individuals, seniors, families, and other organizations. This agreement gave assurance to our advisers that we were not imposing our values on others. But the Department could raise and explore the questions. The Department could educate citizens about the implications of various ethical questions and decisions. Additionally, the Department could seek advice, guidance, and training from persons educated in ethical matters.

We used an evolving list of questions and issues to demonstrate the range of emerging ethical dilemmas. We discussed, for example, how far respect for autonomy goes. How can staff balance state laws on reporting abuse and neglect and supplying services to individuals when a fully competent person refuses services? Why are people so angry about non-compliance with advance directives? We thus learned that older people fear losing control of their lives as they grow older and face death and dying. Some older people describe their quandaries when conveying the dread of calling 911 for fear that their medical providers will ignore their wishes. What is the Department's and social workers' responsibility to honor "do-not-resuscitate" orders in the home? Should staff call for an ambulance anyway? Relatives ask about how to handle the parent's unwillingness to stop driving. Adult sons and daughters ask service providers to sanction their proposals to remove personal items from their parents' home without parental consent because they consider the items dangerous. Some adult children ask whether they can insist that a reluctant parent leave the adult child's home and move to a nursing home.

A consensus was emerging that the Department should begin to assemble information and materials and assist in developing processes to help individuals and staff respond to some of these issues. We struggled to envision the next careful steps. In addition to respecting differences and setting boundaries, the Florida project focused on the "doable" and "obvious" first as a way to succeed. We practiced the adage that nothing succeeds like success, and we needed success in order to overcome residual resistance. So, one way to calm critics was to develop statewide attention to local community issues. Rather than take on the issues at the state level, we suggested that issues be explored and tools developed for willing community partners. We sought community partners who had interests in ethical problems and projects. Moreover, in emphasizing the local community approach, we de-emphasized the "state" as having the role of leader to one of partner.

At that time, the purposes of the Florida initiative were established:

- to assist aging people, their family members, and service providers and other professionals who struggle with ethical challenges that arise in Florida's new aging society;
- to provide information, create awareness, and develop ethics processes useful for community groups and individuals; and
- to focus on questions of ethics at the local level, where the actual situations occur.

Frontier Territory

Without question, the initiative moved the Department into new territory. We were experienced in handling questions of resources, politics, funding, and contracting for long-term-care alternatives to nursing home and hospitals. But we had little experience in the area of policy exploration, and little training on what we considered client "personal choice" matters. Hence, our initial step was a 2-day session hosted by the Department with a large and diverse group of experts in aging from around the state. We included older people who had faced some very complex ethical and moral dilemmas. The expert group reviewed the broad scope of questions and generated ideas for a starting place. They also reviewed the availability of resources in the community to respond to the initiative. It was this group that began to envision some of the products and processes for use in the community.

This group spoke often about the meaning of old age today and in the future. During the 2-day session, they proposed that ethical matters for seniors are characterized through phrases like "personal responsibility." Since then, many have used this particular phrase to describe our purposes. It imparts the sense of autonomy and self-control that many people fear losing. It also fit the current conservative idea that people are responsible for themselves, rather than turning to government to address human problems. However, the phrase "personal responsibility" mutated and eventually became a vision of "shared responsibility," because even if the response is personal, few of us are able to be fully responsible for ourselves. Harry R. Moody (1992) eloquently explains that we are never really independent of others and autonomy is almost always exercised in relation to others. As the initiative developed, individuals began to realize that multiple parties and ideas of shared responsibility were more complete and realistic views of the scope of most ethical problems.

Our next step was to convene several focus groups of older persons and caregivers to discuss case studies and to evaluate their experience in discussing ethical questions in a small group setting. Personal invitations proved to be the most effective way to attract people to these discussion groups, which lasted about an hour and a half and covered three to five cases.

Soon it became clear that people from varied backgrounds were eager to discuss difficult topics. The case study approach provided participants with an initial layer of protection by depersonalizing the discussion to a hypothetical "other." The more people talked and asked questions, the more personal the stories and questions became. Some people realized a need to address living wills, others explored what they ought to expect from adult children. We learned that if we broached a subject that had legal as well as ethical considerations, participants needed a clear understanding of law before they would consider the ethical dimensions of the questions. Perhaps most important, participants told us they did not want media present as they discussed such difficult topics. Many participants enjoyed the experience so much that they asked facilitators to come back for follow-up sessions.

Based on the outcomes of these focus groups and the work of the previous advisory and expert groups, the Department and consultant, Margaret Lynn Duggar and Associates, developed a guide for addressing ethical concerns for use by community organizations. The purpose of *The Field Guide for Community Initiatives on the Ethics and Responsibility of Aging* is to offer "how to" materials for community providers and leadership groups who work with older people, regarding starting an ethics discussion. It promotes dialogue and education about ethical choices. The guide describes structures and processes that allow participants to think through their own choices and decisions. This guide is now available on a Web site developed through the University of Central Florida at *http://grants.cohpa.usf.edu/age-ethics*. It has been used by area agencies, community coalitions, and in workshops to design community events focusing on specific ethics questions. It has also been used as an education tool to introduce the subject of ethics in lay terms to the service provider community. Perhaps that is the guidebook's best feature; it is targeted to individuals and organizations who are just encountering the ethical questions emanating from an aging society.

So it was not surprising that long-term-care providers reported to the Department that some staff and agencies needed more intensive training than a guidebook provides in order to effectively deal with emerging questions of ethics. The Department contracted with the Program in Bioethics for Law, Humanities, and Medicine at the University of Florida to develop a curriculum. The curriculum development process involved consultation with a large and diverse advisory committee including long-term-care providers, physicians, clergy, lawyers, and agency board members. The six-module curriculum can be delivered in six separate components or in a two-day training event. Staff from several groups in Florida, including hospices, community care agencies, area agency on aging staff, and assisted living administrators have completed the training.

The Department then contracted with the Area Agency on Aging, Senior Resource Alliance, in Orlando, Florida to work with the University of Central Florida and a willing group of community providers to demonstrate an idea that had been discussed at several planning meetings. The demonstration model was derived in part from hospital-based ethics committees. Ethics committees in the acute care setting usually address individual case questions and engage in educational activities. The same need for information, education, and awareness of choices occurs in long-term-care settings, but there are few ethics committees in these settings. The Community Ethics Committee would be composed of designated individuals from many aging related organizations. The Committee's purpose was to educate its members and its community about the types of ethical issues aged persons and organizations must face. The demonstration question was whether this would be a meaningful experience and worth the effort. The new project is off to an excellent start operating as a community ethics committee dedicated to formulating education for itself, its member organizations, and the community.

The Community Ethics Committee reviewed 60 exemplary case studies and compiled them into a document for use in discussion and education. The Committee initiated the web page mentioned above as a resource for long-term-care providers and older people. It plans to develop a secure chat room on the Web to create an opportunity to share ideas and consultation via the Internet. As part of the demonstration, the organization which helped develop the Committee, the Senior Alliance Resource, produced a process evaluation, a manual, and a set of recommendations for other groups who wish to read and learn about their experience. The evaluation and recommendations show how a collaborative process can develop across a broad array of disciplines and organizations.

In addition to the activities described above, the Department's Ethics and Aging Initiative spawned several more efforts. Each month the Department publishes a statewide newsletter, "Elder Update," with a circulation of over 100,000 senior households, as well as others. After working with the focus groups and collecting information about ethical issues, the Department began carrying an article each month on an ethics question. Knowledgeable people, who could raise questions and discuss the implications of difficult ethical decisions, wrote the articles. Topics varied: for example, they covered the meaning of "do not resuscitate" orders, questions of sex in the nursing home, and the meaning of old age. Additionally, the Department cosponsored several local conferences on ethical issues in dying in several communities. Later, the Department cosponsored forums and public hearings on the state's advance directives statutes. The Department cohosted these sessions with senior centers and other cosponsors including the Elder Law Section of the Florida Bar, Florida Hospice, and Area Agencies on Aging. Comments gathered through these events were sent to the new, legislatively established Florida End of Life Study Panel. The Department was an appointed member of this panel. We were able to bring ethicists and citizens from around the state to the table to participate in these legislative discussions.

PERSPECTIVE FROM THE OUTSIDE: IS STATEWIDE, STATE AGENCY PUBLIC POLICY EVER AN ETHICS ISSUE?

Resource allocation, health and safety standards, business decisions, and questions of truth-telling are the substance of state policy. Each of these contains potential elements of ethical conflicts and moral questioning. Moral decisions about distributive justice, autonomy, safety, beneficence, business principles, and cost benefit analysis in the face of limited resources are made every day in the typical state work environment.

Resource Allocation

For example, we could ask whether resources are really scarce or if we, as a society, are simply unwilling to obtain and allocate more resources. Even the question of whether resources are truly limited or not is, in some sense, an ethical question. But we rarely frame questions in the language of processes of ethics or value theory. Instead, in Florida what most often drives public agendas and reasoning behind public policymaking is public administration theory, scientific management of social problems, civil as well as raw politics, and a bit of chaos theory. While the production of state policy is replete with moral questions, most often the stage is not set to discuss matters of mores, values, or "habits of the heart."

There are very few public settings or forums for addressing what we value or assessing the meaning of such values. For example, state policy in Florida throughout the 1990s reiterated public goals from the 1970s. If you were to ask our experts then and today, they would say that state policy for the Department of Elder Affairs (state agency for aging) is to assist seniors "to stay in their own home and remain independent whenever possible." This is not just a convenient way to state department purposes, or a holdover of useful phraseology from the 1960s and 1970s when the aging network was built around a populist movement to improve the lives of seniors. The mission of the Department is based on an engrained history of American ideals of individualism and dignity, freedom and independence, and prosperity for all Americans. A Department mission statement that honors these ideals is not really questioned. It is based on our American heritage. "Independence" is our mantra.

However, I seriously doubt whether this really is the Department's present-day mission. Perhaps other states fully engage in weighing their values and principles as they decide their aging department's mission and where to spend their resources. But I suspect that most states are like Florida, assuming and adopting a list of goods and values and subsequent processes and procedures without much inquiry. For example, I suspect most departments and offices on aging across the country assume that "targeting" long-term-care services is an appropriate activity that is beyond questioning. In this scenario, targeting is the prevailing policy of selecting who will get nursing home care and other services developed to help the severely disabled remain independent. Government servants respond to this policy in a manner consistent with usual social science and public administration models. The course of action seems apparent—it aims to target resources to certain clients in the most accountable, cost efficient, and scientific way possible.

Yet, this resource allocation approach really has little to do with a goal of helping the state's seniors remain independent. Targeting is Florida's main operating policy, but it is focused on a very small and narrow group of clients. In the beginning, the Department selected the following targeting goal: the frailest and poorest individuals, who could be diverted from nursing home placement at considerable savings to the state, who would not then incur Medicaid nursing home costs. While this policy seems benevolent, the primary goal was to divert the most costly clients to a less expensive form of care. After experimentation with this criterion, the targeting shifted to those who could "benefit the most from use of the services." Why? Because the poorest and the frailest were costing more in the community than they would have cost the state had they stayed in the nursing home. Today, I'm not sure what that policy really means.

I do know this, though: Leaving this decision about the Department's mission and operating policy to a small number of legislators, agency managers, and state policy analysts constitutes a major moral decision about "who does not get served." Current policy reflects some attempt to consider the collective good when using limited state resources, but it also places cost savings at the core of the policy process. Can we really say the Department mission is to promote the independence of Florida's seniors?

Beyond that question, we might note that the word "rationing" is familiar in health care discussions but is rarely raised in discussions about community-based long-term-care service programs. In philosophical circles, rationing is identified with utilitarian principles. To most people, rationing means denying potentially beneficial services to some people based on some criteria such as age or income level. While "targeting of resources" is the idiom of choice in long-term-care policy debates, philosophical language and principles are rarely discussed. Targeting seems a nobler proposition. It implies setting a goal, as well as a kind of beneficence, to assist a particular individual or group in need.

Yet both actions, rationing and targeting, leave people who have needs without benefit of adequate goods or good will. Both leave a lot of people without assistance. Both achieve the same intended and sometimes unintended consequences. Would the discussion about "targeting" as a central mission in long-term-care policy be elevated to a more public debate if we switched to the word "rationing"?

Over the last two decades, state government has generated scientific management tools designed to target resources to an increasingly small, well-defined group. Devices such as client assessment instruments, improved client data bases, sliding fee scales, activities of daily living studies, performance measures, and service-unit costing methods all reinforce the idea that the state's goal is to target special people for services. Use of these tools assumes that targeting is morally and unquestionably right. Continued use and refinement of these tools reinforce the assumption that targeting is what state government is about when it comes to community-based care for seniors.

It is ironic that state agency advisors were so nervous in 1997 when Florida began its ethics initiative. Their concern was that the "state" or a small group of individuals might impose their values on the citizenry. Yet, a few individuals and the "state" impose public policy of major proportions on the citizenry every day. It is true that our democracy exposes to scrutiny some of our decision-making processes in public arenas such as standard public hearings and brief legislative meetings. More often than not, though, essential values and ethical principles are not discussed in these arenas. Competing values are most often left to the political decision-making processes, many of them obscure, rather than public discussion forums. I suggest it would be beneficial to structure a public discourse, an ethics dialogue, about "who gets service" and "who does not."

Quality or Cost?

Another issue in statewide public policy that is essentially a values question is how to balance quality and costs. It is interesting that, in a sense, this issue parallels the one on targeting. Florida state government operates on utilitarian principles and standards. However, the government, and in this case the Department, speak the language of "right."

The Legislature, the Department, and policy "wonks," myself included, assure the network of service providers that this is the era of competition. The accompanying rhetoric is that public policy should be "best quality for best cost." Yet, daily practice tells us that cost is the state's higher value. At least state government acknowledges the cost of quality, asking for estimates from providers and examining costs for budget and within legislative exercises. But the final judgment is almost always based on lower costs. The Department, like other state agencies, closely monitors its service and client unit costs. A few providers try to hold values discussions and to honor their quality principles and their integrity of service. However, there is little, if any real discussion within state government, or between the Department and providers, about quality issues and the price of not delivering quality. As a consequence, some of the state's directives toward cost control compromise some service providers' principles.

Two examples reveal how conflicts between quality and cost affect health and safety. One is the cost of congregate and home-delivered meals that meet basic requirements of temperature, volume, and recommended daily allowance (RDA) requirements. If the meals are in compliance, but many participants refuse to eat the meal, then the question becomes not just a business decision but a moral one. Should adjustments in costs be made to buy more appetizing meals, thereby serving fewer participants? What about waste of uneaten food? What if some people find the meal acceptable at this low cost level, while others find the food inedible? How many uneaten meals constitute too many? Should the state and federal government continue to compare costs as the primary measure of success? Just how far should a state go in satisfying food preferences?

The second example involves state subsidies for caregivers in the home. Early in the development of community-based long-term-care programs, Florida initiated its Home Care for the Elderly Program, which offered a small financial subsidy to seniors at risk of nursing home placement who had a caregiver in the home. Eligibility requirements were strict and focused on the poor. Also, in order to satisfy the state law, case managers had to certify that the home was "safe" before the recipient could qualify. (Florida has always been a leader in laws and rules governing facility safety.) Now, just imagine these people and their homes. People with problems of activities of daily living, great financial and service needs, and a strong desire to remain at home were also old, the poorest of the poor, and likely to live in an old house which they had occupied for decades. Frequently, their homes could not qualify as "safe." Case managers knew the homes were dangerous because of their broken doors, leaky plumbing, ancient roofs, and lack of air-conditioning. Yet, in order to declare clients qualified, case managers had to report the home safe so that they could assist the clients in their quest to remain independent. The Department's need for documentation placed frontline contract staff directly up against the question of either telling the truth and losing services for their clients or omitting some information and thereby qualifying their clients. Shouldn't state policy periodically be discussed and realistically reassessed for whether it generates such unintended moral dilemmas? Why leave law and rule in place just to satisfy some myth that the state is not participating in neglect of its clients?

The issue is not only truth-telling. It also reflects the conflict between two kinds of beneficence: (1) help people by getting public support and resources, versus, (2) help people by keeping them safe. It could also be viewed as an issue of justice, for example when a service provider denies services to a very disabled senior because her home cannot qualify, even though she needs, wants, and is willing to accept services in the home. The state's policy is fraught with value issues. Surely questions like these deserve a forum in which the state can at least explore the ethical questions centered on quality. The state needs mechanisms to explore the "meaning of quality" and what it is we value within our very pluralistic culture.

Questions of Values

Most often, the beginning points for a department in answering complex problems and issues are, "How shall we fix this?" or "What is the goal?" and not, "What are the underlying values?" Perhaps the first question should not be about our goals, but about what we collectively cherish, treasure, and consider important.

Florida has become expert in strategic planning, goal setting, and refining measurable objectives. We know we are one of the best. But rarely do we retreat one step and question, in any kind of public or overt way, what we really value. Do we value serving fewer people with more service or more people with less service? Would Floridians be willing to assume more costs if they understood the plight of many in the long-term care population? Is that a choice we really have to make? Earlier, I mentioned that maybe we agree too readily that this is an age of dwindling resources. After all, Florida rarely discusses tax increases. Rarely do we assess our rhetoric to determine whether we really have a commitment to assisting older people to remain independent or if we mean "just some older people."

Several people have influenced my thinking about ethics and public policy They offer material for agendas for statewide policy exploration. Some of those people are contributors to this book. Thomas Cole and Martha Holstein (1996) posed a significant question that is potential material for state agency and statewide discussion. They predicted that the next 2 decades would certainly include discussions of the virtues and responsibilities of older people. They considered the issues of age and allocation of resources in America and concluded that, although there have been many efforts to deduce a system of distributive justice, as yet we have no consensus about distribution criteria. They also point out that the moral status of the elderly cannot rest simply on their entitlements, or their roles as abstract bearers of rights or passive recipients of treatment.

Indeed, in Florida we use the phrase "personal responsibility" in government circles, but we have not defined it. Consequently, some use it to mean "autonomy and control of the self, by the self." Others use it almost as code for, "It's not the state's responsibility." We don't have a public forum or discussion underway in Florida about what we mean regarding rights and responsibilities. Such a dialogue seems appropriate.

Larry Polivka's question in chapter 21 of this volume and in previous publications (Polivka, 1997) also deserves a public dialogue. He and Harry R. Moody raise important challenges to our present infatuation with autonomy as the central ethical value. Moody's (1992) argument for negotiated rather than informed consent is probably tacitly accepted most often in cases of individual ethical dilemmas—but the idea of negotiated consent seems appropriate even for statewide public policy. State agencies still struggle with client autonomy, families and providers, liability, media attention to special cases, and the politics of "doing what is right." More public discourse about these questions in the framework of ethics dialogues might make for better answers and fewer convoluted laws and rules.

In reflecting on the place for ethics discussions at the macro policy level, and at a state level, the work of Leo Sandon at the Florida State University Department of Religion is relevant. At the invitation of the state in the early 1980s, Sandon developed an anthology on ethics, aging, and public policy questions drawn from humanities and social sciences texts (Multidisciplinary Center on Gerontology, 1986). This anthology included works by Cicero, Robert Frost, Alan Pifer, Robert Binstock, May Sarton, Bernice and Dale Neugarten, and many more. Sandon adapted a discussion technique called the Aspen model to guide leaders in aging public policy in discussions about ethics. The anthology and two-day seminar provided a stimulating learning model that helped prepare participants for discussion, debate, and reflection on aging issues. In the mid-1980s, this anthology/seminar was set aside so that leaders could grapple with the beginning of the era of budget cuts and the looming age of scarcity. Perhaps it is time to update that instrument and process, and reintroduce public policy leaders to the rigors of an ethics review and discussion. This approach, along with others drawn from the humanities, just might be the origin of extra tools needed in state government circles to accompany the collection of scientific management devices.

Another place to look for modeling an agenda for macro policy issues at a department or state level is *Benchmarks for Fairness for Health Care Reform* by Norman Daniels, Donald Light, and Ronald Caplan (1996). Daniels and colleagues pose essential questions around equal opportunity, a key American value. They suggest that macro policy should address not only the question of opportunity but explore the "fairness" of opportunities. Their work may provide a guide on how to reframe public policy questions in long-term care into questions with ethical structures.

I do not suggest that ethical and moral reasoning are the only considerations for reexamining department and state process to create state policies. But ethics concerns are sufficient reason to contemplate the possibility of increasing public dialogue. There is a place and a need for enhancing current decision processes. An ethics discussion would surely bring new information and viewpoints to the table. A quality ethics dialogue should ensure fewer unintended consequences, because some things could be envisioned and discussed before unwanted and negative activity occurred. From the outside, this is all easier to say and to write than it is to do from the inside. We can trust though, that people who work in this area are seasoned in responding to the most difficult of matters. Ideas find their place and time. Now is the time.

REFERENCES

Cole, T., & Holstein, M. (1996). Ethics and aging. In R. H. Binstock, L. K. George, & V. W. Marshall (Eds.), *Handbook of aging and social sciences* (4th ed., pp. 480–497). Academic Press, Inc.

Churchill, L. R. (1987). *Rationing health care in America: Perceptions and principles of justice.* Notre Dame: University of Notre Dame Press.

Daniels, N., Light, D. W., & Caplan, R. L. (1996). *Benchmarks of fairness for health care reform.* New York: Oxford University Press.

Moody, H. R. (1992). *Ethics in an aging society.* Baltimore: Johns Hopkins University Press.

The Multidisciplinary Center on Gerontology at Florida State University. (1986). In L. Sandon, J. Howell, R. Christie, M. Cowart (Eds), *Ethical Aspects of Aging Policy.* A reader for the Department of Health and Rehabilitative Services Aging and Adult Services Seminar.

Polivka, L. (1997). *Autonomy and dependency in an ethics of care for the frail elderly.* Tampa: Florida Policy Exchange Center at the University of South Florida.

Index

Abuse
  elder
    case, 86–87
    cognitive impairment, 188
  and fraud
    paid family caregivers, 280–282, 294
Accountability, 42–43
Action
  care, 61
Activities of daily living, 5
Acute care
  vs. nursing homes, 70–75
Administrative costs
  paid family caregiving, 282
Adult day services, 166–186
  balance, 177–180
  bonding, 174
  decision-making, 167–171
  discharge, 172–173
  family perspective, 180–182
  homogenous attitudes, 182–186
  intimacy, 177–180
  leaving, 174–176
  limitations, 172
  moral predicaments, 177–180
  overlapping duties, 170–171
  peer interaction, 185
  preferential treatment, 173
  staff/family partnership, 171–174
Adult day services center, 11–12
Aged. *See* Elderly
Ageism, 135
Aging
  cultural differences, 252–253
  dignity, 255–259
  meaning, 25
Aging as fall from grace, 137
Alternative medicine, 255
Alzheimer's disease
  case study, 152–156
  government role, 191
  home care, 187–188
  moral pain, 191
  unique problems, 11
  values, 191
Ambiguous loss, 194
Ancestral home
  migration, 52
Anxiety, 216
Appeals
  new technology, 25
Applied ethics, 3
Assisted living
  geriatric social workers, 148–150
  managed risk contracting
    examples, 230
  risk, 220–221
Assisted living admission material
  managed risk contracting
    examples, 229
Attention, 20
Attitudes
  homogenous
    adult day services, 182–186
Authority
  lack

311

Authority *(continued)*
    frontline long-term-care workers, 113
Autonomy, 5, 20, 41, 53, 56, 267–268, 269
    care plans, 272
    client
        prejudice, 238–239
    death, 202
    lack
        frontline long-term-care workers, 113
    long term care, 19–21, 271–272
    nursing assistants, 273
    nursing home, 71
Autonomy and Long-Term Care, 268
Autonomy in long term care initiative
    collaboration, 22
    everyday ethics, 23
    interdisciplinary perspectives, 21
    lessons, 21–23
    lived experience, 22
    medical ethics, 22–23
    outcomes, 23

Balance
    adult day services, 177–180
Beliefs, 45
Belmont Report, 20
Benchmarking
    ethical, 91–92
Benchmarks for Fairness for Health Care Reform, 310
Beneficence, 204
Biases, 98–109
    personal
        recognition, 100–101
Blurred boundaries, 101–102
Bonding
    adult day services, 174
Boss, Pauline, 194
Boundaries, 98–109
    blurred, 101–102
    case, 84–86
    professional
        respecting, 100–101
Brody, Elaine, 195

Caplan, Arthur, 70
Caplan, Ronald, 310
Care
    action, 61
    broad understanding, 61–67
    definition, 61
    ethic of, 60–68
    meaning, 61
    nature, 61
    phases, 62–64
    process, 62
    standard, 61
Caregivers
    women
        injustice, 9–10
Caregiving, 63
    families, 9–11
    gender injustice, 9–10
    morality, 39
Care plans
    autonomy, 272
Care receivers, 5
Care receiving, 63–64
Caretaking
    prejudice, 239–241
Caring about, 62
Caring for, 63
Caring judgments, 64–65
    guiding, 66
Cartesian self, 54
Case managers
    interorganization issues, 40
    perspectives, 10–11
Case managers meeting, 208–216
    case presentation, 210–216
    outline, 209
Case narratives
    training program, 37–38
Case presentation
    case managers meeting, 210–216
Case study
    Alzheimer's disease, 152–156
    boundary issues, 84–86
    dementia, 171–176, 189–192
        middle-age, 192–195
    elder abuse, 86–87
    ethics, 13–15, 46–48

hazardous duty, 87–88
language deficits, 178–180
partnerships, 89–90
short-term memory loss, 176–177
stroke, 180–182
three generation household, 195–198
trauma, 156–160
widow, 161–163
Cash and Counseling Demonstration and Evaluation (CCDE), 24, 291–292
Cassel, Christine, 21
Cassell, Eric, 53
Casuistry, 28–29
CCDE, 24, 291–292
CCP, 34, 290
CCPAC, 31, 278, 284–285
Change, 69, 136
Character, 103
Chinese
  cultural diversity, 256
Choice
  clients, 45
  consumers, 282
  death, 202
CJE Ethics Guide, 95, 146, 150–151
Clash of Civilizations, 252
CLESE, 28
Client-directed care
  frontline long-term care worker, 116–117
Clients
  autonomy
    prejudice, 238–239
  choice, 45
  information, 41
  intimate relationships, 39–40
  knows best, 24
  satisfaction
    paid family caregivers, 288
  support
    prejudice, 239–241
Clinical settings, 107–108
Clinical work
  unique aspects, 105–106
Coalition for Limited English-Speaking Elderly (CLESE), 28

Cognitive impairment
  elder abuse, 188
  surrogate risk-taking, 232
Cole, Thomas, 309
Collaboration
  autonomy in long term care initiative, 22
Communication, 268–269
  decision-making, 176–177
  honest, 170
Communicative ethics, 73–74
Community, 103
  elders, 1–15
  emphasis, 25
Community Care Program Advisory Committee (CCPAC), 31, 278, 284–285
Community-care program (CCP), 34, 290
Compassion, 136
Compensation
  family caregiving, 119–120
  frontline long-term care worker, 113–114
  home care workers, 58
Complementary medicine, 255
Complex situations, 44–46
Confidentiality, 268
Consent
  informed, 268
  negotiated, 257
Consumer-centered care, 32
Consumers
  choice, 282
  risk taking, 220
    deconstructing, 221–225
  self direction, 24
Context, 39
Continuous quality improvement, 95
Contracting
  managed risk. *See* Managed risk contracting
Core values statement, 96
Costs
  opportunity, 287
  paid family caregiving
    administrative, 282

Costs *(continued)*
  program, 283
  stage agency public policy, 306–308
Cost savings
  home care, 52–53
Council for Jewish Elderly, 8, 94, 145–164
  change, 95–96
  ethics program, 95–97
Counterstory, 139
Countertransference, 101–102
Cross-cultural geriatric ethics, 249–259
Cultural diversity, 127
  aging, 252–253
  insensitivity, 8
  recent history, 253–255

Daily living
  activities of, 5
Danger
  frontline workers, 40
Daniels, Norman, 310
Day services, 11–12
  adult. *See* Adult day services
Day services center
  adult, 11–12
Death, 138–139
  autonomy, 202
  choice, 202
  independence, 202
  individualism, 202
  rational approach, 205
  self-control, 202
Decisional capacity, 150–151
Decision making, 44–46
  adult day services, 167–171
  discharge, 149–150
  health care providers, 100
  limited communication skills, 176–177
  long-term care, 273
  new technology, 25
Deconstructing
  consumer risk taking, 221–225
Delegation
  nurse
    frontline long-term care worker, 117–119
    role conflicts, 118
    standards, 118–119
Demand
  paid family caregivers, 293
Dementia
  case study, 171–176, 189–192
  middle-age, 192–195
  spouse, 194
Demming, Edwards, 95
Denial, 136–137
Dependency workers
  difficult position, 6–7
  shortage, 7
  unions, 7
Depression, 216
Descartes, 53
Determinism, 103
Developmental disabilities, 266–267
Differences
  acknowledgment, 8
Difficult families, 40
Dignity
  aging, 255–259
Dignity of risk, 227
Disabilities
  developmental, 266–267
Discharge
  adult day services, 172–173
  decisions, 149–150
Discrimination, 236
Discussion group
  ethics, 208–216
Disruptive families, 39
Diversity
  elderly, 24
Do no harm, 11, 217
Dying. *See also* Death
  care, 200–206

Elder abuse
  case, 86–87
  cognitive impairment, 188
Elderly. *See also* Aging
  community, 1–15
  diversity, 24
Enforcement
  new technology, 25

Enhancing sense of self
  home care workers, 58
Equal opportunity, 254, 270–271
Ethical benchmarking, 91–92
Ethical clashes, 107
Ethical-clinical analysis
  framework, 106–107
Ethical complications
  home-based care, 4–6
Ethical dilemma
  cause, 106
  resolution, 106–107
Ethical frameworks, 69–75
Ethical importance
  home care, 51–59
Ethical organization
  creation, 79–93
    advantages and disadvantages, 91–93
    cases, 84–91
    defined, 81–82
Ethical self-assessments, 102–103
Ethical theories, 103
Ethic of care, 60–67
Ethics, 43–44
  applied, 1
  case study, 13–15, 46–48
  communicative, 73–74
  cross-cultural geriatric, 249–259
  defined, 96, 102
  discussion group, 208–216
  emerging issues, 23–26
  ethnic
    danger, 259
  everyday, 23, 36, 112
  feminist, 73, 241–242
  fundamental questions, 11
  historical perspective, 19–29
  home care, 31–49
    outcomes, 35–39
    project, 34–35
    themes, 39–43
  long-term care, 267–271
  medical, 22–23
  narrative, 28
  organizational, 94–97
  organizations, 8
  virtue, 28–29, 103
Ethics-centered group
  creation, 83–84
Ethnic ethics
  danger, 259
Ethnicity, 250–252. *See also* Racism
Ethnicity, Ethics and Aging project, 251–253
Everyday ethics, 36, 112
  autonomy in long term care initiative, 23
Everyday Ethics, 70
Exhaustion, 40
Exploitation
  paid family caregiving, 279–280
Extended families, 52

Fall from grace
  aging, 137
Families, 39
  caregiving, 9–11
    paying, 119–120
  decision-making
    adult day services, 168–169
  difficult, 40
  disruptive, 39
  extended, 52
  multicultural, 133–135
  nuclear, 52
  nursing home, 71–75
  perspective
    adult day services, 180–182
Family caregivers
  paid. *See* Paid family caregivers
Family Maternal Leave Act, 276
Family/staff partnership
  adult day services, 171–174
Feministic ethics, 73, 241–242
Field Guide for Community Initiatives on the Ethics and Responsibility of Aging, 302
Flexibility, 139–140
Florida Ethics and Aging Initiative, 299–304
  frontier territory, 301–304
  history, 299–301
Fluidity, 140

Formalist approach
  racism, 235–237
Frail elderly, 52
Fraser, Nancy, 64
Fraud and abuse
  paid family caregivers, 294
  paid family caregiving, 280–282
Free will, 103
Friedman, Marilyn, 269–270
Frontline long term care worker, 111–120
  authority
    lack of, 113
  autonomy
    lack of, 113
  caught in middle, 113
  client-directed care, 116–117
  emerging trends, 115–120
  ethical concerns, 113–115
  nurse delegation, 117–119
  pay, 113–114
  racism, 114
  working conditions, 113–114
Frontline workers, 36
  danger, 40
  isolation, 40

Gender identity, 134–135
Gender injustice
  caregiving, 9–10
Generational identity, 134–135
Georgetown mantra, 11
Geriatric ethics
  cross-cultural, 249–259
Geriatric social work, 145–164
Geriatric social workers
  assisted living, 148–150
  home care, 148–150
Good death, 200–206
Government role
  Alzheimer's disease, 191
Guilt, 40

Hardwig, John, 203
Harm
  defined, 218
Hazardous duty
  case, 87–88
HCBS
  safety, 217–233
  providers' role, 225–226
Health care providers
  decisions, 100
Health threats
  living environment, 149
Hermeneutics, 28
Holstein, Martha, 309
Home
  ancestral
    migration, 52
  loss
    self erosion, 55–57
    personal space, 55
  self, 53–55
  sense of self, 54
Home-and community-based services (HCBS)
  safety, 217–233
  providers' role, 225
Home care, 4–6, 187–198
  Alzheimer's disease, 187–188
  cost savings, 52–53
  difficulties, 53
  ethical complications, 4–6
  ethical importance, 51–59
  ethics, 31–49
    outcomes, 35–39
    project, 34–35
  geriatric social workers, 148–150
  intrinsic limitations, 57–58
  managed risk contracting
    examples, 231
  multigenerational households, 132–141
  transition, 42–43
Home care workers, 6–8
  case study, 13–15
  difficult position, 6–7
  enhancing sense of self, 58
  intrusion, 58
  pay, 58
  racism, 7, 40
  shortage, 7
  turnover, 58

unions, 7
worker cooperatives, 7
Homogenous attitudes
  adult day services, 182–186
Hospice, 90
HouseBound Aide and Attendance Allowance Program
  Veterans Administration, 289–290
Households
  multigenerational
    home care, 132–141
Human rights, 254
Huntington, Samuel, 252

Identity, 135–139
  gender, 134–135
  generational, 134–135
Identity politics, 252
Illinois Department on Aging, 8, 34
Independence
  death, 202
Independent living, 266–267
Individual, 103
  atomist concept, 73
Individualism
  death, 202
Information
  clients, 41
Informed consent, 268
Informed risks, 220
Informed risk taking
  ingredients, 226
Injustice
  women caregivers, 9–10
Insensitivity
  cultural diversity, 8
Institutionalized care
  symbolic meaning, 55–56
Instrumental reason, 264
Interdependence, 128
Interdisciplinary perspectives
  autonomy in long term care initiative, 21
Interorganization issues
  case managers, 40
Intimacy
  adult day services, 177–180

Intrusion
  home care workers, 58
Isolation, 184, 216
  frontline workers, 40

Jecker, Nancy, 203
Joint Commission on Accreditation of Healthcare Organizations, 96
Judgments
  caring, 64–65
  guiding, 66
  moral, 64
  political, 64
  psychological, 64
  technical, 64
  value, 104
Justice
  social, 259

Kane, Rosalie, 70, 272
Knowledge
  moral, 74

Language deficits
  case study, 178–180
Light, Donald, 310
Limited communication skills
  decision-making, 176–177
Lived experience
  autonomy in long term care initiative, 22
Living environment
  health threats, 149
Long-term care. *See also* Nursing homes
  autonomy, 271–272
  current system, 265–266
  decision-making, 273
  ethics, 267–271
  perceptions, 266–267
  science, 263–274
Long Term Care Initiative, 20–21
Long term care initiative
  autonomy, 19–21
Long-term-care worker
  frontline. *See* Frontline long-term-care worker

Loss
  ambiguous, 194
  home
    self erosion, 55–57
  short-term memory
    case study, 176–177

Managed care, 24–25
Managed risk contracting, 219, 226–228
  examples, 228–231
    assisted living, 230
    assisted living admission material, 229
    home care, 231
    Oregon, 227
    proponents, 228
  steps, 227
Matter of Principles, 26
McCurdy, David, 34
Medicaid home care waivers, 6
Medical ethics
  autonomy in long term care initiative, 22–23
Medicare home health care programs, 265
Memory loss
  short-term
    case study, 176–177
Migration
  ancestral home, 52
Milwaukee County Department of Aging
  case managers meeting, 208–216
Mobility
  social, 52
Model of man, 65
Moody, Harry R., 309
Moral ecology, 92
Morality
  caregiving, 39
Moral judgments, 64
Moral knowledge, 74
Moral pain
  Alzheimer's disease, 191
Moral philosophy, 53
Moral predicaments
  adult day services, 177–180
Moral problems, 65
Moral responsibilities
  continually reflective, 82
Moral wrong, 243
Multicultural families, 133–135
Multigenerational households
  home care, 132–141
Mutual agreement, 45

Narrative competence, 141
Narrative ethics, 28
NASW, 104
NASW Code of Ethics, 150–151
National Association of Social Workers (NASW), 104
National Commission for the Protection of Human Subjects of Biomedical and Behavioral Research, 19–20
National Elder Abuse Incidence Study, 188
National Research Act, 19–20
Needs interpretation, 64
Negotiated consent, 257
Negotiated risk, 160, 219
  contracting, 226–228
  steps, 227
Negotiation, 268–269
New technology
  decisions
    principles, 25
Nonmaleficence, 204
Nonprofit agency
  organizational ethics, 94–97
Nuclear families, 52
Nurse delegation
  frontline long-term care worker, 117–119
  role conflicts, 118
  standards, 118–119
Nurses aides
  training, 118
Nursing assistants
  autonomy, 273
Nursing homes
  autonomy, 71

family, 71–75
need, 52
vs. acute care, 70–75

Older persons. *See* Elderly
Opportunity costs, 287
Oregon
  managed risk contracting, 227
Organizational ethics
  nonprofit agency, 94–97
Organizations
  ethics, 8
Outcomes
  autonomy in long term care initiative, 23

Paid family caregivers, 10, 119–120, 276–285
  administrative costs, 282
  alternatives, 284–285
  benefits, 287–289
  defined, 287–289
  demand, 293
  disadvantages, 278–284
  exploitation, 279–280
  fraud and abuse, 280–282, 294
  program costs, 283
  quality, 293–294
  research, 289–291
  safety, 288
  supply, 288
Pain
  moral
    Alzheimer's disease, 191
Paraprofessional care workers, 111–120
Park Ridge Center for the Study of Health, Faith, and Ethics (PRC), 2
Partnerships
  case, 89–90
  staff/family
    adult day services, 171–174
Past, 56–57
Patients. *See* Clients
Pay
  family caregiving, 119–120
  frontline long-term care worker, 113–114

home care workers, 58
Peer interaction
  adult day services, 185
Perceptions
  values, 101
Personal bias
  recognition, 100–101
Personal responsibility, 309
Personal space
  home, 55
Phenomenology, 27, 73, 241–242
Philosophy
  moral, 53
Point of view
  relational
    prejudice, 241–243
Political judgments, 64
Politics
  identity, 252
Polivka, Larry, 309
PRC, 2
Preferential treatment
  adult day services, 173
Prejudgments, 103
Prejudice, 234–247
  client autonomy, 238–239
  patient support, 239–241
  reflection, 246–247
  relational point of view, 241–243
  social view, 243–246
Principlism, 253, 259
  limitations, 26–27
Principles, 103
Principles of Biomedical Ethics, 26
Process
  care, 62
Professional boundaries
  respecting, 100–101
Program costs
  paid family caregiving, 283
Psychological judgments, 64
Publicity
  new technology, 25
Public policy, 297–310
Public resources
  scarcity, 4–5

Quality
  paid family caregivers, 293–294
  stage agency public policy, 307–308
Quality improvement
  continuous, 95
Quality of life, 150

Racial conflicts, 127
Racism, 234–247, 250–252, 254
  formalist approach, 235–237
  frontline long-term care worker, 114
  home care workers, 7, 40
Rational approach
  death, 205
Rationing, 305
Reality check, 149
Reasonableness
  new technology, 25
Reflection
  prejudice, 246–247
Relational point of view
  prejudice, 241–243
Relationship
  therapeutic
    client's terms, 105–106
Research
  paid family caregivers, 289–291
Resentment, 126–127
Resource allocation, 5–6, 20
  stage agency public policy, 302–306
Responsibilities
  moral
    continually reflective, 82
Responsibility
  personal, 309
Retirement Research Foundation
    (RRF), 20
Rights
  human, 254
  risk-taking, 219–221
Right to flourish, 271
Risk chart, 146–147
Risks
  avoidance, 221–222
    negative effects, 224–225
  clarification, 232–233
  consumers
    deconstructing, 221–225
  defined, 219
  informed, 220, 226
  likelihood, 223
  negotiated, 160, 219
  to others, 223
  quantification, 223–224
  rights, 219–221
  severity, 222
Robert Wood Johnson Foundation
    (RWJF), 24
Role conflicts
  nurse delegation, 118
RRF, 21
RWJF, 24

Sacrifices, 9
Safety, 41, 72
  HCBS, 217–233
    providers' role, 225
  paid family caregivers, 288
  perspectives, 42
Sandon, Leo, 309–310
Sandwich generation, 195
Satisfaction
  clients
    paid family caregivers, 288
Self
  Cartesian, 54
  enhancing sense of
    home care workers, 58
  home, 53–55
  sense of
    home, 54
Self-assessments
  ethical, 102–103
Self-control
  death, 202
Self-direction
  consumers, 24
Self-erosion
  home loss, 55–57
Self-gratification, 139
Self-identity, 54
Self-sufficiency, 55
Sense of belonging, 56
Sense of self

home, 54
Sexism, 135
Short-term memory loss
  case study, 176–177
Social justice, 259
Social mobility, 52
Social role, 72
Social view
  prejudice, 243–246
Social work
  geriatric, 145–164
Social workers
  geriatric
    assisted living, 148–150
    receiving home care, 122–131
Space
  personal
    home, 55
Spirituality, 103
Spouse
  dementia, 194
Staff/family partnership
  adult day services, 171–174
Stage agency public policy, 302–310
  cost, 307–308
  quality, 307–308
  resource allocation, 302–307
  values, 308–310
Standard
  care, 61
Story telling, 139–140
Stroke
  case study, 180–182
Supply
  paid family caregivers, 288
Support
  clients
    prejudice, 239–241
Surrogate risk-taking
  cognitive impairment, 232

Technical judgments, 64
Telephone calls, 272
Terminal care, 200–206. *See also* Death
Therapeutic relationship
  client's terms, 105–106
Three generation household

case study, 195–198
Trauma
  case study, 156–160
Treatment refusal, 42
Trust, 45–46
Turnover
  home care workers, 58

Unions
  home care worker, 7
University of Central Florida, 302–303

Value judgments, 104
Values, 45, 96
  Alzheimer's disease, 191
  conflicts, 179
  core, 96
  defined, 96
  perceptions, 101
  stage agency public policy, 308–310
Veterans Administration
  HouseBound Aide and Attendance
    Allowance Program, 289–290
Virtue ethics, 28–29, 103
Vladeck, Bruce, 265–266
Voice, 103
Vulnerability, 65–67
  acknowledgment, 66
  weakness, 66

Weakness
  vulnerability, 66
Western philosophers, 53
Widow
  case study, 161–163
Women caregivers
  injustice, 9–10
Worker cooperatives
  home care worker, 7
Worker exploitation
  paid family caregivers, 294–295
Working conditions
  frontline long-term care worker,
    113–114
Wounded healer, 122–131
Wrong
  moral, 243

www.ingramcontent.com/pod-product-compliance
Ingram Content Group UK Ltd.
Pitfield, Milton Keynes, MK11 3LW, UK
UKHW021839210426
5322IPUK00021B/364